Sports Derm

Sports Dermatology

Brian B. Adams, MD, MPH
*Associate Professor of Dermatology, University of Cincinnati,
Director of Dermatology, Veterans Administration Medical Center,
Cincinnati, Ohio, USA*

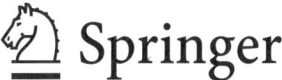

Brian B. Adams, MD, MPH
Associate Professor of Dermatology
University of Cincinnati
Director of Dermatology
Veterans Administration Medical Center
Cincinnati, OH 45208
USA

Library of Congress Control Number: 2005932038

ISBN-10: 0-387-28837-6
ISBN-13: 978-0387-28837-6

Printed on acid-free paper.

© 2006 Springer Science+Business Media, LLC
All rights reserved. This work may not be translated or copied in whole or in part without the written permission of the publisher (Springer Science+Business Media, LLC, 233 Spring Street, New York, NY 10013, USA), except for brief excerpts in connection with reviews or scholarly analysis. Use in connection with any form of information storage and retrieval, electronic adaptation, computer software, or by similar or dissimilar methodology now known or hereafter developed is forbidden.
The use in this publication of trade names, trademarks, service marks, and similar terms, even if they are not identified as such, is not to be taken as an expression of opinion as to whether or not they are subject to proprietary rights.
While the advice and information in this book are believed to be true and accurate at the date of going to press, neither the authors nor the editors nor the publisher can accept any legal responsibility for any errors or omissions that may be made. The publisher makes no warranty, express or implied, with respect to the material contained herein.

Printed in the United States of America.   (BS/EB)

9 8 7 6 5 4 3 2 1

springer.com

This book is dedicated to my loving family in Cincinnati (Jilda and Charlotte), who have adapted for months to life punctuated by my unyielding presence in front of either computer, even on vacations. It is also dedicated to my mother and father, whose polarized views of the world in terms of education and sports are truly the genesis of this book and my daily activities. My brothers and sisters have been unending sources of support and competition; I learn every day from all of you. To my brother Daniel, your courage and strength in sports and life challenge me to become a better person. To my grandparents and uncles, I think of you each day, and your interwoven love of athletics, medicine, and scholarship shines through in this book. To my friends, thanks for making me laugh during the construction of this work and for your continued support.

Preface

Millions of people participate in sporting activities every day. During these activities, the most common injuries affect the skin. Cutaneous conditions afflict all athletes from the recreational neophyte to the professional. For years, dermatologists, primary care physicians, orthopedic surgeons, coaches, athletes, parents, public health officials, and the media have inundated me with questions and consultations regarding the diagnosis, treatment, and prevention of simple and occasionally complex skin diseases related to sports. Epidemics of antibiotic resistant bacterial skin infections in high school, college, and professional teams throughout the country have prompted extensive media coverage.

In my capacities as a researcher and clinical care physician, I have worked with high school and college teams, professional athletes, and the "weekend warriors." The breadth of skin disease surpasses even the myriad sports that exist. Conditions ranging from innocuous skin injuries to skin disease that can bench a nationally ranked wrestling team occur at alarming rates. To help educate medical professionals, I have written multiple case reports and several review articles in peer-reviewed journals, but these venues have their limitations. Review articles and book chapters that discuss sports-related dermatoses are too general and often offer only cursory information. Enormous interest blossomed from my national lectures (at the American Academy of Dermatology annual meeting and at University departments) and media presentations over the past few years and gave me the impetus to explore a novel adventure.

Experiencing the dearth of information in the literature and recognizing the enormous interest in this incipient field, I ventured to construct a book that served to fill that void. As such, this book exhaustively reviews and summarizes the various skin disorders resulting from sports participation. The common and unusual disorders related to sports are reviewed in detail. Each sports-related skin condition is discussed with attention to the following subheadings: epidemiology, clinical presentation, diagnosis, treatment, and prevention. I have separated the sports-related dermatoses into categories including infections, benign and malignant neoplasms, inflammatory reactions, traumatic conditions, and environmental hazards. Clinicians will be able to review myriad conditions affecting athletes of a specific sport and, at the same time, have the ability to investigate the many sports affected by a specific skin condition. Two separate indices direct the reader by disease and sport. Photographs of the sports-related dermatoses will help the clinician visualize the different clinical morphologies apparent in athletes. In many cases, the use of summary tables will help the clinician organize their thinking regarding prevention and treatment of various infectious conditions. Hopefully using these tables, the clinician will be able to choose the most appropriate treatment and prevention plan for their specific athlete population. All recent advances and up-to-date information are included; evidence-based medicine is a key feature of this book.

This book is the first of its kind and it will be the resource book for the latest information on sports dermatology. Sports discussed in this book include all the sports on the Olympic programme, nearly all of the recognized sports by the International Olympic Committee, and several recreational sporting activities.

Individuals using this book will find that they can quickly locate current data on sports-related dermatoses. This book is intended for clinicians who deal with sports-related skin injuries such as dermatologists, primary care sports medicine specialists, athletic trainers, orthopedic surgeons, public health officials, and other physicians who wish to keep up with the current advances in the diagnosis, treatment, and prevention of sports-related skin conditions. Those individuals who are fascinated by and committed to sports and its impact on the well-being of the athlete will find this book to be all they ever need in order to care for their athletic patients' skin complaints.

Brian B. Adams, MD, MPH

Acknowledgments

I would like to thank my Chairman of the Department of Dermatology at the University of Cincinnati, Diya F. Mutasim, MD, for his unending encouragement and numerous photographs used in this book. I would also like to thank Hugh M. Gloster, MD, for the photographs of skin cancers used this book. Also a thank you to Toby Mathias, MD, whose photos of foosball appear in this book. I am indebted to Jennifer Finnicum whose line drawings appear in this book.

Brian B. Adams, MD, MPH

Contents

Preface vii
Acknowledgments ix
Nomenclature xiii

Section I Sports-Related Skin Infections

1 Bacterial Skin Infections 3
2 Viral Skin Infections 35
3 Fungal Skin Infections 57
4 Atypical Mycobacterial Skin Infections 81
5 Parasitic Skin Infections 84

Section II Sports-Related Aberrant Growths

6 Athlete's Nodules 95
7 Sunburns and Skin Cancer 106

Section III Sports-Related Inflammatory Reactions

8   Allergic Contact Dermatitis 127
9   Irritant Contact Dermatitis 164
10 Pruritus and Urticaria 180
11 Exercise-Induced Angioedema/Anaphylaxis 195

Section IV Sports-Related Traumatic Conditions

12 Friction Injuries to the Skin 203
13 Friction Injuries to the Hair 241
14 Pressure Injuries 245

15	Traumatic Injuries to the Nails and Toes	262
16	Combined Factors (Pressure, Friction, Occlusion, and Heat)	282

Section V Sports-Related Conditions Induced by the Environment

17	Chemical Deposition	293
18	Anabolic Steroids	297
19	Thermal Reactions	300
20	Encounters with Animals	311

Index 339

Nomenclature

Bulla   A clear fluid-filled lesion that is greater than one centimeter in size.
Erosion   A well-defined lesion of partially lost epidermis.
Macule   A flat lesion less than one centimeter that cannot be felt.
Nodule   A solid deep lesion that can be felt.
Papule   A raised lesion less than one centimeter that can be felt.
Patch   A flat lesion greater than one centimeter that cannot be felt.
Plaque   A raised lesion greater than one centimeter that can be felt.
Pustule A raised lesion comprised of purulent material that may be white, yellow, or green.
Ulcer   A well-defined lesion of complete loss of epidermis.
Vesicle A clear fluid-filled lesion that is less than one centimeter in size.

Section I Sports-Related Skin Infections

1. Bacterial Skin Infections

Chapter 1 on bacterial skin infections is the first of five chapters in the section on sports-related skin infections. These skin conditions are among the most prevalent seen in a medical practice dealing with athletes. The importance of bacterial skin infections is underscored by the fact that they can result in individual athlete disqualification and significant team disruption.

The athlete's skin is ideally suited for infection. The athlete's activities facilitate microorganism entry into the epidermis. The facilitation results from two different processes. First, supersaturation of the stratum corneum (the first layer of protection of the skin) due to sweating and soaked clothes allows easy passage of the microorganism through the epidermis. Second, most athletes experience abrasions and cuts that allow entrance of the microorganism through the epidermis.

Sporting activities and their venues place athletes at risk. Skin-to-skin contact inherent in many sports encourages the spread of microorganisms throughout the team. Athletes in both contact and noncontact sports frequently share equipment and towels, thus allowing spread of fomites among team members. Many studies have documented the presence of bacteria, viruses, fungi, atypical mycobacteria, and parasites on playing surfaces and on surfaces of athletes' locker rooms and showers. Because of these factors, epidemics have occurred in virtually every sport with skin-to-skin contact.

The clinician caring for athletes must be able to recognize the myriad types of skin infection. Several of these infections are relatively sport-specific, such as ringworm in wrestlers (so-called *tinea corporis gladiatorum*). Other infections can occur in athletes participating in any sport, such as jock itch (otherwise known as *tinea cruris*). Sports clinicians must understand when public health measures are necessary and if athlete disqualification is required. Duration of disqualification is equally important. Treatment and prevention measures in athletes often are quite different compared to the measures implemented for nonathletes.

Chapter 2 reviews viral skin infections in the athlete. Most of these infections can result in the athlete's disqualification from practice and competition. The conditions range from the mundane common warts to herpes gladiatorum and herpes rugbeiorum, which can cause significant individual morbidity and team or league disruption. Chapter 3 discusses fungal skin infections, which constitute the most common group of all skin infections. The conditions range from the seemingly ordinary tinea pedis to disqualifying conditions such as tinea corporis gladiatorum.

Chapter 4 examines the epidemics caused by atypical mycobacteria in swimmers. Chapter 5 reviews the parasitic skin infestations of athletes.

Chapter 1 focuses on the myriad bacterial infections of the athlete's skin. These infections fall into two categories, those resulting from (1) Gram-positive organisms and those resulting from (2) Gram-negative organisms. Gram-positive organisms frequently infect not only the skin but also the hair. *Pseudomonas aeruginosa* produces all the Gram-negative skin infections in the athlete. In addition, *P. aeruginosa* can infect the athlete's hair, nails, and skin of the ear. It is critical for the sports clinician to rapidly identify and treat these conditions. Careful foresight and prevention are critical to prevent further infections in the affected athlete and other team members.

Gram-Positive Infections

Impetigo

Epidemiology

Impetigo occurring in rugby players is termed *scrum strep* and can result in epidemics. Five scrum players on one team in England developed the condition. One of these players also required admission to the hospital and subsequently developed acute glomerulonephritis (Ludlam and Cookson, 1986). Fifty-seven percent of an indoor soccer team and nearly 21% of all participants in a 22-team tournament in Europe developed impetigo (Falck, 1996).

In one epidemic among the University of North Carolina football team, 37% of the team developed superficial bacterial infections. Investigators identified a nephritogenic *Streptococcus* (M-type 2), although clinical nephritis did not occur (Glezen et al., 1972). Data from the National Collegiate Athletic Association injury surveillance system (NCAAISS) notes that in the years 1991 to 2003, impetigo composed 14% of all skin infections in collegiate wrestlers.

Marine recreational waters also transmit *Staphylococcus aureus*. One study showed that individuals with *S. aureus* infection were 18 times more likely to have been exposed to seawater than were those who did not have skin infection (Torregrossa and Casuccio, 2001). Another study supported this finding by noting that athletes who developed *Staphylococcal* skin infection were four times more likely to have been exposed to seawater than were those not exposed (Charoenca and Fujioka, 1995). The mean age of the affected swimmers was 4.5 years. Therefore, surfers, swimmers, snorkelers, sailors, and divers theoretically are at risk for infection. Canoeists have also developed furuncles.

In addition to skin-to-skin contact, the abrasions acquired by athletes (e.g., rugby and football players and wrestlers) increase the risk for developing disease. *Staphylococcus aureus* or *Streptococcus* species cause impetigo.

Clinical Presentation

Early lesions are characterized by well-defined, erythematous papules. Typical and classic lesions represent older lesions and are characterized by erythematous papules and plaques with honey-colored crust with or without pustules (Figures 1-1 and 1-2, see color plate for Figure 1-1). A more unusual variety

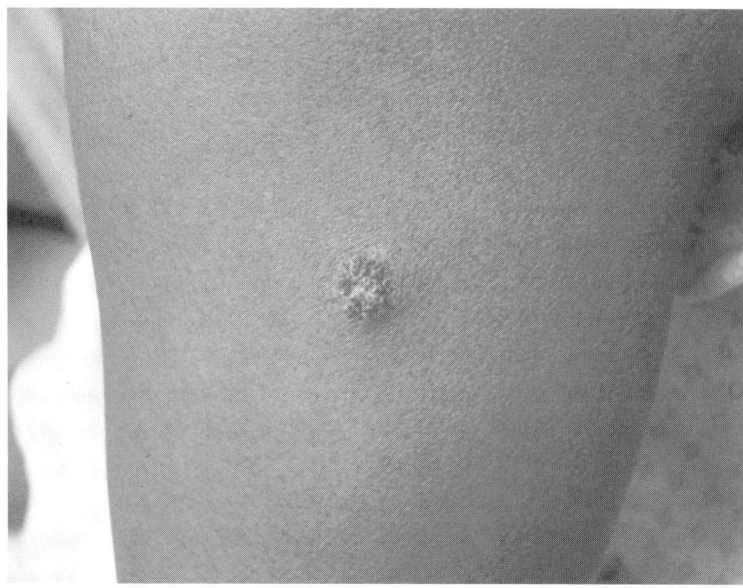

Figure 1-1. Well-defined, erythematous, centrally crusted papule characteristic of impetigo located on an arm. (See color plate.)

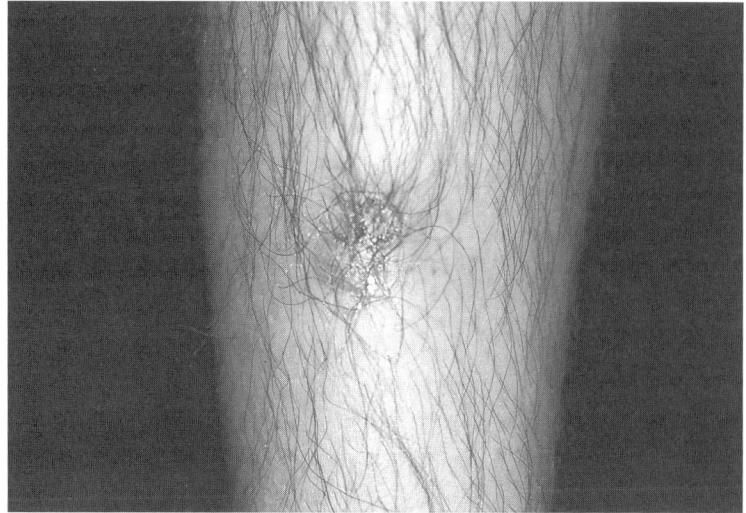

Figure 1-2. Impetigo may enlarge to several centimeters.

presents with discrete, clear, fluid-filled vesicles that coalesce into larger bullae (Figure 1-3). Lesions occur on the exposed skin that comes in close contact with competitors' skin. As a result, the face and upper extremities experience the most lesions. The lower extremities become infected in athletes who participate in sports such as wrestling and rugby (and football when shorts are worn during practice).

Regional lymphadenopathy and pharyngitis occur. Concomitant positive streptococcal throat cultures have been noted in rugby players with impetigo. Complications include poststreptococcal glomerulonephritis. When this complication occurs in rugby players, it is termed *scrum kidney.*

Diagnosis

The diagnosis can be challenging, especially for early lesions, but is generally made clinically. The differential diagnosis includes acne vulgaris, atopic dermatitis, folliculitis, herpes gladiatorum, and tinea corporis gladiatorum.

Culture confirms the diagnosis and should absolutely be performed during epidemics. Culture also identifies methicillin-resistant *S. aureus* (MRSA) infection. Throat cultures should be considered. Clinicians also should consider nasal and crural swabs to identify any latent bacterial colonization. Urinalysis and

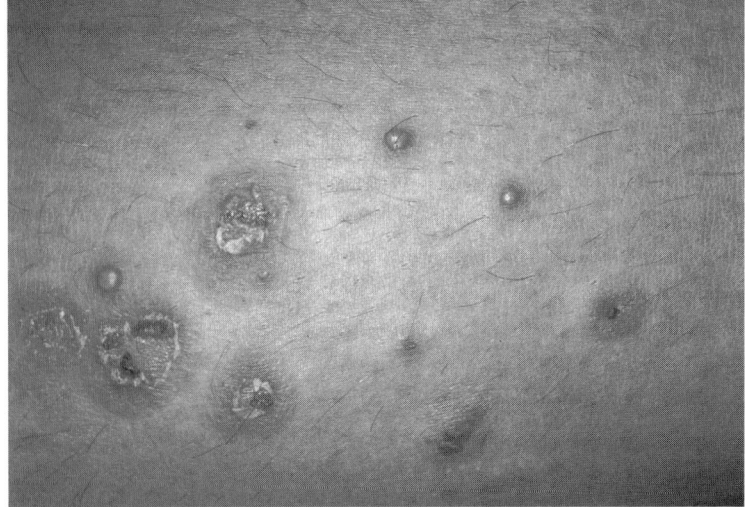

Figure 1-3. Impetigo may create tiny or medium-size blisters or pustules. Resolving lesions reveal a crust where the blister was located.

serum complement levels (C3) are indicated if a *Streptococcus* species is cultured. Post-streptococcal nephritis may occur up to 3 weeks after skin infection.

Treatment

Warm-water soaks must be applied three times per day for 5 to 10 minutes until clear. Localized and few lesions may require only topical mupirocin twice per day for 10 days. Extensive disease necessitates oral dicloxacillin 500 mg three times per day or cephalexin 500 mg three times per day for 10 to 14 days in addition to topical antibiotics. Penicillin-allergic patients may take erythromycin or clindamycin. Patients with MRSA respond to topical mupirocin. In vitro studies show that mupirocin inhibits growth of MRSA and even linezolid-resistant *S. aureus*. The first-line therapy for extensive lesions of MRSA may also require oral trimethoprim/sulfamethoxazole or clindamycin for at least 14 days. Second-line therapy includes tetracycline, vancomycin, linezolid, or dactinomycin. Some clinicians recommend povidone-iodine liquid soap or 4% chlorhexidine gluconate liquid detergent.

National Collegiate Athletic Association wrestling rules mandate that for infected athletes to compete, they must have taken oral antibiotics for at least 72 hours and must not have any new lesions for 48 hours before the match. After satisfying these two criteria, wrestlers must cover any visible lesions with a nonpermeable dressing that will not dislodge. Although the NCAA has standard guidelines, each state's high school association has different guidelines, and the disqualification standard often resides at the discretion of the individually treating physician.

Prevention

Athletes must avoid sharing equipment, towels, ointments, and tape. Clinicians and staff should not dispense ointments from common containers. Athletes or the support staff must clean clothes and equipment daily. Clinicians should not forget to clean equipment such as sensor wires used in fencing. Bleach and water, at a temperature of at least 71°C, must be used for laundering. Athletes must shower with antibacterial soap as soon as possible after the sports activity. Athletic programs should provide this antibacterial soap in the shower areas. Injured skin should be covered immediately, and athletes should wear loose-fitting clothing to decrease the exposed skin area. Body shaving should be discouraged in contact sport athletes (Table 1-1).

Moisture-wicking, synthetic clothing is ideal and keeps the athlete cool, even when the athlete is wearing long pants and long sleeves. Athletes should thoroughly shower before getting into communal hot tubs. These hot tubs are required to have automatic disinfection feeders and filtration and recirculation equipment. Whirlpools without these accessories must be emptied and disinfected after each athlete's use. Trainers must have easy access to hand cleanser

Table 1-1. Prevention Techniques to Prevent Bacterial Skin Infection Epidemics

Frequent, if not daily, skin checks by athletes and trainers
Daily showers immediately after practices or competition
Routine antibacterial soap use in the showers
Frequent handwashing by trainers and affected athletes
Universal availability of alcohol-based, waterless, soap cleansers
Regular laundering of equipment and clothing
Mandatory no-sharing policy for equipment and personal items
Required personal towels
Meticulous covering of all wounds
Periodic formal education for the athletes, coaches, and trainers

for use between examining athletes. Investigators have failed to document the presence of pathogenic bacteria on wrestling mats, but caution suggests that wrestling mats be thoroughly cleaned (Table 1-2).

Athletes with positive nasal or crural cultures require application of topical mupirocin to each nares and to the perianal area twice per day for 1 week. This application should be repeated every 4 to 6 months to keep the growth of *S. aureus* in check. Athletes can continue to practice if the impetigo lesion can be securely bandaged. The clinician should bench the athlete during epidemics or if the lesion cannot be safely secured.

Folliculitis

Epidemiology

Although any athlete can develop furunculosis, wrestlers frequently acquire folliculitis (Table 1-2). *Staphylococcus aureus* causes folliculitis.

Clinical Presentation

Discrete, small, peripherally erythematous pustules present in follicular orifices (Figure 1-4, see color plate). They can occur anywhere on the body, especially the back and buttocks.

Diagnosis

The diagnosis can be challenging, especially for early lesions, but is generally made clinically. The differential diagnosis includes acneiform folliculitis, *Pityrosporum* folliculitis, hot tub folliculitis, and molluscum.

Culture confirms the diagnosis and should absolutely be performed during epidemics. The clinician must brush the swab in the pustular material and not simply on the surface of lesions. The clinician should rub the lesion with an alcohol pad and then use a no. 11 or 15 blade to lance the pustule for proper culture. Culture also identifies MRSA infection. Clinicians should consider nasal and crural swabs to identify any latent bacterial colonization.

Treatment

Warm-water soaks must be applied three times per day for 5 to 10 minutes until clear. Localized and few lesions may require only topical mupirocin

Table 1-2. Evidence for Transmission of *Staphylococcus* by Fomites

Equipment Type	Epidemic Study	Level of Evidence
Fencing sensor wires	CDC, 2003	+
Whirlpools	Kazakova	+
	Begier	+++
	Bartlett	+++
	Seidenfeld	——
	Lindenmayer	——
Weights	Kazakova	+
Towel sharing	Kazakova	+
	Begier	——
	Seidenfeld	——
	Sosin	——
	Lindenmayer	——
Equipment sharing	Begier	——
	Seidenfeld	——
	Sosin	——
	Lindenmayer	——
Tape sharing	Seidenfeld	——
Elbow pad use	Sosin	+++
	Seidenfeld	++
	Bartlett	+++
Athletic tape use	Sosin	+++
	Bartlett	+++
Skin lubricant use	Bartlett	+++

+, suggested link; ++, increased risk but not statistically significant; +++, statistically significant increased risk; ——, no statistical association.

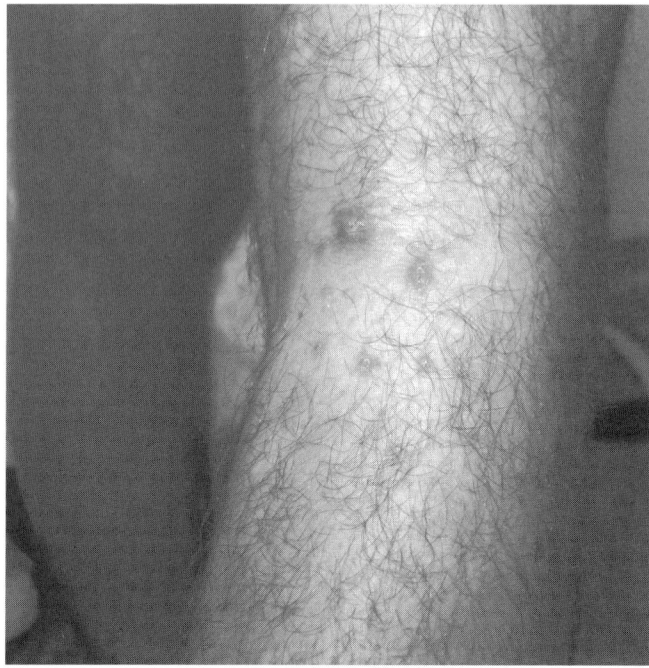

Figure 1-4. Well-defined, scattered, red, follicular papules and pustules that are classic for folliculitis occurring under occlusive knee pads. (See color plate.)

twice per day for 10 days. Extensive disease necessitates oral dicloxacillin 500 mg three times per day or cephalexin 500 mg three times per day for 10 to 14 days in addition to topical antibiotics. Penicillin-allergic patients may take erythromycin or clindamycin. Patients with MRSA infection respond to topical mupirocin. In vitro studies show that mupirocin inhibits growth of MRSA and even linezolid-resistant *S. aureus*. First-line therapy for extensive lesions of MRSA may also require oral trimethoprim-sulfamethoxazole or clindamycin for at least 14 days. Second-line therapy includes tetracycline, vancomycin, linezolid, or dactinomycin. Some clinicians also recommend povidone-iodine liquid soap or 4% chlorhexidine gluconate liquid detergent.

National Collegiate Athletic Association wrestling rules mandate that for infected athletes to compete, they must have taken oral antibiotics for at least 72 hours and must not have any new lesions for 48 hours before the match. After satisfying these two criteria, wrestlers must cover any visible lesions with a nonpermeable dressing that will not dislodge. Although the NCAA has standard guidelines, each state's high school association has different guidelines and the disqualification standard often resides at the discretion of the individually treating physician.

Prevention

Athletes must avoid sharing equipment, towels, ointments, and tape. Clinicians and staff should not dispense ointments from common containers. Athletes or the support staff must clean clothes and equipment daily. Clinicians should not forget to clean equipment such as sensor wires used in fencing (Table 1-2). Bleach and water, at a temperature of at least 71°C, must be used for laundering. Athletes must shower with antibacterial soap as soon as possible after the sports activity. Athletic programs should provide this antibacterial soap in the shower areas. Injured skin should be covered immediately, and athletes should wear loose-fitting clothing to decrease the exposed skin area. Body shaving should be discouraged in contact sport athletes (Table 1-1).

Moisture-wicking, synthetic clothing is ideal and keeps the athlete cool, even when the athlete is wearing long pants and long sleeves. Athletes should thoroughly shower before getting into communal hot tubs. These hot tubs are required to have automatic disinfection feeders and filtration and recirculation equipment. Whirlpools without these accessories must be emptied and disinfected after each athlete's use. Trainers must have easy access to hand cleanser to be used in-between seeing athletes. Athletes should thoroughly shower before getting into communal hot tubs. Investigators have failed to document the presence of pathogenic bacteria on wrestling mats, but caution suggests that wrestling mats be thoroughly cleaned (Table 1-2).

Athletes with positive nasal or crural cultures require application of topical mupirocin to each nares and to the perianal area twice per day for 1 week. This application should be repeated every 4 to 6 months to keep the growth of *S. aureus* in check. Athletes can continue to practice if the follicultitis lesion can be securely bandaged. The clinician should bench the athlete during epidemics or if the lesion cannot be safely secured.

Furunculosis

Epidemiology

Many authors have documented epidemics in Olympic, professional, collegiate, high school, and club athletes. Although any athlete can develop furunculosis (boils), fencers, canoeists, rafters, swimmers, and football, rugby, and basketball players seem particularly susceptible. One case of MRSA furunculosis in a weightlifter is reported.

Club

Methicillin-resistant *S. aureus* infected 7% of members of a fencing club in Colorado. The mean age of the infected fencers was 31 years (range 11–51 years). Three fencers were hospitalized. Extensive epidemiologic investigation did not reveal the vector of this infection, although fencers shared equipment and the facility had no showers. Sensor wires, used to identify touches by the opponent, were not regularly cleaned even though the wires were routinely shared (Table 1-2) (Centers for Disease Control and Prevention [CDC], 2003).

Professional

Five professional football players (9%) from one team developed MRSA furunculosis during the season. All isolated MRSA carried the gene for Panton-Valentine leukocidin and the gene complex for mec type IVa resistance, which differs from the resistance seen in nosocomially acquired organisms. All lesions occurred at sites of turf burns. Linemen were 10 times more likely than quarterbacks or backfielders to develop lesions. Interestingly, the risk of infection increased with the increasing weight of the lineman. These professionals lost 17 days of practice and game time (Kazakova, 2005).

This professional football epidemic prompted a close inspection of the players' daily activities. Turf burns occurred two to three times per week per player, and players rampantly shared towels on the playing field (three players per towel). The players did not shower before they used the communal whirlpool, trainers did not have accessible handwashing, and weights were not periodically cleansed (Table 1-2).

Another epidemic of professionals occurred when one third of a rugby team in England developed MRSA furunculosis in 1996 (Stacey et al., 1998).

Collegiate

Several college football teams have experienced epidemics. One of the earliest reports of an *S. aureus* epidemic occurred at Dartmouth College in 1963. Nine percent of the team acquired furunculosis and cellulitis. The following year, 33% had the disease. After intervention, 4% of the team had furuncles in 1965 (Pollard, 1967). More recently, 7% of the University of Georgia football team contracted MRSA furunculosis. Seven of 10 college football players in Pennsylvania and two college football players in California required hospitalization because of MRSA infection.

In 2003, MRSA infected 10% of a Connecticut College team and resulted in hospitalization of 2% of the team (Begier et al., 2004). Epidemiologic investigations revealed that cornerbacks and wide receivers were 17.5 and 11.7 times more likely than other players to develop furunculosis, respectively. Turf burns, cosmetic body shaving, and use of the whirlpool increased the risk of infection by seven, six, and 12 times, respectively. The presence of methicillin-sensitive *S. aureus* in athletes' nares and sharing of personal items (towels, equipment, deodorant, or soap) were not associated with infection (Table 1-2). No soap was available in the showers, and towels were inadequately laundered.

High School

Multiple high school teams in Texas, Kentucky, Illinois, and Indiana have endured epidemics of furunculosis. Thirty-six percent of a Texas football team contracted furunculosis in 1982. More cases occurred in strong contact players (linebackers, center, etc.) than in noncontact players. Athletes who wore elbow pads appeared to develop more infections than athletes who did not use the pads, although this difference was not statistically significant. No correlations existed between infection and use of the whirlpool or sharing of towels, equipment, or tape (Table 1-2) (Seidenfeld and Martin, 1983).

One study extensively examined the football and basketball teams from a Kentucky high school in 1989. *Staphylococcus aureus* infected 28% of the football players and 14% of the basketball players. In this study, prior skin injury (e.g., turf burns) or use of athletic tape increased the risk of infection by two to three times. Varsity athletes and athletes who used elbow pads and who came into contact with other athletes' furuncles appeared especially infection prone. Contact with towels and equipment, except elbow pads, did not increase an athlete's risk of infection (Table 1-2) (Sosin et al., 1989).

Another study of Illinois high school football players revealed that 18% of the team developed furuncles. Of all furunculosis cases, 60% were linemen and 40% were cornerbacks and defensive ends. The presence of a prior open wound and contact with shared skin lubricants, elbow pads, whirlpool baths, and athletic tape all seemed to increase the likelihood of infection (Table 1-2) (Bartlett et al., 1982). Soap in the showers was available to the athletes only 60% of the time.

Finally, at least 40% of a wrestling team contracted furunculosis in 1993 and 1994. Clinicians demonstrated MRSA in 22% of the wrestling team. The percentage of time the extremities were uncovered during practice, use of the whirlpool, acquisition of mat burns, and sharing of clothing or towels were not associated with the risk of infection (Table 1-2). One of the high school wrestlers ultimately required hospitalization (Lindenmayer et al., 1998).

Recreational

River rafting or canoeing guides have developed many furunculosis lesions. As many as 50% of guides acquired furuncles in the summer of 1982 in

Tennessee, South Carolina, and North Carolina. Employees of the same companies who were not involved in water activities did not develop the disease. Frequent minor skin wounds obtained while rafting and close skin contact with other rafters increased the risk of infection (Decker et al., 1986). *Staphylococcus aureus* causes furunculosis.

Clinical Presentation

Once the athlete is infected, the condition rapidly progresses to tender lesions (within 1–2 days). Furuncles present as tender, approximately 1 cm to several cm, well-defined, erythematous, occasionally fluctuant nodules distributed primarily on the extremities (Figure 1-5).

In the earliest known epidemic, Dartmouth College football players presented with lesions on the legs (59%), arms (26%), head and neck (12%), and buttocks (3%) (Pollard, 1967). In the Connecticut College football epidemic, 92% of the lesions occurred on the extremities, with the distribution equally divided between the arms and legs (Begier et al., 2004). In the Illinois high school epidemic, 89% of the furuncles developed on the extremities and 80% occurred on skin typically not covered by the uniform (Bartlett et al., 1982). The fencers involved in the MRSA epidemic also developed lesions on the abdomen, axilla, and buttock. Rafters exhibit lesions exclusively on the legs. Tens of athletes have required hospitalization, reflecting the seriousness of this skin infection.

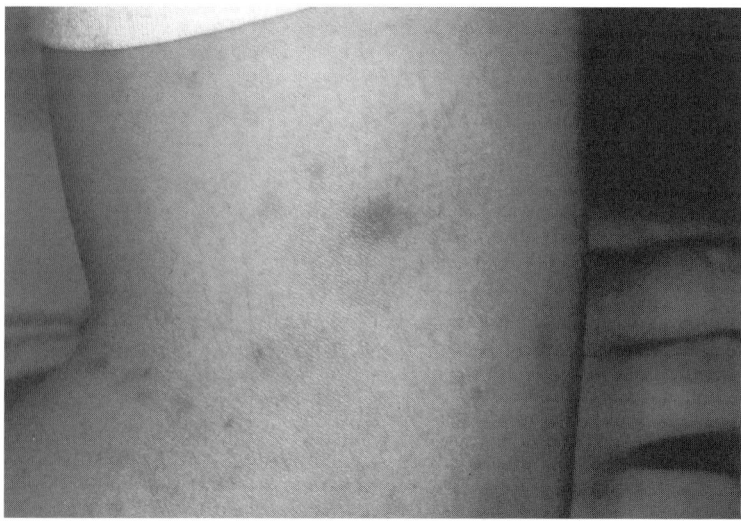

Figure 1-5. Well-defined, erythematous, tender nodules typify furunculosis.

Diagnosis

The diagnosis can be challenging, especially for early lesions, but is generally made clinically. The differential diagnosis includes ruptured epidermoid cyst, acne vulgaris, folliculitis, herpes gladiatorum, tinea corporis gladiatorum, and erythema nodosum (when on the leg).

Culture confirms the diagnosis and should absolutely be performed during epidemics. The clinician must brush the swab in the pustular material and not simply on the surface of lesions. The clinician should rub the lesion with an alcohol pad and then use a no. 11 or 15 blade to lance the pustule for proper culture. Culture also identifies MRSA infection. Clinicians should also consider nasal and crural swabs to identify any latent bacterial colonization.

Staphylococcus aureus does not colonize the nares infrequently in athletes (normal adults carry *S. aureus* in the nose 30%–50% of the time). In a professional football epidemic, 42% of the players and staff had positive *S. aureus* cultures (none were MRSA). Investigators also cultured *S. aureus* from the whirlpools and taping gel used by the trainers. In the Connecticut College football epidemic, none of the athletes exhibited MRSA in nasal cultures, but investigators discovered methicillin-sensitive *S. aureus* in 43% of the nasal cultures from players (Begier et al., 2004). During the rafting epidemic, 89% of rafters had positive nasal *S. aureus* cultures (Decker et al., 1986). This study of rafters also noted frequent positive *S. aureus* cultures after swabbing the surface of the raft upon which the rafters rested their legs. Fifty-five percent of the rafts demonstrated positive *S. aureus* cultures after use. These investigators also found that 29% of the rafts kept in storage for 72 hours still exhibited positive *S. aureus* cultures.

The mere presence of methicillin-sensitive *S. aureus* in the nares is of questionable importance as a cause for epidemics. For example, in the high school epidemic in Kentucky, the percent positive nasal cultures of *S. aureus* did not differ between control groups and the teams with furunculosis epidemics (Sosin et al., 1989). In the rugby MRSA epidemic, only one of the five infected players had a positive nasal culture. Investigators could not culture MRSA from any of the communal lubricant ointments (Stacey et al., 1998).

Treatment

Warm-water soaks must be applied three times per day for 5 to 10 minutes until clear. Localized and few lesions may require only topical mupirocin twice per day for 10 days. Extensive disease necessitates oral dicloxacillin 500 mg three times per day or cephalexin 500 mg three times per day for 10 to 14 days in addition to topical antibiotics. Penicillin-allergic patients may take erythromycin or clindamycin. Patients with MRSA respond to topical mupirocin. In vitro studies show that mupirocin inhibits growth of MRSA and even linezolid-resistant *S. aureus*. First-line therapy for extensive lesions of MRSA may also require trimethoprim-sulfamethoxazole or clindamycin for at least 14 days. Second-line therapy includes tetracycline, vancomycin, linezolid, or dactinomycin. Some clinicians also recommend povidone-iodine liquid soap or 4% chlorhexidine gluconate liquid detergent.

National Collegiate Athletic Association wrestling rules mandate that for infected athletes to compete, they must have taken oral antibiotics for at least 72 hours and must not have any new lesions for 48 hours before the match. After satisfying these two criteria, wrestlers must cover any visible lesion with a nonpermeable dressing that will not dislodge. Although the NCAA has standard guidelines, each state's high school association has different guidelines, and the disqualification standard often resides at the discretion of the individually treating physician.

Prevention

Although the results regarding the influence of equipment on the development of furunculosis is not conclusive, it seems most prudent for athletes to avoid sharing equipment, towels, ointments, and tape. Clinicians and staff should not dispense ointments from common containers. Athletes or the support staff need to clean clothes and equipment daily. Clinicians should not forget to clean equipment, such as sensor wires used in fencing (Table 1-2). Bleach and water, at a temperature of at least 71°C, must be used for laundering. Athletes must shower with antibacterial soap as soon as possible after the sports activity. Athletic programs should provide this antibacterial soap in the shower areas. Injured skin should be covered immediately, and athletes should wear loose-fitting clothing to decrease the exposed skin area. Body shaving should be discouraged in contact sport athletes (Table 1-1).

Moisture-wicking, synthetic clothing is ideal and keeps the athlete cool, even when the athlete is wearing long pants and long sleeves. Athletes should thoroughly shower before getting into communal hot tubs. These hot tubs are required to have automatic disinfection feeders and filtration and recirculation equipment. Whirlpools without these accessories must be emptied and disinfected after each athlete's use. Trainers must have easy access to hand cleanser to be used between seeing athletes. Investigators have failed to document the presence of pathogenic bacteria on the wrestling mats, but caution suggests that wrestling mats be thoroughly cleaned (Table 1-2).

During an epidemic at Dartmouth College, investigators intervened by fogging the locker and training rooms three times per week with a organotin antimicrobial solution. They also rinsed the laundry area and mopped the floors with the solution. Postintervention cultures noted a greater than 97% reduction in bacterial counts on the athletic department floors, benches, and lockers (Pollard, 1967).

Athletes with positive nasal or crural cultures require application of topical mupirocin to each nares and to the perianal area twice per day for 1 week. This application should be repeated every 4 to 6 months to keep the growth of *S. aureus* in check. Athletes can continue to practice if the furunculosis lesion can be securely bandaged. The clinician should bench the athlete during epidemics or if the lesion cannot be safely secured.

Erythrasma

Epidemiology

No studies are available, but most clinicians believe the disease is common in athletes. Athletes' groins are warm, dark, occluded, and macerated with sweat, conditions that make them ideal areas for microorganism growth.

Clinical Presentation

Corynebacterium minutissimum causes the well-defined, erythematous, minimally scaling plaques in the axilla or groin characteristic of erythrasma (Figure 1-6).

Diagnosis

The differential diagnosis includes tinea cruris, maceration intertrigo, seborrheic dermatitis, inverse psoriasis, and candidiasis. The diagnostic device

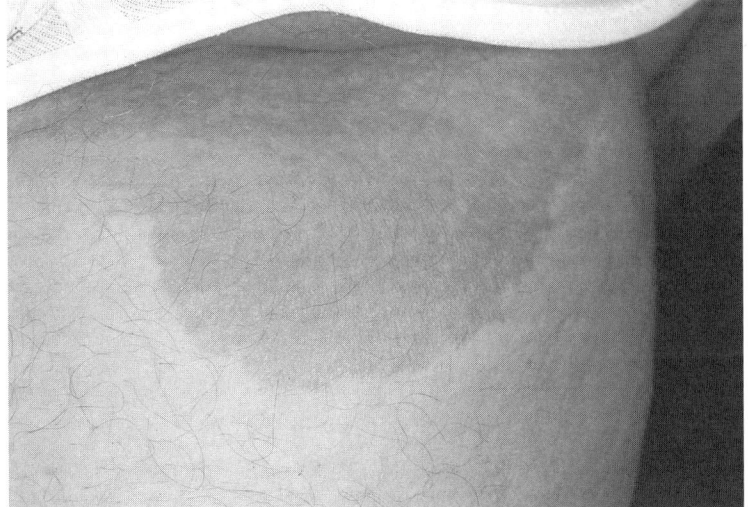

Figure 1-6. *Corynebacterium* infection on the medial upper thigh causes erythrasma, extending into the groin.

of choice is the Wood's lamp, which in a dark room reveals a brightly fluorescent coral-red color.

Treatment

A study in 1968 showed that using antibacterial soaps for 30 seconds twice during the shower significantly cleared erythrasma compared to placebo soap (Dodge et al., 1968). Tetracycline or erythromycin orally 250 mg three times per day should clear the eruption in 7 to 10 days. Topical antibiotics such as clindamycin and erythromycin may not clear the eruption as quickly.

Prevention

Athletes must wear moisture-wicking (such as Dri-fit) underwear to keep the groin and axillae as dry and cool as possible. Prophylactic use of topical clindamycin by athletes during the season may prevent outbreaks. Routine use of antibacterial soaps in the groin and axillae may prevent erythrasma.

Pitted Keratolysis

Epidemiology

This condition is also known as *sweaty sock syndrome.* Investigators examining 184 competitive athletes discovered the incidence of pitted keratolysis was 14% (Wohlrab et al., 2000). Basketball players, tennis players, and runners are specifically noted with this condition. The two main risk factors appear to be occlusive footwear and exertional hyperhidrosis of the foot. Several Gram-positive organisms, including *Micrococcus* and *Corynebacterium*, purportedly cause pitted keratolysis.

Clinical Presentation

The affected foot reveals well-defined craterlike pits on the sole, particularly on the weightbearing aspects (Figure 1-7). A distinct foul odor is present.

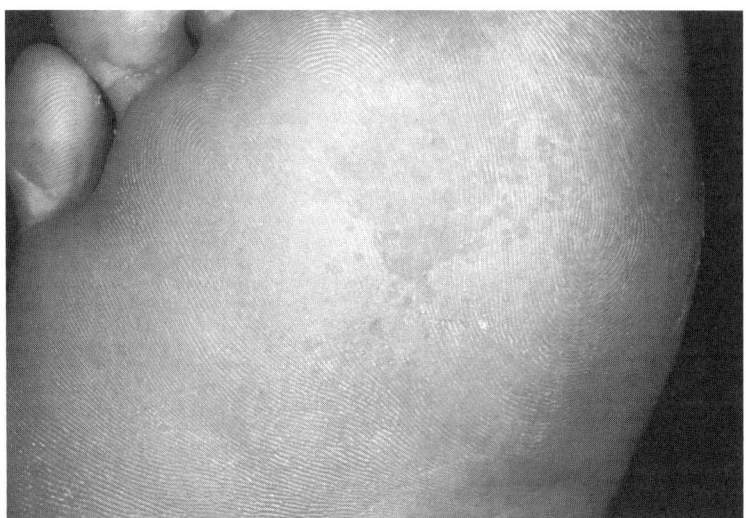

Figure 1-7. Characteristic pits cover the weightbearing aspect of the sole in pitted keratolysis.

Diagnosis

The diagnosis is generally straightforward but can be easily confused with tinea pedis and warts. The characteristic pits and the fact that the lesions can be made more obvious by submerging the affected area in water help to differentiate pitted keratolysis. It is important to note that the athlete can easily become secondarily infected because of the disturbed epidermal barrier.

Treatment

Topical therapies include clindamycin and erythromycin solution, lotion, or gel. Benzoyl peroxide is not only antimicrobial but also drying. Unfortunately, the athlete with the plentiful pits often experiences pain with use of benzoyl peroxide. Aluminum subacetate (Domeboro) soaks three times per day for 5 to 10 minutes is helpful. Superinfection must be treated with topical mupirocin (Bactroban) or oral dicloxacillin or cephalexin.

Prevention

Chronic moisture in the sock and shoe promotes the growth of causative organisms. Athletes can apply aluminum chloride to their feet before exercising to decrease the amount of sweating. Excellent advances in clothing technology allow the athlete to don synthetic, moisture-wicking socks. These socks keep the foot dry and cool. Companies manufacture socks for a variety of situations, including, but not limited to, socks that are lightweight, insulated, and extra padded.

Bikini Bottom

Epidemiology

Recreational and competitive swimmers develop this condition after prolonged exposure to wet, tight-fitting swimming suits. This condition also is noted in female volleyball players who sweat profusely in tight-fitting suit shorts. Women primarily experience this condition because of the styles of their suits.

Clinical Presentation

The occlusive and wet nature of the suits creates several tender, erythematous papules and nodules on the inferior aspects of the buttock (Figure 1-8).

Diagnosis

The clinician who fails to make the connection between sports participation and infection may have difficulty making the diagnosis. The clinical features and the history of wet, tight-fitting shorts or suits clinches the diagnosis.

Treatment

Athletes must avoid wet, tight-fitting shorts and take systemic antibiotics for 1 week. Topical antibiotics such as clindamycin and erythromycin can be effective. Athletes often prefer the gel and lotion preparations of topical antibiotics.

Prevention

Athletes should keep their buttocks as dry as possible. Athletes must change out of wet suits during long periods of inactivity out of the

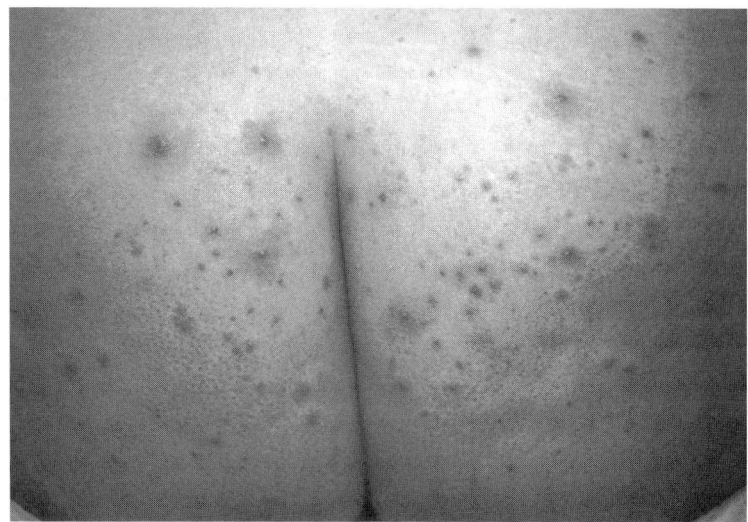

Figure 1-8. Follicular papules and pustules beneath the bikini characterize bikini bottom.

water. Daily prophylactic topical antibiotics during the season are recommended.

Erysipeloid

Epidemiology

This condition is also known as *fish handler's disease*, *shrimp picker's disease*, *crab poisoning*, and *blubber finger*. *Erysipelothrix rhusiopathiae*, the Gram-positive rod organism that causes the condition, can be found in fresh or salt water environments and is hearty. The organism survives normal processing of fish (salting, drying, pickling) and for up to 12 hours in direct sunlight. Divers, fishers, and swimmers contract the disease.

Clinical Presentation

This disease most commonly presents 1 to 7 days after a puncture wound sustained while the person was handling marine animals. It frequently occurs on the hand. The condition appears as a central area of erythema and edema surrounded by a halo of clearing. Peripheral to the clearing, however, is a well-defined, erythematous, violaceous plaque. Occasionally the lesion develops blisters. Complications include systemic infection with subsequent endocarditis, but in general there are no constitutional symptoms or lymphadenopathy.

Diagnosis

The diagnosis should be considered for aquatic athletes with localized infection. The lesion should be cultured (requires a special media consisting of 1% glucose). It is important to perform a cardiac examination and obtain blood cultures when systemic involvement is suspected. The differential diagnosis includes erysipelas (which usually has lymphadenopathy, unlike erysipeloid), cellulitis, and *Vibrio* infection.

Treatment

Untreated disease resolves spontaneously in 3 weeks. Therapy with penicillin, erythromycin, or a first-generation cephalosporin results in rapid resolution. Warm-water soaks should be applied to the wound for 5 to 10 minutes three or four times per day.

Prevention

Divers and fishermen must take great care not to sustain puncture wounds while they are handling marine animals. Gloves are quite helpful in preventing puncture wounds.

Gram-Negative Infections

Green Foot

Epidemiology

Only one case in a basketball player is reported (LeFeber and Golitz, 1984). The occlusive and sweaty nature of basketball shoes may allow the growth of *Pseudomonas* on shoe surfaces.

Clinical Presentation

Pseudomonas may cause asymptomatic green discoloration of the feet and toenails. The green color does not scrape or wipe off.

Diagnosis

The clinician who fails to make the connection between sports participation and the skin eruption may have difficulty making the diagnosis. Culture of the athletic shoes reveals the causative organism. Cultures of the skin may be negative.

Treatment

The reported athlete washed his basketball shoe and let it dry out before he used it a second time. The green color resolved within 1 month.

Prevention

Athletes must avoid wearing wet, sweaty basketball shoes. Daily application of 20% aluminum chloride to the foot decreases plantar hyperhidrosis and makes the shoes less hospitable to *Pseudomonas* colonization.

Diving Suit Dermatitis

Epidemiology

Several case series of this condition in scuba divers ranging in age from 12 to 58 years are reported (Lacour et al., 1994; Mantoux et al., 2003; Saltzer et al., 1997). *Pseudomonas aeruginosa* (serotypes O:10 and O:6—different from hot tub folliculitis) causes diving suit dermatitis. Diving suits occlude, resulting in superhydration of the epidermis. Furthermore, tight suits facilitate skin abrasions from the salt in sea water. These two factors decrease the protective value of the outer layer of the skin. *Pseudomonas* may originally reside in the water reservoir used to wash the suit, and the neoprene microalveoli create an ideal warm, moist microenvironment for the microorganism.

Clinical Presentation

Infected divers develop diffuse, scattered, erythematous papules and pustules on the trunk and extremities. On rare occasions divers exhibit fever, headache, and malaise.

Diagnosis

The differential diagnosis includes other types of folliculitis caused by acne, *Staphylococcus*, *Pityrosporum*, and steroids and other dermatoses such as bug bites, scabies, and swimmer's itch. Culture of the pustules or the diving suit confirms the diagnosis and provides serotyping of the organism.

Treatment

Unlike hot tub folliculitis, diving suit dermatitis requires oral antibiotics (ciprofloxacin 500 mg twice per day). The diving suit should be washed with 0.45% lactic acid.

Prevention

Diving suits must be thoroughly cleaned after each use. Divers should shower immediately after diving.

Hot Tub Folliculitis

Epidemiology

Any athlete is at risk for developing hot tub folliculitis, also known as *Pseudomonas* folliculitis. Several epidemics have been reported in football and racquetball players, athletes undergoing rehabilitation, snowmobilers, and waterslide enthusiasts. A national survey of states over a 10-year period revealed 72 different outbreaks of *Pseudomonas* folliculitis (Spitalny et al., 1984). Thirty-three percent of these nationwide outbreaks occurred at health or athletic clubs. In the same study, 14 racquetball players developed hot tub folliculitis in their club in Michigan. One study noted hot tub folliculitis in 47 people who used two whirlpools over a 2-month period (Shaw, 1984).

More than 80% of all cases of hot tub folliculitis have involved hot tubs or whirlpools, but nearly 20% have involved swimming pools (Chandrasekar et al., 1984). It appears that swimming pools that have very warm water can be risky. Ninety-three percent of swimmers (117 people) developed *Pseudomonas* from one swimming pool (Fox and Hambrick, 1984; Thomas et al., 1985), and 88% of a group of snowmobilers developed the condition from one swimming pool (Hopkins et al., 1981).

The largest epidemic of *Pseudomonas* folliculitis occurred at a water park. In Utah, 590 swimmers developed *Pseudomonas* folliculitis after enjoying a waterslide one day in April 1983 (CDC, 1983).

Pseudomonas aeruginosa O:11 is the most common serotype causing whirlpool folliculitis (Spitalny et al., 1984). Types O:6, O:1, O:4, O:9, and O:10 also are noted. Several factors allow the overgrowth of this organism. *Pseudomonas* proliferates at high temperatures (Sausker, 1987). High temperatures, turbulence, and heavy usage decrease chlorine levels and allow *Pseudomonas* to flourish. Turbulence may slough skin cells from the body that provide carbon debris for *Pseudomonas* growth (Green, 2000). Ammonia may contribute to the growth of *Pseudomonas*. When the pH of the water is >5, ammonia mixes with free chlorine and makes monochloramine, which is 1/13 as effective as chlorine in killing *Pseudomonas* (Silverman and Nieland, 1983). A correlation exists between the quantity of organisms and the severity of the folliculitis (Fox and Hambrick, 1984).

Host factors facilitate the entry of *Pseudomonas*. The high temperatures of the hot tub dilate follicular openings, and the water macerates the stratum corneum. Abrasions and lacerations inherent in athletes' skin are other avenues for *Pseudomonas* entry (Green, 2000). The prolonged period the injured athlete spends in the whirlpool also increases the risk for infection (Chandrasekar, 1984). It has been shown experimentally that a supersaturated stratum corneum (as one would expect to find in an athlete sitting in a hot tub) markedly enhances the growth of *Pseudomonas* (Silverman and Nieland, 1983). A very high attack rate between 90% and 100% for hot tub folliculitis in swimmers is documented (Hopkins et al., 1981; Thomas et al., 1985).

The cause of hot tub folliculitis is not without controversy. The inability to demonstrate *Pseudomonas* in histologic specimens has created speculation that some cases of hot tub folliculitis instead are caused by an exotoxin released by the organisms. In addition, cultures of pustules can reveal *Pseudomonas*, but not universally (Silverman and Nieland, 1983).

Clinical Presentation

The average incubation period is 49 hours (range 1–5 days). The infected athlete complains about pruritic, generalized, erythematous papules and pustules (Figure 1-9). Green pustules in an injured football player are reported (Green, 2000). The eruption occurs on any part of the body that was submerged and may concentrate on the skin beneath the bathing suit. The palms and soles are spared. Some athletes have noted a higher propensity of lesions in the axillae, groin, and

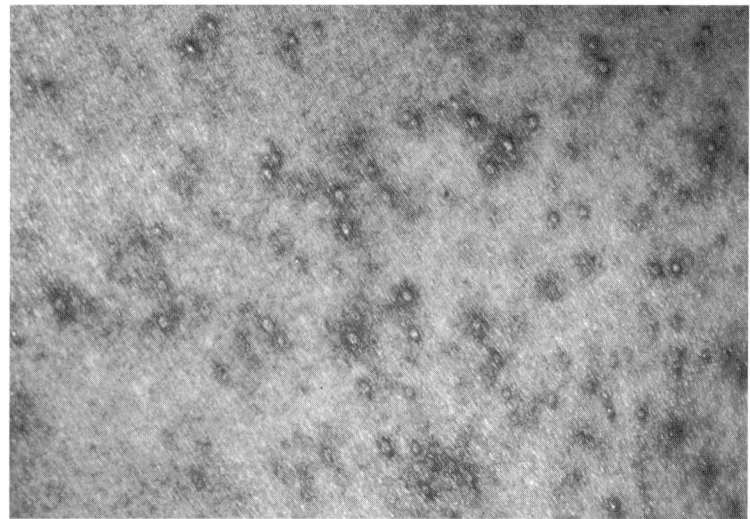

Figure 1-9. In hot tub folliculitis, erythematous papules and pustules develop on any submerged surface.

breasts as a result of apocrine involvement (Sausker, 1987). The median duration of the rash is 7 days (range 4–14 days) (Spitalny et al., 1984).

Systemic findings are not uncommon. Infected individuals can develop headache (42%), myalgias (34%), sore eyes (31%), fatigue (30%), and fever (26%) (CDC, 1983). Pharyngitis, lymphadenopathy, nausea, vomiting, and abdominal cramps are other associated signs and symptoms. Sepsis has occurred in at least one case (Goette and Fowler, 1984).

Diagnosis

The diagnosis is based on the distinctive clinical morphology, distribution, and association of whirlpool use. The differential diagnosis includes other types of folliculitis caused by acne, *Staphylococcus*, *Pityrosporum*, and steroids and other dermatoses such as bug bites, scabies, and swimmers itch (Fox and Hambrick, 1984; Hopkins et al., 1981; Silverman and Nieland, 1983). Culture of the pustules confirms the diagnosis and provides serotyping of the organism. Cultures of the hot tubs or pool water also may be positive (Fox and Hambrick, 1984; Silverman and Nieland, 1983; Thomas et al., 1985).

Treatment

Therapy is not needed; in fact, therapy is associated with recurrences (Green, 2000). The eruption is self-limited and resolves in 1 week. Oral therapy should be considered if the athlete is immunocompromised. Antihistamines may control the pruritus.

Prevention

The key to prevention includes adequate chlorination of whirlpools. Investigators have not been able to culture *Pseudomonas* from whirlpools that were adequately chlorinated so that standard coliform levels were negative (Shaw, 1984). If coliforms are present, the likelihood of culturing *Pseudomonas* from the pool increases. Some people have substituted bromine for chlorine to disinfect whirlpools. Unfortunately, one study showed that 25% of cultures from one whirlpool using bromine were positive for *Pseudomonas* even though the test for safe water (coliforms) was negative. Operators using brominated pools may incorrectly assume that the whirlpool is safe based on the negative coliform test. The free chlorine level should be at least 0.6 mg/L and the pH kept between 7.2 and 7.8.

Adequate chlorination does not guarantee that the whirlpool will be free of *Pseudomonas*. In 16% of the epidemics reported by state epidemiologists, chlorine levels in the pool were acceptable (Fox and Hambrick, 1984; Spitalny et al., 1984). The water in hot tubs should be changed frequently (Chandrasekar, 1984), and athletes should not enter the hot tub if the water is cloudy or foul smelling (Fox and Hambrick, 1984). The number of athletes in the pool at any given time must be limited. Showering 30 minutes after exposure to infected water does not appear to reduce the incidence of disease (CDC).

Pools with known presence of *Pseudomonas* require hyperchlorination so that the chlorine level is maintained at 5 mg/L for 3 days (Thomas et al., 1985).

Pseudomonas *Hot-Foot Syndrome*

Epidemiology

This unusual dermatologic condition was noted in 40 children who had used a community pool in Canada in 2001 (Fiorillo et al., 2002). The median age of the affected children was 6 years. *Pseudomonas aeruginosa* appears to cause this unusual skin condition.

Clinical Presentation

The condition occurred 10 to 40 hours after pool exposure. The first symptom in all patients was intense pain on the soles, followed within hours by marked edema, erythema, and excruciating pain on the soles prohibiting weight-bearing activities. Clinically the children had well-defined, violaceous, somewhat dusky, 1- to 2-cm nodules on the soles of the feet. Some individuals also developed fever, nausea, and malaise.

Diagnosis

The diagnosis may be challenging. The clinical presentation and the history of swimming pool use should be helpful. Culture and biopsy may be necessary to confirm the diagnosis. The differential diagnosis includes neutrophilic eccrine hidradenitis (also known as *idiopathic palmoplantar hidradenitis*, which can occur in athletes), and panniculitis. Lack of histologic findings of eccrine involvement, lack of recurrences, and positive cultures help to distinguish this condition from neutrophilic eccrine hidradenitis.

Treatment

In most swimmers, the condition clears with symptomatic therapy only. All symptoms resolve within 2 weeks.

Prevention

In the first report of this condition, the authors were able to culture *Pseudomonas* from the index swimming pool. Maintaining safe chorine levels, changing water filters, and smoothing rough pool surfaces may be prudent actions to decrease epidemics. Swimmers should avoid pools that have a known overgrowth of *Pseudomonas.*

Otitis Externa

Epidemiology

Some authors have noted that otitis externa (otherwise known as *swimmer's ear*) occurs in swimmers five times more often than in nonswimmers (Strauss and Dierker, 1987). Divers also are at risk. *Pseudomonas aeruginosa* or *S. aureus* produce swimmer's ear. Prolonged exposure to water causes maceration of the epidermis in the external auditory canal and dissolution of the sebum that protects the epithelium. Cerumen plugs and partial blocked canals related to individual anatomy can increase maceration of the epithelium along the external auditory canal (Strauss and Dierker, 1987). The pH of the canal is altered by this saturation and increases the potential for infection. Minor trauma (or chronic and excessive cleaning of the canal) experienced by swimmers is an additional risk factor for *Pseudomonas* infection in the ear canal.

Clinical Presentation

The incubation period of disease, after exposure to water, ranges from a few hours to several days. The infected swimmer complains of pain (occasionally severe) and pruritus, especially with chewing or movement of the pinna. Fever, lymphadenopathy, malaise, and ear drainage are possible associated symptoms and signs. Chronic cases are associated with decreased hearing.

Diagnosis

The diagnosis is made based on the typical clinical presentation and the history of swimming, although some cases develop days after aquatic exposure. Otoscopic evaluation reveals an erythematous and edematous external auditory canal that may be filled with debris and exudate.

Treatment

Treatment of mild cases includes liquid antibiotic ear drops (such as neomycin) twice per day and liquid steroids that are commercially found in combination. Topical steroids can significantly decrease pain and inflammation. A considerable percentage of people are allergic to neomycin; therefore, contact allergy should be considered in athletes who use this regimen, appear to improve, and then worsen. Oral analgesics and antiinflammatory agents also should be considered.

Acetic acid 2% in propylene glycol can be applied three times per day and should desiccate the area and restore the relative acidic microenvironment that prevents *Pseudomonas* growth. The clinician may need to carefully remove the debris from the external auditory canal. More severely affected patients with systemic symptoms require oral anti-*Pseudomonas* medications in addition to oral systemic steroids. The infection should be cleared before athletes return to the pool.

Prevention

Swimmers should dry their ears after swimming. Acetic acid 2% in propylene glycol application after swimming appears to decrease the incidence of swimmer's ear (Basler et al., 2000). Swimmers also can prevent otitis externa by wearing earplugs or a swimming cap. Swimmers with recurrent bouts should be carefully examined for anatomic anomalies.

Vibrio *Infection*

Epidemiology

This condition is caused by *Vibrio vulnificus*, a Gram-negative rod that proliferates in warm saline water. The organism is found in coastal water and populates certain surfaces of marine animals, such as shark teeth and sea urchin needles. Divers, fishermen, and swimmers are most at risk for *Vibrio* infection.

Clinical Presentation

The disease most commonly presents 1 to 3 days following a puncture wound sustained while the person was handling marine animals. Infection frequently occurs on the hand. The aquatic enthusiast develops a painful, erythematous, edematous plaque that may blister and necrose (Figure 1-10). Rapid spread of cellulitis occurs. Rarely fever, chills, and sepsis result (Auerbach, 1987).

Diagnosis

The diagnosis should be considered for aquatic athletes with localized infection. The lesion should be cultured (requires a special media consisting of 1% glucose). It is important to perform a cardiac examination and obtain blood cultures when systemic involvement is suspected. The differential diagnosis includes cellulitis, erysipelas, and erysipeloid infection.

Treatment

Warm-water soaks should be applied to the wound for 5 to 10 minutes three or four times per day. Tetracycline can be used for uncomplicated local skin

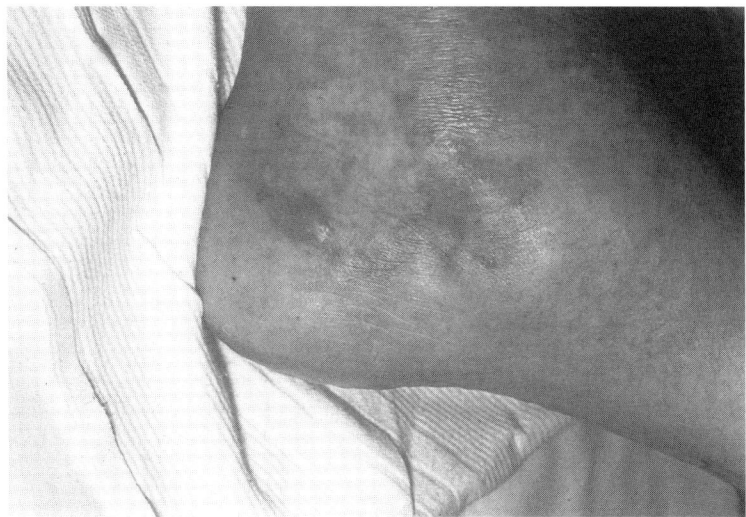

Figure 1-10. Well-defined, erythematous, necrotic plaques most often located on the extremities exemplify *Vibrio* infection.

infections. Imipenem, third-generation cephalosporins, amikacin, and gentamicin are among the treatment options for systemic disease.

Prevention

Divers and fishermen must take great care not to sustain puncture wounds while they are handling marine animals. Gloves and boots are quite helpful in preventing puncture wounds.

Tropical Ulcers

Epidemiology

Seven members of an English rugby team developed tropical ulcers while playing in Fiji (Webb, 1992). *Fusobacterium ulcerans* appear to play a role in the genesis of tropical ulcers.

Clinical Presentation

The disease develops within 2 weeks after athletes sustain minor abrasions while in endemic areas (e.g., the tropics). In the reported case series, most lesions developed on the knees, although some occurred on the hand and wrist. Multiple, well-defined, shallow, painless ulcers with indurated edges develop in the involved areas.

Diagnosis

The diagnosis should be considered for athletes who recently traveled to the tropics in whom abrasions from sporting activities do not heal and progress to ulcers. Cultures are necessary and may reveal bacteria causing a superinfection.

Treatment

Warm-water soaks should be applied to the wound for 5 to 10 minutes three or four times per day. Oral penicillin and cotrimoxazole have been effective.

Prevention

Athletes traveling to endemic areas should take great care to protect exposed skin. Abraded skin should be immediately and carefully cleaned.

Bibliography

Auerbach PS. Natural microbiologic hazards of the aquatic environment. Clin Dermatol 1987;5:52–61.

Basler RSW, Basler GC, Palmer AH, et al. Special skin symptoms seen in swimmers. J Am Acad Dermatol 2000;43:299–305.

Bartlett PC, Martin RJ, Cahill BR. Furunculosis in a high school football team. Am J Sport Med 1982;10:371–374.

Begier EM, Frenette K, Barrett NL, et al. A high-morbidity outbreak of methicillin-resistant Staphylococcus aureus among players on a college football team, facilitated by cosmetic body shaving and turf burns. Clin Infect Dis 2004;39:1446–1453.

Centers for Disease Control and Prevention (CDC). An outbreak of Pseudomonas folliculitis associated with a waterslide—Utah. MMWR Morb Mortal Wkly Rep 1983;32:425–427.

Centers for Disease Control and Prevention (CDC). Methicillin-resistant staphylococcus aureus infections among competitive sports participants: Colorado, Indiana, Pennsylvania, and Los Angeles County, 2000–03. MMWR Morb Mortal Wkly Rep 2003;52:793–795.

Chandrasekar PH, Rolston KVI, Kannangara DW, et al. Hot tub-associated folliculitis due to Pseudomonas aeruginosa Arch Dermatol 1984;120:1337–1340.

Charoenca N, Fujioka RS. Association of Staphylococcal skin infections and swimming. Water Sci Tech 1995;31:11–17.

Decker MD, Lybarger JA, Vaughn WK, et al. An outbreak of Staphylococcal skin infections among river rafting guides. Am J Epidemiol 1986;124:969–976.

Dodge BG, Knowles WR, McBride ME, et al. Treatment of erythrasma with an antibacterial soap. Arch Dermatol 1968;97:548–552.

Falck G. Group A streptococcal skin infections after indoor association football tournament. Lancet 1996;347:840–841.

Fiorillo L, Zucker M, Sawyer D, et al. The Pseudomonas hot-foot syndrome. N Engl J Med 2001;345:335–338.

Fox AB, Hambrick GW. Recreationally associated Pseudomonas aeruginosa folliculitis. Arch Dermatol 1984;120:1304–1307.

Glezen WP, DeWalt JL, Lindsay RL, et al. Epidemic pyoderma caused by nephritogenic streptococci in college athletes. Lancet 1972;1:301–304.

Goette DK, Fowler V. Hot-tub acquired Pseudomonas septicemia. J Assoc Mil Dermatol. 1984;10:40–41.

Green JJ. Localized whirlpool folliculitis in a football player. Cutis 2000;65:359–362.

Hopkins RS, Abbott DO, Wallace LE. Follicular dermatitis outbreak caused by Pseudomonas aeruginosa. Public Health Rep 1981;96:246–249.

Kazakova SV, Hageman JC, Matava M, et al. A clone of methicillin-resistant Staphylococcus aureus among professional football players. N Engl J Med 2005;352:468–475.

Lacour JP, El Baze P, Castanet J, et al. Diving suit dermatitis caused by Pseudomonas aeruginosa: two cases. J Am Acad Dermatol 1994;31:1055–1056.

LeFeber WP, Golitz LE. Green foot. Pediatr Dermatol 1984;2:38–40.

Lindenmayer JM, Schoenfeld S, O'Grady R, et al. Methicillin-resistant Staphylococcus aureus in a high school wrestling team and the surrounding community. Arch Intern Med 1998;158:895–899.

Ludlam H, Cookson B. Scrum kidney: epidemic pyoderma caused by a nephritogenic streptococcus pyogens in a rugby team. Lancet 1986;2:331–333.

Mantoux F, Hass H, Lacour JP. Wet suit-related Pseudomonas aeruginosa dermatitis in a child. Pediatr Dermatol 2003;20:458–459.

Pollard JG. The Staphylococcus plagues a football team. J Am Coll Health Assoc 1967;15:234–238.

Saltzer KR, Schutzer PJ, Weinberg JM, et al. Diving suit dermatitis: a manifestation of pseudomonas folliculitis. Cutis 1997;59:245–246.

Sausker WF. Pseudomonas aeruginosa folliculitis ("splash rash"). Clin Dermatol 1987;5:63–67.

Seidenfeld S, Martin D. Staphylococcus aureus infections in a high school football team. Austin, TX: Bureau of Epidemiology, Texas Preventable Disease News, week 13, 1983.

Shaw JW. A retrospective comparison of the effectiveness of bromination and chlorination in controlling Pseudomonas Aeruginosa in spas (whirlpools) in Alberta. Can J Public Health 1984;75:61–68.

Silverman AR, Nieland ML. Hot tub folliculitis: a familial outbreak of Pseudomonas folliculitis. J Am Acad Dermatol 1983;8:153–156.

Sosin DM, Gunn RA, Ford WL, et al. An outbreak of furunculosis among high school athletes. Am J Sport Med 1989;17:828–832.

Spitalny KC, Voot RL, Witherell LE. National survey on outbreaks associated with whirlpool spas. Am J Public Health 1984;74:725–726.

Stacey AR, Endersby KE, Chan PC, et al. An outbreak of methicillin resistant Staphylococcus aureus infection in a rugby football team. Br J Sport Med 1998;32:153–154.

Strauss MB, Dierker RL. Otitis externa associated with aquatic activities (swimmer's ear). Clin Dermatol 1987;5:103–111.

Thomas P, Moore M, Bell E, et al. Pseudomonas dermatitis associated with a swimming pool. JAMA 1985;253:1156–1159.

Torregrossa MV, Casuccio A. Correlation between staphylococcal skin infections and sea bathing: a case-control study. Ann Ig 2001;13:19–24.

Webb J, Murdoch DA. Tropical ulcers after sports injuries. Lancet 1992;339:129–130.

Wohlrab J, Rohrbach D, Marsch WC. Keratolysis sulcata (pitted keratolysis): clinical symptoms with different histological correlates. Br J Dermatol 2000;143:1348–1349.

2. Viral Skin Infections

This second chapter on sports-related skin infections summarizes the aspects of viral diseases as they pertain to athletes. Technically smallpox has been eradicated from the world, so the case of smallpox in a boxer in 1948 is not discussed in detail but is mentioned here for historical perspective. A Norwegian boxer developed the pustular eruption of smallpox on his head, neck, and right arm after he came in contact with an English competitor's contaminated boxing gloves. This case probably is one of the first reported skin infections in athletes.

Athletes with viral infections are particularly susceptible to pain, loss of practice time, and disqualification. Of all dermatologic conditions occurring in the athlete, viral infections, specifically herpes simplex infection, are among the most likely to cause morbidity, intense worry, and significant team disruption. In some cases, the virus spreads by skin-to-skin contact, whereas other times the virus is transmitted to the skin from inanimate objects. Even without contact, the athlete may develop recurrent herpes virus infection upon exposure to the elements.

Early identification, rapid treatment, and ultimately prevention are essential activities for clinicians in order to decrease disruption in practices and competitions. Epidemics can also be thwarted. This chapter specifically addresses herpes simplex infection occurring in noncontact and contact sports, verrucae (warts), and molluscum contagiosum.

Herpes Labialis (Noncontact Sports)

Epidemiology

Exposure to prolonged ultraviolet (UV) irradiation increases the risk of reactivating prior herpes simplex virus (HSV) infection. One study determined that the sun induced HSV in approximately 20% of the population during the summer months and in up to 40% of patients younger than 30 years (Ichihashi, 2004). Thus, all outdoor athletes who fail to protect their lips are at potential risk for developing herpes labialis. A few studies that examined the epidemiology of HSV concentrated on skiing. Twelve percent of skiers with a known history of HSV developed lesions during 1 week of skiing (Mills et al., 1987).

Several studies determined the amount of UV irradiation to which outdoor athletes are exposed is several times the amount needed to induce a burn. Winter athletes whose sport occurs in the snow and at high altitudes experience an even higher risk. Snow reflects a large amount of UV irradiation, thus multiplying the level of UV exposure to winter enthusiasts. Furthermore, athletes at high elevation must contend with more intense irradiation because less UV is filtered out by the atmosphere. One study showed that a skier at 11,000 feet in Vail,

Colorado, received the same intense UV B radiation as a beachgoer in Orlando, Florida. Other at-risk athletes include snowboarders, snowmobilers, tobogganers, and athletes participating in other outdoor sports.

Scuba divers suffer from herpes labialis for other reason (Potasman and Pick, 1997). During drills that simulate emergency situations, divers may frequently share mouthpieces of the pressurized air regulator, and a great deal of saliva tends to develop around the mouthpiece. Because these transitions among divers occur in less than 3 seconds, HSV likely survives on the mouthpiece during this brief time. Athletes who share protective mouthpieces are at risk for acquiring herpes labialis from other athletes with active infection (Table 2-1). Herpes simplex virus type 1 (HSV-1) causes most cases of oral herpes labialis.

Clinical Presentation

Athletes with herpes labialis (primary infection or reactivation) often complain of a stinging or burning sensation in the area that eventually develops skin lesions (so-called *prodrome*). After 1 to 4 days, a painful erythematous papule develops in the same location as the prodrome. In one study, the median time to lesion development after a person arrived to ski was 3.5 days (Mills et al., 1987). The papule soon develops grouped vesicles upon an erythematous base. After several days, the lesion becomes crusted and resolves slowly (Figure 2-1). Systemic findings are not unusual in the setting of oral herpes labialis, especially in the primary form. Athletes may suffer sore throat, fever, myalgias, arthralgias, and lymphadenopathy.

Diagnosis

The diagnosis often is straightforward and can be made based on clinical findings alone. In indeterminate cases, Tzanck smear, direct immunofluorescence (DFA), or culture may be necessary. Tzanck smear provides the most rapid result but can be technically challenging even for seasoned dermatologists. Direct immunofluorescence provides rapid results (often within just a few

Table 2-1. Evidence-Based Support for Viral Infection Epidemics

Viral Infection	Associated Sport or Activity
Herpes labialis	Skiing, scuba diving
Herpes simplex	Rugby, wrestling
Molluscum	Cross-country running, swimming
Verrucae	Rowing, swimming, showering

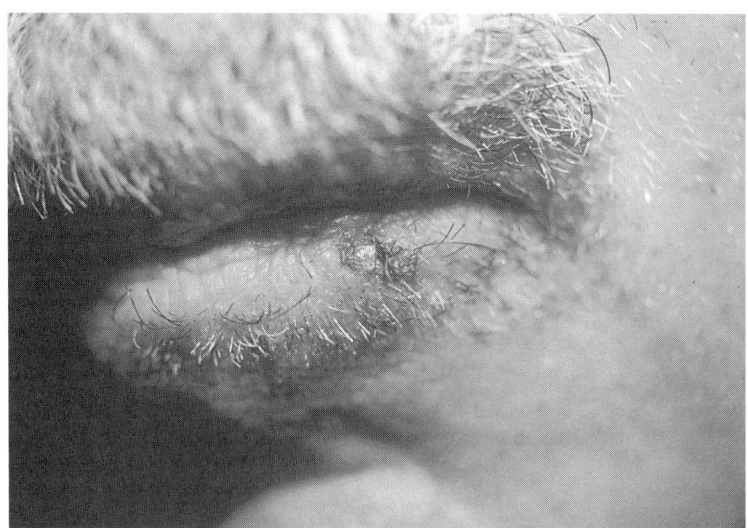

Figure 2-1. Typical herpes labialis lesion that might be seen in an outdoor athlete exposed to intense ultraviolet radiation (e.g., a skier).

hours), but the test is not universally available at all laboratories. Culture is the gold standard for identifying the presence of HSV infection, but the culture may take 1 to 2 days to become positive.

Treatment

Because most of the infections resulting from participation in noncontact sports actually are reactivated herpes labialis, the dosing regimen for this type of infection is most appropriate (Table 2-2). Oral acyclovir 200 mg can be given

Table 2-2. Dosing Regimens for Treatment of Recurrent Herpes Labialis, Herpes Gladiatorum, or Herpes Rugbeiorum

Medication	Dose (mg)	Frequency	Duration (days)	Cost
Acyclovir	200	5 times/day	5	Low
Famciclovir	500	bid	5	High
Valacyclovir	2000	bid	1	Medium

five times per day for 5 days. More expensive but easier dosing regimens, which likely translate into increased compliance, include famciclovir and valacyclovir. The dose of oral famciclovir is 500 mg twice per day for 5 days. A study revealed that an effective dosage of valacyclovir is 2 g twice per day for only 1 day. This simple dosing regimen is as effective as the other regimens and likely will result is high athlete compliance.

Prevention

Athletes with active herpes labialis are clearly contagious. Unfortunately, athletes may shed the virus asymptomatically and unwittingly transmit the HSV to other athletes. Under no circumstance other than emergent should infected athletes share protective mouthpieces. Scuba divers, who may be required to share mouthpieces in emergency situations or during practice drills, must be excluded from diving if they have active herpes labialis.

Skiers, snowboarders, snowmobilers, tobogganers, and other winter outdoor enthusiasts must protect their lips with sunscreen. Many commercially available lip balms with sun protective factor (SPF) are available. The balms are compact and are easily carried in pockets. Sweating decreases the effectiveness of sunscreen, so it must be reapplied frequently. A double-blind, placebo-controlled study demonstrated that, after UV exposure to the lips, 71% of unprotected individuals developed HSV lesions, whereas none of those who wore sunscreen developed lesions (Rooney et al., 1991).

Pharmacologic therapy for herpes labialis has been studied in skiers. Skiers who took acyclovir 400 mg twice per day beginning 12 hours before anticipated sun exposure were significantly less likely to develop HSV lesions (Spruance et al., 1988).

Herpes Simplex (Contact Sports)

Epidemiology

All athletes participating in sports with close, intense skin-to-skin contact are susceptible to acquiring HSV infection (otherwise know as *fever blisters*) from other athletes. The two most studied athletes are rugby players and wrestlers, although on rare occasions lesions are noted in soccer players during heading maneuvers (Table 2-1). Macerated skin from sweating and traumatic skin injuries inherent to both wrestling and rugby facilitate infection by HSV.

Rugby

Rugby players have prolonged and concentrated skin-to-skin contact during the act of the scrum, wherein the players link arms, encircle the ball, and attempt to take possession of the ball. Members of the scrum have abrasive contact with each other for 30 to 45 seconds repeatedly during games. *Herpes rugbeiorum* (HR) (or *scrum pox)* is the term designated for HSV infection in rugby players. The epidemiology of HR is much less studied than that of herpes gladiatorum (HG), but epidemics clearly can occur among rugby players. Interestingly, the forwards (who are members of the scrum) are the players whose position places them at greatest risk for developing HR. Other position players may become infected but are less likely to because of relatively less skin-to-skin contact. On one team, four of the eight rugby forwards were infected (the left and right prop, the lock, and one of the second row) (White and Grant-Kels, 1984). Another study in England demonstrated that nearly half of the rugby clubs had skin disease, and 95% of the infected players were forwards (Shute et al., 1979). Another study demonstrated that 38% of a rugby team developed HR (Skinner et al., 1996).

Wrestling

Herpes gladiatorum is the term designated for HSV infection in wrestlers. Wrestlers have arguably the most intense skin-to-skin contact during matches. Most clinicians accept the term herpes gladiatorum; however, some authors disapprove because of the term's incorrect etymology (Laur et al., 1979). They indicate that gladiators are distinctly different from wrestlers and suggest incorporating the Latin term for wrestler, preferring the term *herpes luctator*. The literature is replete with the HG designation, however, so the condition is henceforth described in this book as herpes gladiatorum.

The epidemiology of HG probably is the best studied of all cutaneous sports ailments. Seventeen completed prevalence studies have reported a wide spectrum of results. The lowest reported prevalence is 2.6% and the highest is 40.5% (Becker et al., 1988; Belongia et al., 1991; Brenner et al., 1994; Dyke et al., 1965; Porter and Baughman, 1965; Wheeler and Cabaniss, 1965). The median prevalence (which likely represents the true estimate) is 20%. The large range reflects the dissimilar manner in which the studies were performed. For instance, the lowest prevalence of 2.6% was determined in a study of athletic trainers who were asked to recall the number of high school and college athletes who had been infected. Because of recall bias, selection bias, and the very small fractional survey return rate, the true prevalence likely was underestimated. Based on data from the National Collegiate Athletic Association injury surveillance system (NCAAISS), 39% of all skin infections in collegiate wrestlers between 1991 and 2003 were caused by HSV. Shingles (another *Herpes* virus) composed 3% of the skin infections.

An interesting HSV exposure method involves an injured athlete whose need to use the whirlpool may place the athlete at risk for developing HSV. One study showed that HSV may survive on plastic spa surfaces at temperatures above 100°F for 4.5 minutes. Transmission to an athlete undergoing rehabilitation may be facilitated by the athlete's skin abrasions (Nerurkar et al., 1983).

Most of the clinical work on HSV infection in contact sports has involved HG. There is no reason to suspect that the principles of diagnosis, treatment, or prevention of HSV would be different among the various contact sports. Herpes gladiatorum is caused by HSV-1, although not all studies report typing the virus.

Clinical Presentation

Once HSV is located on an athlete's skin, its incubation period ranges from a few days to several weeks. Athletes first experience a prodrome characterized by burning, stinging, itching, or pain in the area that eventually develops a skin lesion. The appearance of HG varies and depends primarily on the age of the lesion (Table 2-3). Very early lesions have a nonspecific clinical appearance and are well-defined erythematous papules. As the lesion matures, it develops the characteristic grouped vesicles upon an erythematous base (Figures 2-2 through 2-4, see color plate for Figure 2-2). As the individual lesion resolves, crust develops on top. The lesion eventually heals, with or without therapy.

It is important for clinicians to realize that athletes know the presence of HSV results in disqualification. To avoid detection, athletes may secondarily alter the clinical morphology of the lesion. They may attempt to use sandpaper or household bleach to mask the appearance of blisters or suspicious papules.

The distribution of HG and HR results from the skin-to-skin contact inherent in both rugby and wrestling. In both sports, the most common locations of HSV infection are extramucosal sites. The head and neck account for 75% of all HG lesions. The extremities are the next most common location of lesions, followed by the trunk (Adams, 2001; Anderson, 2003; Dworkin et al., 1999). In rugby, the most common location for infection is on the head and neck (representing more than two thirds of all lesions), but the shins, hip and hands also can be infected (Skinner et al., 1996; White and Grant-Kels, 1984).

Systemic symptoms are not unusual, especially in cases of primary HSV infection. Athletes may complain of fever, sore throat, malaise, myalgias, arthralgias, and swollen lymph glands.

Complications of either HG or HR are not inconsequential. Several organ systems are affected. Athletes participating in both sports report eye complica-

Table 2-3. Clinical Appearance of Lesions of Herpes Gladiatorum or Herpes Rugbeiorum Based on Duration

Clinical Appearance	Age of Lesion (days)
Red papule	1–2 (very early)
Grouped blisters	2–6
Crusted papule	5–14

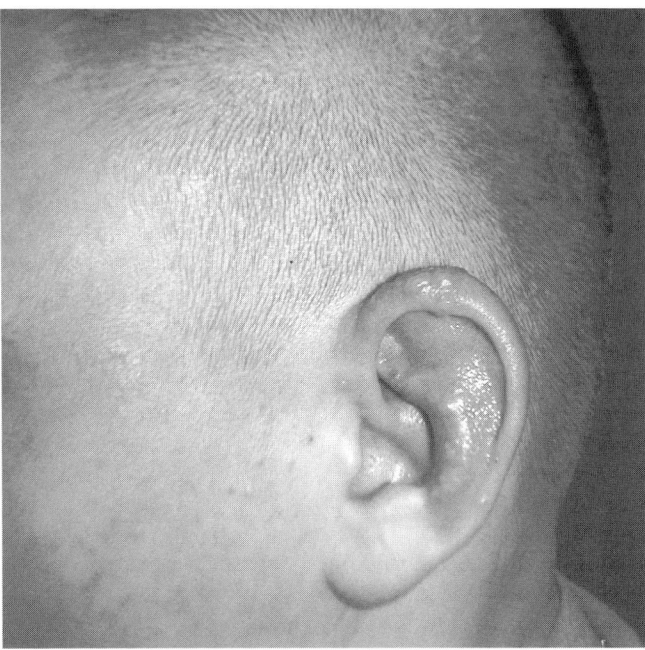

Figure 2-2. Grouped vesicles on an erythematous base are characteristic of herpes gladiatorum or herpes rugbeiorum. The ears are commonly affected in wrestlers. (See color plate.)

tions. Involvement of the eye, including herpes conjunctivitis, blepharitis, and keratitis (Holland et al., 1992; Rosenbaum et al., 1990; Selling and Kibrick, 1964), has been noted in 8% of wrestlers with HG (Holland et al., 1992). Likewise, more than half of reported patients with HR developed ophthalmologic complications, including keratoconjunctivitis and blepharitis (Skinner et al., 1996; White and Grant-Kels, 1984). Although these ophthalmic findings generally resolve, permanent impairment has been noted (Keilhofner and McKinsey, 1988). The risk of ocular recurrence is greater than 33% within 5 years. Recurrence may affect the cornea even though the initial infection involved only the eyelid (Mast and Goodman, 1997). One wrestler developed a monoarticular arthritis from which HSV was cultured (Shelley, 1980); this complication has not been documented in rugby players. Neurologic involvement has been reported in HR. One rugby player with HR developed HSV-related meningitis and sacral ganglionitis with perineal and lower extremity paresthesias (White and Grant-Kels, 1984).

The distribution of lesions supports the prevailing idea that HSV infections in sports are not transmitted through inanimate objects such as wrestling mats. If the mat played a role, more lesions on the lower extremities would be expected.

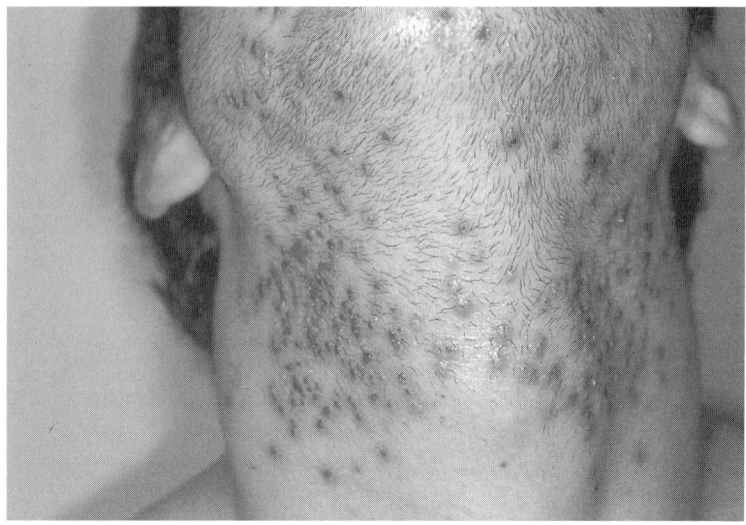

Figure 2-3. Primary herpes gladiatorum infection can be extensive and frequently occurs on the neck.

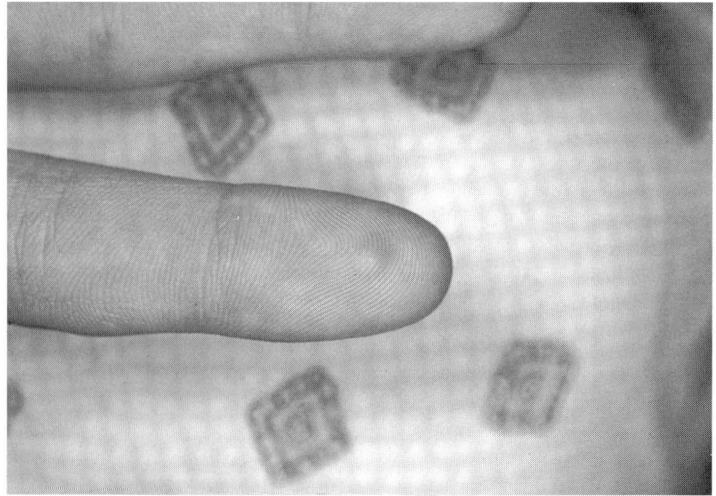

Figure 2-4. Herpes gladiatorum can be quite subtle and difficult to diagnose, especially in atypical locations. A very high index of suspicion helps prevent misdiagnosis.

However, most lesions occurring on the head and neck correspond to the cross-face maneuvers and locking-up position of wrestlers. Maceration resulting from sweating and the abrasions obtained facilitate HSV infection. Abrasive shirts and unshaven beards are other purported reasons for easy transmittal of HSV (Strauss et al., 1989).

Transmission of HG or HR is enhanced by the fact that infected individuals may shed virus for days before the infection becomes obvious. Once infected, an athlete is a carrier and may insidiously infect others before outward signs of blisters are apparent. One study showed that the probability of HSV transmission in the setting of wrestlers was 33%.

Diagnosis

The diagnosis can be challenging because very early lesions are difficult to distinguish from acne vulgaris, atopic dermatitis, molluscum contagiosum, tinea corporis gladiatorum, and impetigo (Table 2-4). Furthermore, adulterated or very late lesions do not demonstrate the diagnostic grouped vesicles on an erythematous base. In indeterminate cases, Tzanck smear, culture, DFA, or polymerase chain reaction (PCR) may be necessary.

Tzanck smear provides the most rapid result but can be technically challenging even for seasoned dermatologists. One study showed that practicing dermatologists were only 67% correct in using the Tzanck smear (Grossman and Silvers, 1992). Culture is the gold standard for identifying the presence of HSV infection, but the culture make take 1 to 2 days to become positive. Direct immunofluorescence provides rapid results (often within just a few hours), but the test is not universally available at all laboratories. Advances in PCR technology allow rapid and precise detection of HSV. The enzyme-linked viral inducible system (ELVIS) test is highly sensitive and specific, with positive and negative predictive values of 99% and 99%, respectively (La Rocco, 2000). Although PCR theoretically is the ideal test, its cost and availability limit its use at the "mats." Until national collegiate and state high school associations commit financial resources to making rapid yet affordable tests, such as the DFA, available at wrestling competitions, epidemics at the high school and collegiate levels will continue.

Because DFA may not detect very early lesions of HSV, the clinician must base the diagnosis on a constellation of findings, including a prodrome history, suspicious lesions, and associated systemic findings.

Table 2-4. Differential Diagnosis of Herpes Gladiatorum

Acne vulgaris
Atopic dermatitis
Impetigo contagiosum
Molluscum contagiosum
Tinea corporis gladiatorum

Treatment

Unlike the infections resulting from participation in noncontact sports, contact sport infections with HSV are either newly acquired or reactivated HSV. The original dosing regimen for reactivated HSV was oral acyclovir 200 mg given five times per day for 5 days. Although oral acyclovir is the most inexpensive of all oral antiviral agents for treatment of HG or HR, dosing at five times per day decreases patient compliance. More expensive but easier dosing regimens, which likely translate to increased compliance, include famciclovir and valacyclovir (Table 2-2). The dose of oral famciclovir is 500 mg twice per day for 5 days. In the case of newly acquired HSV lesion, the athlete should take the oral antiviral agent for 1 week. A study revealed that the dosage of valacyclovir is 2 g twice per day for only 1 day. Although this dosing pattern has not been specifically tested in sports-acquired infections, this simple dosing regimen is as effective as the other regimens and likely will result in high athlete compliance. Valacyclovir is a relatively safe medication that has been used in athletes, with no known untoward side effects. This medication should be used with caution in individuals with kidney disease or immunosuppression.

No data support a length of time during which athletes are contagious after treatment with oral antiviral agents. Use of acyclovir decreases viral shedding to 4 days. As a reasonable extrapolation, athletes can safely return to their skin-to-skin contact sport after 4 days of oral antiviral therapy. This recommendation should help thwart team and league epidemics. No studies have examined topical antiviral agents in terms of HG or HR, so these agents should not play a role in the therapy of athletes.

Prevention

No evidence indicates that wrestling mats play a role in transmission of HSV to other athletes. Therefore, the need to perform time-consuming daily washing and cleansing of mats is not supported. However, the practice seems prudent and continues, especially with the recommendation of clinicians. It also seems prudent that athletes routinely and immediately shower after practice and competition, although no evidence-based medicine supports this practice. Athletes must wear sandals while using communal showers. Weak evidence supports the wearing of protective gloves while athletes use weightlifting equipment to decrease the transmission of infectious agents. Athletes should not share protective equipment, towels, razors, or clothing. These items must be cleansed regularly (Table 2-5).

Several companies produce skin protection substances in the form of foams that athletes apply to their skin or trainers and coaches apply to equipment and mats. These skin protectants and wrestling gear and mat cleansers purportedly kill the microorganisms that afflict the wrestler. To my knowledge, no study has investigated these claims, and clinicians should skeptically evaluate the claims made by the manufacturers.

2. Viral Skin Infections   45

Table 2-5. General Primary Prevention of Communicable Skin Infections in Athletes

---
Avoid sharing protective equipment, clothing, towels, razors
Encourage regular cleansing of towels and equipment
Use protective gloves when using weightlifting equipment
Take immediate shower after practice and competition
Wear sandals in the locker room and showers

The keys to thwarting epidemics in teams and leagues are extensive surveillance coupled with rapid institution of oral therapy. Daily practices are ideal times to examine the athletes' skin. Coaches, trainers, and athletes themselves should join forces to ensure that all lesions are detected as early as possible. The ultimate control of epidemics in contact sports will come when a specifically trained clinician is assigned to each school or, if funding is an issue, a group of schools. At present, especially on the high school level of sports activity, a medley of clinicians cares for the athletes on a team. In most states, wrestlers must present a completed evaluation and authorization form to the precompetition official. However, the policy is not consistent, and no uniform or logical diagnostic approach or treatment and prevention plan is available. In addition, the individuals who disqualify or qualify athletes need not be clinicians with any particular expertise in the area.

One interesting study illustrates this quandary. In one area of the United States, more than 90% of wrestlers with a questionable communicable skin disease were incorrectly allowed to return to wrestling. Physicians incorrectly diagnosed 92% of wrestlers (who ultimately were culture positive for HSV) as having impetigo, tinea corporis gladiatorum, and eczema 70%, 10%, and 10% of the time, respectively. Furthermore, viral cultures were completed during the initial evaluation for only 20% of the infected wrestlers. Because of these misdiagnoses, three counties in Washington state experienced an epidemic in which 5% of all wrestlers were infected with HSV (Dworkin et al., 1999).

On the other hand, the NCAA has highly specific guidelines for wrestling coaches, athletes, and clinicians (Table 2-6). No specific guidelines exist for collegiate-level rugby. An athlete with HG may not compete unless (1) all lesions are dried and covered with an adherent crust and (2) the wrestler has been undergoing oral antiviral therapy for at least 120 hours. Wrestlers with a primary outbreak cannot have systemic symptoms of HG, and those with both primary and recurrent infections must not have sustained new blisters 72 hours before the skin check. The NCAA ensures that athletes adhere to these stipulations by requiring the presence of a physician or a certified athletic trainer at the precompetition skin check. No such requirement exists for high school precompetition skin checks, where a nonclinician usually determines qualification. As a result, competitors without contagious skin disease may be unduly barred from competition. Conversely, athletes with transmissible cutaneous infections who erroneously are allowed to compete can infect with epidemic potential.

Once identified, athletes with contact-related HSV should be treated immediately. If the number and location of lesions permit simple bandaging tech-

Table 2-6. Guidelines for Return to Competition for Athletes with Herpes Gladiatorum Based on National Collegiate Athletic Association Guidelines

1. All lesions must be dried with an adherent crust, and
2. The wrestler must have been undergoing oral antiviral therapy for 120 hours, and
3. No systemic symptoms of herpes gladiatorum, and
4. No new blisters within 72 hours of precompetition skin check-in

- Evidence-based data suggest however 96 hours is sufficient
- Valacyclovir's one-time dosing allows competition 96 hours later

niques, athletes can continue to practice. However, in most states, bandaging a lesion during competition is unacceptable and the wrestler is disqualified. If the number and location of lesions do not permit bandaging techniques, the athlete must be benched until oral antiviral therapy has been given for 4 days.

Because the athlete may asymptomatically shed HSV, epidemics still may sprout despite satisfactory surveillance. Oral pharmacologic prevention may help prevent epidemics and obviate the challenging scenario of asymptomatic carriers. A double-blind, placebo-controlled study examined the effectiveness of oral valacyclovir in preventing HG. The study examined two different categories of wrestlers: those who had a primary HSV infection more than 2 years ago and those who had a primary HSV infection less than 2 years ago. Wrestlers who had primary lesions more than 2 years ago and took valacyclovir 500 mg once per day did not develop HG, whereas 33% of wrestlers who took placebo developed HG. Wrestlers with a primary HSV lesion less than 2 years ago who were in the valacyclovir group developed HG 21% of the time, whereas the placebo group developed HG 33% of the time. Although rigorous statistical analyses reveal no differences between the active drug and placebo groups ($p = 0.192$ and $p = 0.68$, respectively), the study was underpowered. A study with greater numbers likely would demonstrate clinical and statistical differences between placebo and active drug (Anderson, 1999).

During the second portion of the season and the study, all wrestlers were given valacyclovir 1 g per day. No wrestlers whose original HG occurred more than 2 years ago developed HSV lesions, and only 8% of wrestlers whose original HG occurred less than 2 years ago developed HSV lesions. Use of daily oral prophylaxis for herpes in athletes participating in contact sports is relatively safe and likely will decrease transmission and prevent epidemics.

One study in Europe evaluated the effectiveness of using an intracellular cytoplasmic detergent-treated virus particle vaccine. After a rugby team experienced an epidemic in which 38% of its players were infected with HSV, the vaccine was given to the entire team and five sociosexual contacts of the players. Based on HR data, at least 10% of the rugby players are expected to develop recurrences during the season. Surprisingly, none of the players developed any HR even 3 years after they received the vaccine (Skinner et al., 1996).

To truly prevent epidemics, the National Federation of State High School Associations (NFHS), state high school associations, and high schools themselves should invest time, energy, and funds to (1) designate one properly trained professional to evaluate all suspicious lesions from one school or region and complete required forms, (2) designate one properly trained professional to officiate at the precompetition check-in, (3) institute guidelines for the adequate diagnosis, treatment, and prevention of herpes in contact sports, and (4) encourage universal adoption of these recommendations. The current NCAA guidelines should be amended as evidence-based data become available.

Molluscum Contagiosum

Epidemiology

Two studies have examined the epidemiology of molluscum contagiosum among athletes. One large study of 7500 children showed that swimmers had a 7.5% incidence of infection (twice that of nonswimmers), which was highly statistically different from that of a control group of nonswimmers (Niizeki et al., 1984). In another study, 8% of 1400 cross-country runners had molluscum contagiosum (Table 2-1) (Mobacken and Nordin, 1987).

Molluscum contagiosum has been reported in multiple contact (rugby players and wrestlers) and noncontact sports (gymnasts) (Cyr, 2004; Halstead and Bernhardt, 2002). Based on data from the NCAAISS, 0.3% of all skin infections in collegiate wrestlers between 1991 and 2003 were caused by molluscum. Although any athlete may acquire the virus, the aforementioned athletes seemed particularly susceptible. In contact sports, the lesions are spread through intense skin-to-skin contact and by autoinoculation. Macerated skin from sweating and traumatic skin injuries inherent to both wrestling and rugby athletes facilitate infection by molluscum contagiosum. Presumably gymnasts, runners, and swimmers acquire their infection as a result of contact with equipment and the apparent hostile microenvironment in which the athletes place their extremities. I have seen numerous molluscum lesions in collegiate women volleyball players. The diving trauma and the tight-fitting occlusive shorts worn by the players facilitate autoinoculation once a solitary molluscum is present.

Clinical Presentation

Molluscum contagiosum, caused by a virus in the Poxviridae family, generally are asymptomatic, small (1–6mm), well-defined white or skin-colored umbilicated (having a central dell) papules (Figures 2-5 and 2-6, see color plate). They occasionally become pruritic and develop surrounding erythema that can be intense and eczematous. The lesions may be grouped and

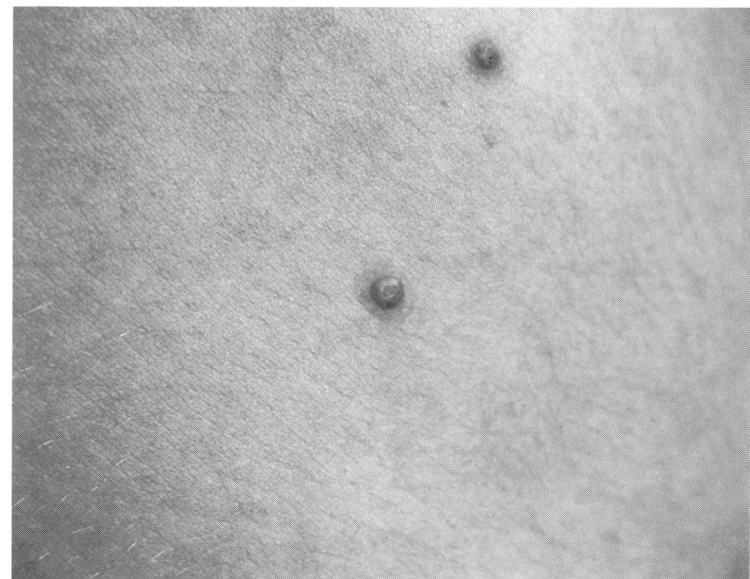

Figure 2-5. Molluscum contagiosum is characterized by a white well-circumscribed papule with a central dell. (See color plate.)

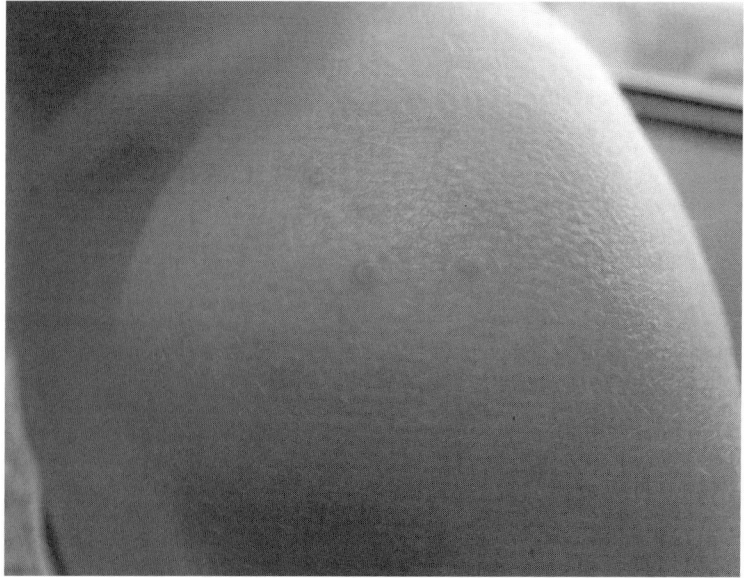

Figure 2-6. Very small lesions of molluscum contagiosum not uncommonly mimic folliculitis in athletes. (See color plate.)

occasionally number in the hundreds, but most often athletes have fewer than 20. The lesions can be found on the hands, forearms, and face of athletes and can be quite contagious, as its name implies. Molluscum contagiosum in athletes can have an atypical presentation with small nonumbilicated papules that resemble folliculitis.

In one study of swimmers, the majority of lesions were found on the trunk (50%) and axillae (32%) and corresponded to the areas where the children held the kickboards (Niizeki et al., 1984). A study of nearly 1400 cross-country runners noted that nearly all the lesions were located on the anterior aspects of the knees and thighs (Mobacken and Nordin, 1987). The authors supposed that distribution correlated to the method of transmission. They believed that sharing of towels, soaps, and brushes or skin-to-skin contact in the sauna and benches could have caused the outbreak. Alternatively, the runners may have acquired the virus through contact with branches, bushes, or barbed wire while they were running through the woods.

Diagnosis

The diagnosis is most often straightforward and made purely on morphologic grounds. The main differential diagnosis includes acne vulgaris, folliculitis, infected eczema, and verrucae. One study noted that athletes with molluscum were commonly misdiagnosed as having folliculitis (first most common) and infected eczema (second most common). The characteristic color and central dell set the molluscum apart but are not universally apparent, especially in some early lesions. Molluscum lacks the pinpoint black dots of verrucae.

Treatment

Lesions often spontaneously resolve in several months to 1 year. This is a long period, and most athletes choose to or must have their lesions treated with destructive methods. Curettement is the surest and most rapid method to remove molluscum. A sharp commercially available curette can be used. Alternatively, the scoop at the end of a tongue depressor that is broken longitudinally can be used (Figure 2-7, see color plate). Unfortunately, bleeding may occur and necessitate pressure or application of aluminum chloride for hemostasis (which stings). Liquid nitrogen destruction also works, but can be painful and does not remove the molluscum as rapidly and dramatically as does curettement. Chemical destructive methods include clinician-painted trichloroacetic acid or cantharidin, which once applied causes a blister to develop within 1 day, after which the molluscum is removed. If rapid resolution is not necessary and many lesions are present, topical imiquimod under an occlusive dressing may be effective. Tretinoin and tazarotene also have been used.

50 Sports Dermatology

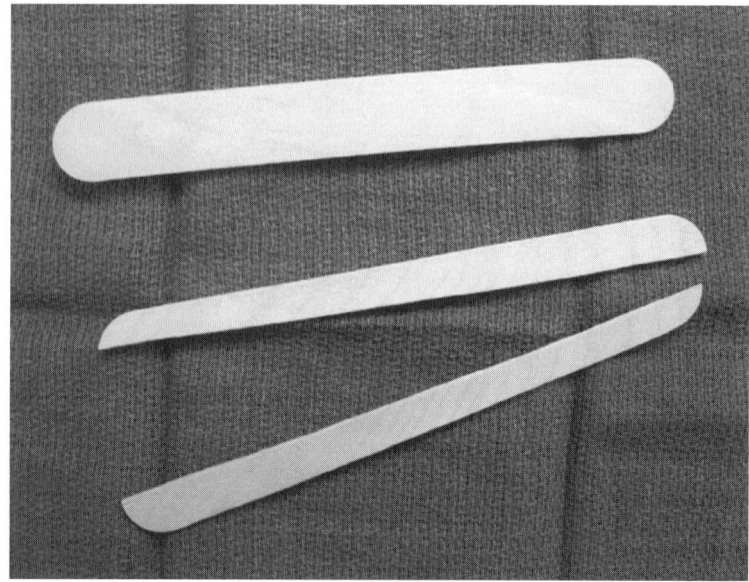

Figure 2-7. A tongue depressor can double as a makeshift curette when a formal surgical instrument is unavailable. The tongue depressor should be broken longitudinally and the rounded end used as the "scooper." (See color plate.)

National Collegiate Athletic Association wrestling guidelines require curettage or removal of molluscum before the athlete participates in meets or tournaments. Single or localized lesions can be covered with Op-site or Bioclusive and subsequently Pro-Wrap and stretch tape, thus allowing the wrestler to compete in the tournament. Some state high school associations do not permit use of bandaging as an adequate means of protection during meets or tournaments (Table 2-7).

Cross-country runners whose competition includes travel through the woods should cover their knees and thighs. Swimmers should ensure that the kickboards are thoroughly cleaned. Infected swimmers should not use the kickboards.

Athletes should not share equipment, such as gloves and masks, during sports such as baseball, hockey, fencing, or softball, or knee or elbow pads during volleyball or wrestling (Table 2-5).

Table 2-7. Return to Competition for Athletes with Molluscum and Verrucae

Skin Infection	Disqualification if
Molluscum	Diffuse lesions not removed, or Solitary or clustered lesions not covered
Verrucae	Multiple lesions not adequately covered, or Multiple facial lesions not covered by mask

Prevention

To prevent the epidemic spread of molluscum to other teammates, athletes should practice several measures. Athletes should routinely and immediately shower after practice and competition. Athletes should wear sandals while using communal showers. Weak evidence supports the wearing of protective gloves while athletes use weightlifting equipment to decrease the transmission of infectious agents. Athletes should not share protective equipment, towels, razors, or clothing. These items must be cleansed regularly.

In addition to the primary prevention methods, secondary prevention should consist of routine and close inspection of the athletes by themselves and by the athletic trainers. All infected athletes must be treated as soon as lesions are identified. Some lesions may be pinpoint, and careful attention should be paid to identifying and treating these very small lesions surrounding large lesions. Athletes with cutaneous infection who are identified, treated, and isolated (or bandaged) early will not transmit the microorganism to unsuspecting fellow athletes.

Warts (Verrucae)

Epidemiology

At least one study has examined the prevalence of warts among swimmers. More than 10% of the girls had warts on their feet, and nearly 5% of the boys had warts on their feet (Gentles and Evans, 1973). Warts can occur in any athlete. Warts are transmitted through skin-to-skin contact and potentially through fomites. The lesions are less contagious than molluscum. Among the contact sports, wrestlers and football players have developed warts. Athletes without significant skin-to-skin contact are at increased risk from swimming pool decks, weightlifting and gymnastic equipment, and locker room and shower floors. Such athletes include swimmers, weightlifters, and gymnasts. Three studies have specifically examined sports' risk factors in the development of warts. Interestingly, no studies have examined skin-to-skin contact transmission of warts.

A case-control study was designed to examine the relationship between swimming and warts. The authors determined that swimmers were 1.81 times more likely to have warts compared to nonswimmers, although the difference was not statistically significant (Penso-Assathiany et al., 1999). One study discovered that hand warts were significantly ($p < 0.05$) more common in members of the crew team (25%) compared with the track team (10%) (Roach and Chretien, 1995). The authors believed that the crew team was at increased risk for warts because they were less likely to wear gloves while lifting weights and suffered more hand trauma while practicing on weight machines and on the river. Theoretically, this additional trauma allows the virus entry through the skin. One might also wonder about the role of rowing equipment (e.g., oars) used both on the rowing machine and on the river.

One study examined locker room and communal shower floors (Johnson, 1995). Twenty-seven percent of swimmers who used the communal showers developed warts on the plantar aspect of their feet, whereas only 1.5% of individuals who walked on the locker room floor but did not use the showers had warts ($p = 0.001$) (Table 2-1).

Macerated skin from sweating and traumatic skin injuries inherent to athletes facilitate infection. An important feature of wart infection in athletes is that autoinoculation is possible through the trauma inherent in sports activities. Furthermore, calluses that are inherent to almost any sport may harbor warts (Adams, 2002). Several subtypes of human papilloma virus cause warts.

Clinical Presentation

Warts have different classifications partly related to the body area affected. Periungual warts occur around the nail; plantar warts occur on the soles; and common warts and verruca plana may appear on many parts of the body. Warts are characterized by well-defined, rough-surface, papillomatous papules ranging in size from a few millimeters to several centimeters, depending on the anatomic site and duration of infection (Figure 2-8). Verruca plana are flat verrucous papules (Figure 2-9).

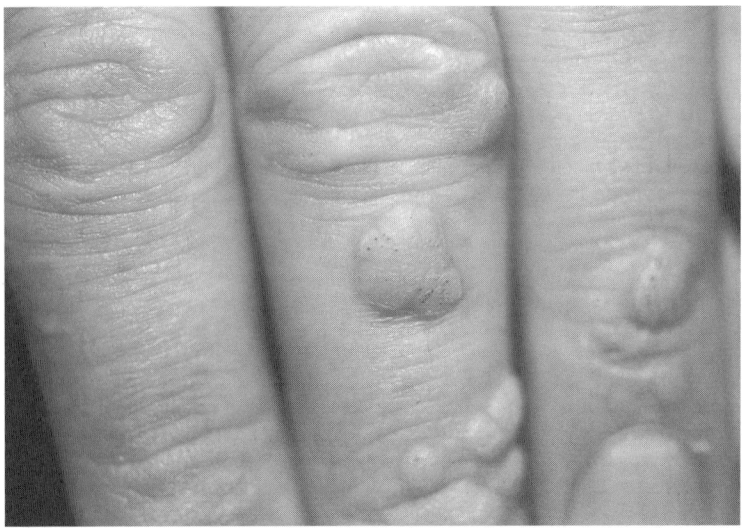

Figure 2-8. Thick verrucous papules characterize warts. Note the faint pinpoint black capillary thromboses.

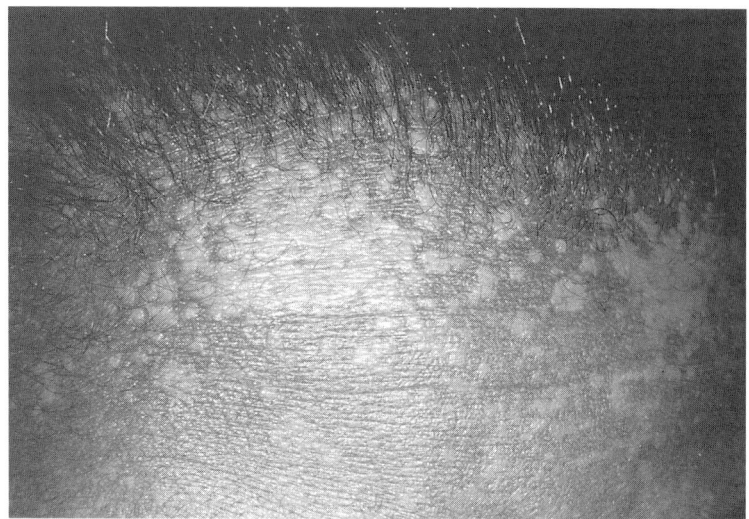

Figure 2-9. Another variant of warts includes flat warts or verruca plana.

Warts on the sole are not exophytic; rather, they exhibit inward growth resulting in frequent pain once they are sufficiently large. Occasionally the pain inhibits an athlete's activity. In one case, a collegiate tennis player was referred to the emergency room, where extensive radiologic tests were performed to evaluate for a stress fracture (Esterowitz et al., 1995). Once a plantar wart was identified as the cause and treated, the patient was able to play pain-free. Nonplantar warts are generally not painful but can inhibit the natural flow of athletic activity.

Diagnosis

The diagnosis is often straightforward if the lesions are filiform and are not related to calluses. Lesions related to calluses or located on the foot can be easily confused with calluses or corns if the clinician does not inspect the area carefully. The clinician may need to pare, using a sharp instrument such as a no. 15 surgical blade, to reveal the typical "black seeds" that represent the capillary thromboses. Upon paring, corns demonstrate a central core, whereas calluses demonstrate very thick epithelium with no alteration of the normal markings of the skin. Verruca plana are not as hyperkeratotic and can be confused with nonpigmented seborrheic keratoses.

Treatment

Warts must be treated because they have contagious potential and can cause discomfort that ultimately may affect an athlete's ability to perform. All hyperkeratotic warts should initially be pared with a sharp instrument (this procedure alone most often allows the ailing athlete to return to practice). Mechanical and chemical means then can be used to destroy warts. Destruction using liquid nitrogen, laser, or curettement is effective but can lead to residual pain, especially with the first two modalities. Very large warts may require multiple visits to ensure adequate removal. The athlete or athletic trainer should regularly pare down the hyperkeratosis between visits for destruction. Athletes may also use salicylic acid patch preparations between visits.

Chemical methods include application of salicylic acid, cantharidin, and trichloroacetic acid. The two latter medications can cause blistering, so the athlete should be forewarned. Topical immunomodulating agents have been developed that may be a significant aid, especially for athletes. Topical imiquimod can be applied to the wart under an adhesive bandage. This method is effective in removing warts with relatively less pain than destructive means. The pitfall to this method is the longer duration of therapy. Adequate paring of the lesion along with thorough soaking of the lesion in water before topical application also are necessary.

Recalcitrant warts can be treated with injected *Candida,* mumps antigen, or bleomycin. This approach must be performed carefully by an individual with expertise. Oral cimetidine 30–400 mg/kg per day also can be used.

Guidelines for a wrestler's participation in competition are available for NCAA athletes. Athletes with single or a few scattered lesions should be treated before the meet or tournament. Wrestlers who have multiple warts on the face that cannot be adequately covered by a mask or who have multiple warts on the body that cannot be adequately covered will be disqualified (Table 2-7).

Prevention

Athletes should practice several measures to decrease the spread of verrucae. Athletes should routinely and immediately shower after practice and competition. Athletes should wear sandals while using communal showers. Weak evidence supports the wearing of protective gloves while athletes use weightlifting equipment to decrease the transmission of infectious agents. Athletes should not share towels, razors, or clothing. Athletes should not share equipment such as gloves and masks during sports such as baseball, hockey, fencing, or softball, or knee or elbow pads during volleyball or wrestling. These items must be cleansed regularly (Table 2-5).

In addition to the primary prevention methods, secondary prevention should consist of routine and close inspection of the athletes by themselves and by the athletic trainers. Athletes with cutaneous infection who are identified, treated, and isolated (or bandaged) early will not transmit the microorganism to unsuspecting fellow athletes.

Bibliography

Adams BB. Sports dermatology. Adolesc Med 2001;2:305–322.
Adams BB. Dermatologic disorders of the athlete. Sports Med 2002;32:309–321.
Anderson BJ. The effectiveness of valacyclovir in preventing reactivation of herpes gladiatorum in wrestlers. Clin J Sport Med 1999;9:86–90.
Anderson BJ. The epidemiology and clinical analysis of several outbreaks of herpes gladiatorum. Med Sci Sports Exerc 2003;35:1809–1814.
Becker TM, Kodsi R, Bailey P, et al. Grappling with herpes: herpes gladiatorum. Am J Sports Med 1988;16:665–669.
Belongia EA, Goodman JL, Holland EJ, et al. An outbreak of herpes gladiatorum at a high-school wrestling camp. N Engl J Med 1991;325:906–910.
Brenner IKM, Shek PN, Shepard RJ. Infection in athletes. Sports Med 1994;17:86–107.
Chan El, Brandt K, Horsman GB. Comparison of Chemicon SimulFluor direct fluorescent antibody staining with cell culture and shell vial direct immunoperoxidase staining for detection of herpes simplex virus and with cytospin direct immunofluorescence staining for detection of varicella-zoster virus. Clin Diagn Lab Immunol 2001;8: 909–912.
Cyr PR. Viral skin infections. Phys Sportsmed 2004;32:33–38.
Dworkin MS, Shoemaker PC, Spitters C, et al. Endemic spread of herpes simplex virus type I among adolescent wrestlers and their coaches. Pediatr Infect Dis J 1999; 18:1108–1109.
Dyke LM, Merikangas UR, Bruton OC, et al. Skin infections in wrestlers due to herpes simplex virus. JAMA 1965;194:153–154.
Esterowitz D, Greer K, Cooper PH, et al. Plantar warts in the athlete. Am J Emerg Med 1995;13:441–443.
Gentles JC, Evans EGV. Foot infections in swimming baths. Br Med J 1973;3:260–262.
Grossman MC, Silvers DN. The Tzanck smear: can dermatologists accurately interpret it? J Am Acad Dermatol 1992;27:403–405.
Halstead ME, Bernhardt DT. Common infections in the young athlete. Pediatr Ann 2002;31:42–48.
Holland EJ, Mahanti RL, Belongia EA, et al. Ocular involvement in an outbreak of herpes gladiatorum. Am J Ophthalmol 1992;114:680–684.
Ichihashi M, Nagai H, Matsunaga K. Sunlight is an important causative factor of recurrent herpes simplex. Cutis 2004;74:14–18.
Johnson LW. Communal showers and the risk of plantar warts. J Fam Pract 1995;40: 136–138.
Keilhofner M, McKinsey DS. Herpes gladiatorum in a high school wrestler. Mo Med 1988;85:723–725.
La Rocco MT. Evaluation of an enzyme-linked viral inducible system for the rapid detection of herpes simplex virus. Eur J Clin Microbiol Infect Dis 2000;19:233–235.
Laur WE, Posey RE, Waller JD. Herpes gladiatorum. Arch Dermatol 1979;115:678.
Mast EE, Goodman RA. Prevention of infectious disease transmission in sports. Sports Med 1997;1:1–7.

Mills J, Hauer L, Gottlieb A, et al. Recurrent herpes labialis in skiers. Am J Sports Med 1987;15:76–78.

Mobacken H, Nordin P. Molluscum Contagiosum among cross-country runners. J Am Acad Dermatol 1987;17:519–560.

Nerurkar LS, West F, May M, et al. Survival of herpes simplex virus in water specimens collected from hot tubs in spa facilities and on plastic surfaces. JAMA 1983;250:3081–3083.

Niizeki K, Kano O, Kondo Y. An epidemic study of Molluscum Contagiosum. Dermatologica 1984;169:197–198.

Penno-Assathiany D, Flahault A, Roujeau JC. Verrues, piscine et atopi. Ann Dermatol Venereol 1999;126:696–698.

Porter PS, Baughman RD. Epidemiology of herpes simplex among wrestlers. JAMA 1965;194:150–152.

Potasman I, Pick N. Primary Herpes labialis acquired during scuba diving course. J Travel Med 1997;4:144–145.

Roach MC, Chretien JH. Common hand warts in athletes: association with trauma to the hand. J Am Coll Health 1995;44:125–126.

Rooney JF, Bryson Y, Mannix ML, et al. Prevention of ultraviolet-light-induced herpes labialis by sunscreen. Lancet 1991;338:1419–1422.

Rosenbaum GS, Strampfer MJ, Cunha BA. Herpes gladiatorum in a male wrestler. Int J Dermatol 1990;29:141–142.

Selling B, Kibrick S. An outbreak of herpes simplex among wrestlers (herpes gladiatorum). N Engl J Med 1964;270:979–982.

Shelley WB. Herpetic arthritis associated with disseminate herpes simplex in a wrestler. Br J Dermatol 1980;103:209–212.

Shute P, Jeffries DJ, Maddocks AC. Scrum-pox caused by herpes simplex virus. Br Med J 1979;2:1629.

Skinner GR, Davies J, Ahmad A, et al. An outbreak of herpes rugbeiorum managed by vaccination of players and sociosexual contacts. J Infect 1996;33:163–167.

Spruance Sl, Freeman DJ, Stewart JC, et al. The natural history of ultraviolet radiation-induced herpes simplex labialis and response to therapy with oral and topical formulations of acyclovir. J Infect Dis 1991;163:728–733.

Spruance SL, Hamill ML, Hoge WS, et al. Acyclovir prevents reactivation of herpes simplex labialis in skiers. JAMA 1988;260:1597–1599.

Strauss RH, Leizman DJ, Lanese RR, et al. Abrasive shirts may contribute to herpes gladiatorum among wrestlers. N Engl J Med 1989;320:598–599.

Wheeler CE, Cabaniss WH. Epidemic cutaneous herpes simplex in wrestlers (Herpes Gladiatorum). JAMA 1965;194:993–997.

White WB, Grant-Kels JM. Transmission of herpes simplex virus type 1 infection in rugby players. JAMA 1984;252:533–535.

3. Fungal Skin Infections

This chapter is the last of the three chapters that discuss the most common skin infections that can result in individual disqualification and significant team disruption. Like the first two chapters, not all of the conditions discussed in this chapter are reasons for disqualification. At the same time, the myriad diseases caused by dermatophytes can create discomfort and a ripe environment for serious secondary superinfection. Dermatophytes are ubiquitous and normally are found in the environment and on the human body (especially the feet and groin) in nonathletes. Athletes may be particularly at risk because of a number of risk factors.

Most dermatophytes enjoy optimal growing where the environment is warm, moist, and dark. Because athletes often are active and sweating, the epidermis is an ideal fungal environment. Furthermore, areas covered excessively by clothing (e.g., groin and feet) not only are superhydrated but also are dark. Therefore, it should not be surprising that the feet and groin are among the most common locations of dermatophyte infection in the athlete. Athletes' skin under protective gear may be at particular risk.

In addition to offering the optimal microenvironment for dermatophytes, athletes' skin is ideal for dermatophyte infection because the skin facilitates entry of the microorganism. This facilitation results from two different processes. First, supersaturation (from sweating) of the stratum corneum (the first layer of protection of the skin) allows easier passage for the microorganism through the epidermis. Second, most athletes experience abrasions and cuts that allow additional entrance of the dermatophyte through the epidermis. Finally, athletes experience increased risk because of unique contacts with dermatophytes. Many athletes have close skin-to-skin contact that permits the transmission of dermatophytes between competitors. Athletes' feet often are exposed to environments that have heavy infestations of dermatophytes, namely, pool decks and shower and locker room floors.

Dermatophyte infections result in different clinical morphologies depending on the body part affected. It is important for the clinician taking care of athletes to recognize the different types of dermatophyte skin infection. The clinician must understand when public health measures and athlete disqualification are necessary. Duration of disqualification is equally important. Treatment and prevention measures often are quite different compared to the measures implemented for nonathletes.

Some dermatophyte infections are sport specific (e.g., tinea corporis gladiatorum) whereas other fungi do not discriminate among sporting events (e.g., tinea cruris). This chapter specifically discusses dermatophyte infections of the feet, nails, and groin and the areas affected by tinea corporis gladiatorum.

Tinea Pedis

Epidemiology

Although any athlete is at risk for developing tinea pedis, the majority of the epidemiologic studies of tinea pedis has focused on swimmers, runners, and locker room and shower users; fewer studies have investigated other sports. Clearly athletes develop tinea pedis more than nonathletes. No statistical differences based on gender are observed. One study of nearly 100,000 people showed that athletic children and adults ages 64 years and younger were nearly two times more likely to develop tinea pedis than their nonathletic counterparts (Caputo).

Users of Communal Showers and Locker Rooms

Without commenting on the specific type of athletic activity performed, some authors have noted a high prevalence of tinea pedis in athletes using communal showers and locker rooms. Studies report the range of tinea pedis in communal bathing areas is between 16% and 37% (Gentles, 1956, 1957; Gentles et al., 1975).

Basketball Players

One study specifically examined basketball athletes and found that 39% had tinea pedis, which is statistically higher than in nonathletes. Basketball players were more than two times more likely to develop tinea pedis than nonathletes (Kamihama et al., 1997).

Judo Practitioners

One cross-sectional analysis showed that judo practitioners have a high prevalence of tinea pedis (Badillet et al., 1982). One study specifically examined judo practitioners and found that 23% had tinea pedis, which was not statistically greater than in nonathletes. Judo practitioners were as likely to develop tinea pedis as nonathletes (Kamihama et al., 1997).

Runners

One study that specifically examined runners found that 56% had tinea pedis, which was statistically greater than in nonathletes. Runners were more than four times more likely to develop tinea pedis than nonathletes (Kamihama et al., 1997). Two studies have examined marathon runners. Twenty-two percent of the runners in the International Marathon of Montreal had culture-positive tinea pedis (Mailler and Adams, 2004). A study of fewer marathoners revealed a somewhat higher infection rate of 31% (Lacroix et al., 2002). Increasing age and use of communal showers were predictive of positive cultures.

Soccer Players

One study specifically examined soccer players and found that 44% had tinea pedis, which was statistically greater than in nonathletes. Soccer players were 2.6 times more likely to develop tinea pedis than nonathletes (Kamihama et al., 1997).

Swimmers

The range of prevalence of tinea pedis in swimmers is vast, but the median of 21% probably is a fair estimate. One small prevalence study showed that 57% of swimmers had tinea pedis (English and Gibson, 1959). However, another very large study of nearly 4000 bathers noted a prevalence of 20% (Gip, 1967). Other studies of several hundred swimmers supported the lower prevalence, with values of 21.5% (Gentles and Evans, 1973; Gentles et al., 1974), 15% (Attye et al., 1990), and 13% and 22% (Bolanos, 1991). One study specifically examined swimmers and found that 55% had tinea pedis, which was statistically greater than in nonathletes. Swimmers were four times more likely to develop tinea pedis than nonathletes (Kamihama et al., 1997).

An interesting study cultured the common floor surfaces at a swimming pool, specific parts of the pool deck, and its associated locker rooms. The study noted that, unrelated to the number of swimmers at the pool, 77% of the positive cultures were obtained during the spring and summer. The springboard of the pool was loaded with dermatophytes, accounting for nearly half of all the dermatophytes isolated. Nearly one third of the total isolates came from the grates (Detandt and Nolard, 1988). Another study showed a mean contamination of 54 dermatophytes per square millimeter in poolside areas where people walked barefoot (Detandt and Nolard, 1995).

Water Polo Players

One study specifically examined water polo players and found that 53% had tinea pedis, which was statistically greater than in nonathletes. Water polo players were 3.7 times more likely to develop tinea pedis than nonathletes (Kamihama et al., 1997).

Hockey

Of note, one study examined 28 professional hockey players on one team and did not find any cases of dermatophyte infection (Mohrenschlager et al., 2001).

Three main genera of dermatophytes cause skin infection: *Trichophyton*, *Epidermophyton*, and *Microsporum*. *Trichophyton* is the main cause of tinea pedis, with *Trichophyton mentagrophytes* and *Trichophyton rubrum* composing nearly all the causative species. One small study was able to isolate only *T. mentagrophytes* in swimmers (English and Gibson, 1959). A study of nearly 4000 bathers found that 75% of the dermatophytes on the feet were *T. mentagrophytes*. *Trichophyton rubrum* and *Epidermophyton* species were found in 3% and 6% of cases, respectively (Gip, 1967). Another study of nearly 300 athletes revealed that *T. mentagrophytes* more commonly caused tinea pedis than did *T. rubrum* in swimmers and basketball players (Attye et al., 1990; Bolanos, 1991; Gentles and Evans, 1973; Kamihama et al., 1997). *Sporothrix schenckii*, which results in deep mycosis and typically does not cause superficial infections, has been cultured from swimming pool floors.

The distribution of dermatophytes is curious because, in the population at large, *T. rubrum* dominates as the most common dermatophyte in tinea pedis at >4:1 (Kemna and Elewski, 1996). The reason that swimmers and basketball players display the reverse ratio is unclear. One study of marathon runners also observed this reverse ratio: 50% of the runners with tinea pedis had *T. mentagrophytes*, whereas only 35% had *T. rubrum* (Lacroix et al., 2002). Other sports, such as judo, soccer, and water polo, resemble the general population with regard to the distribution of dermatophytes causing disease (Kamihama et al., 1997).

Candida also can cause tinea pedis. In one study of swimmers, *Candida* composed 12% of the positive cultures (Bolanos, 1991).

A study of pool surfaces and locker rooms revealed that 55% of all dermatophytes were *T. rubrum*, 42% were *T. mentagrophytes*, and 3% were *Epidermophyton floccosum* (Detandt and Nolard, 1988).

Clinical Presentation

There are three clinical morphologies of tinea pedis. The classic type of tinea pedis is characterized by somewhat ill-defined, scaling, minimally to moderately erythematous plaques in a moccasin-like pattern on the sole of the foot (Figure 3-1). Another clinical type is the interdigital variety. Moist (macerated), scaling, minimally to intensely erythematous plaques are present between the toes (Figure 3-2). These two types are caused by *T. rubrum*. The last type of tinea pedis is clinically characterized by intensely pruritic, scaling, moderately erythematous, vesicular papules and plaques often on the instep of the sole; this type is caused by *T. mentagrophytes* (Figure 3-3).

All varieties may become secondarily infected with bacteria. In this scenario, pustules may be seen and the intensity of erythema enhanced. This condition can lead to significant time away from practice and competition.

An important aspect of tinea pedis that the clinician must remember is that athletes may be asymptomatic carriers of dermatophytes. Studies have shown

3. Fungal Skin Infections 61

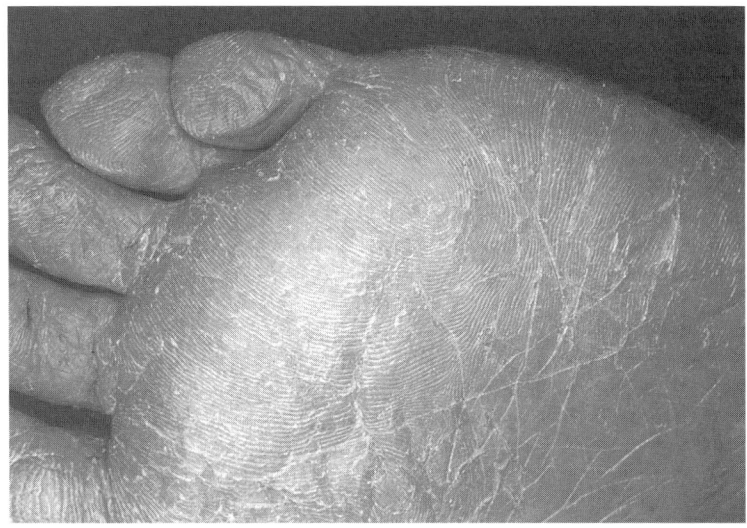

Figure 3-1. Classic form of tinea pedis in a moccasin-like pattern.

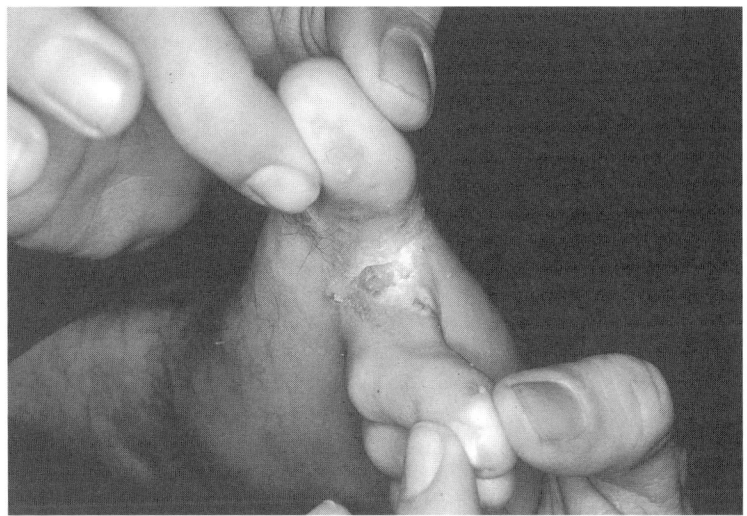

Figure 3-2. Interdigital variant of tinea pedis marked by maceration.

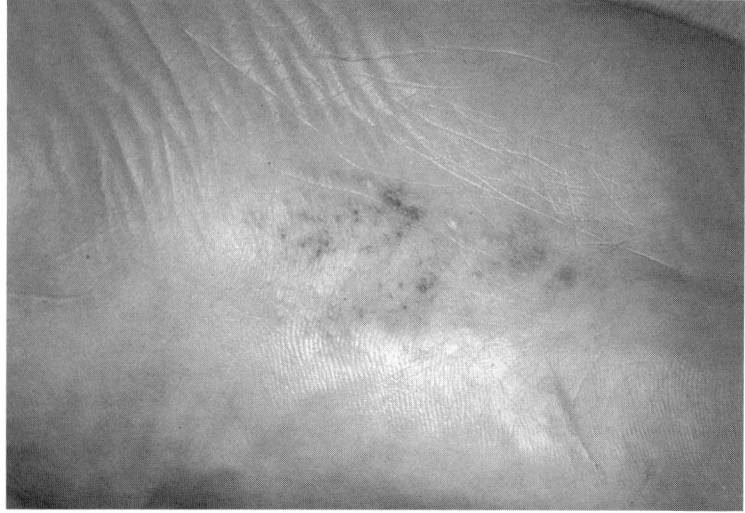

Figure 3-3. Vesicular tinea pedis can be intensely pruritic.

that a considerable number of athletes shed dermatophytes without obvious clinical disease, such as marathon runners (27%–48%) (Lacroix et al., 2002; Mailler and Adams, 2004), judokas (15%) (Badillet et al., 1982), and swimmers (36%) (Attye et al., 1990). These athletes may unwittingly transmit the organisms to other athletes in the shower, locker room, or pool deck or while sharing equipment.

Diagnosis

The diagnosis is generally straightforward but can easily be confused with subacute dermatitis unrelated to an infection (e.g., contact dermatitis to shoewear). Psoriasis and pitted keratolysis also must be considered. To confirm the diagnosis, potassium hydroxide examination and/or culture should be performed. The clinician should scrape an adequate amount of scale onto a glass slide for microscopic evaluation. Another glass slide or a plastic table knife makes an ideal scraper. Under low-power magnification, long branching hyphae are seen traversing the cell borders (Figure 3-4, see color plate). The clinician should send the scrapings for culture to confirm or speciate the microorganism.

Tinea pedis may be secondarily infected with *Staphylococcus* or *Pseudomonas*. Cultures may be necessary to confirm the diagnosis. Wood's lamp examination may yield a greenish color indicative of a pseudomonal superinfection.

Treatment

Topical therapy twice per day for several weeks (often at least 1 month) is necessary, although claims abound that 1 week is sufficient. The fungicidal (i.e., not the fungistatic) type of topical cream is preferred and includes the allylamines. My preference is to use ciclopirox because it not only is fungicidal but also is antibacterial. Some studies suggest that use of these antifungal agents once per day for 1 week clears only 60% of tinea pedis in the first week (Bakos et al., 1997; van Heerden and Vismer, 1997). After 2 weeks, 74% to 87% is clear. Maximal clearance appears to occur after approximately 3 weeks, with 90% clearance. The fungistatic azoles appear to have a much slower onset of action, although ultimately both topical fungicidal and fungistatic agents have similar cure rates (Millikan et al., 1988). Topical aluminum chloride 30% has also been shown to effectively treat tinea pedis. Its efficacy relates to its ability to dry and create a microenvironment that is inhospitable for the dermatophyte (Leyden and Kligman, 1975).

Oral antifungal therapy with itraconazole 200 mg once per day or terbinafine 250 mg once per day for 2 weeks should be used for athletes with severe tinea pedis. Careful attention should be paid to the athlete's preexisting medication list. Several medications are contraindicated if the athlete is taking either oral terbinafine or itraconazole. Results of liver function tests and complete blood counts should be normal before and 1 month after therapy is started. Concomitant topical therapy should be used twice per day.

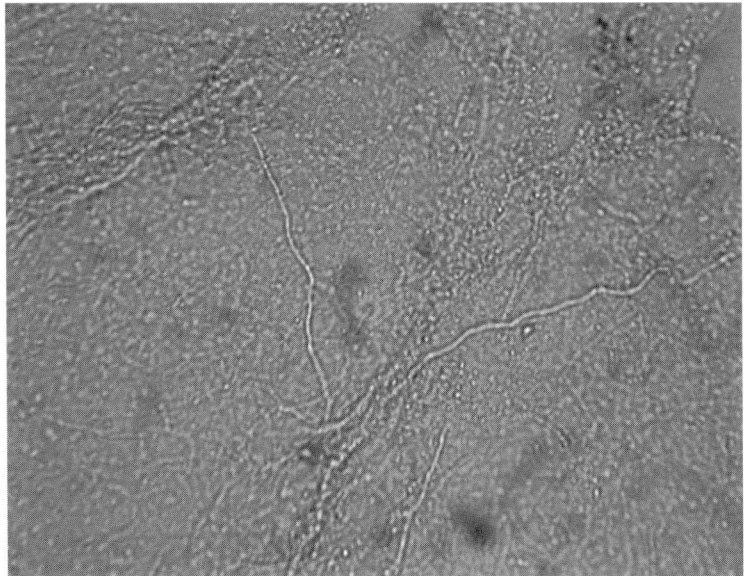

Figure 3-4. Microscopic examination of scale shows multiple hyphal structures traversing the normal cells of the skin (corneocytes). (See color plate.)

Additional topical therapy is required in some situations. Sometimes the scale of tinea pedis becomes thick and hyperkeratotic, and topical antifungal preparations may not be able to penetrate this thick scale. Application of urea 40% cream along with the topical antifungal agent is necessary twice per day. Occasionally athletes with vesicular or weeping lesions may need to soak their feet twice per day in a footbath containing warm water and Domeboro crystals. Soaking with a mixture of vinegar and water also may be drying and therapeutic. The clinician often needs to encourage this soaking process when the athlete's tinea pedis is secondarily infected with bacteria. Finally, not uncommonly the athlete complains of intense pruritus and erythema. As long as the athlete is using the appropriate antifungal therapy, the clinician should not hesitate to prescribe a moderate-potency topical corticosteroid, such as triamcinolone 0.1% ointment, for this specific clinical presentation.

No recommendations regarding tinea pedis are available from the National Collegiate Athletic Association (NCAA). The NCAA guidelines on skin infections have some latitude, however, and college athletes with exposed feet during competition should ensure prompt therapy of their tinea pedis. The NCAA (NCAA, 2005) guidelines on skin infections begin by stating in general that "infectious skin conditions that cannot be adequately protected should be considered cause for medical disqualification from practice and competition."

Prevention

Clearing dermatophytes from athletes' feet is difficult, so prevention is paramount (Table 3-1). First, athletes should wear synthetic moisture-wicking socks that keep the feet dry even as the athletes sweat profusely. Second, athletes need to immediately remove these "advanced socks" and their shoes and take a shower. Showers (and the locker room floor and pool deck) are not without their own peril. Several studies have noted a high prevalence of dermatophytes in these areas (Detandt and Nolard, 1988; English and Gibson, 1959; Gentles, 1956, 1957). Investigators cultured samples taken from a pool twice per day every other week for 1 year. Dermatophytes were cultured from the pool or locker rooms each time the areas were sampled (Detandt and Nolard, 1988).

Table 3-1. Preventative Measures for Tinea Pedis and Tinea Unguium

Synthetic moisture-wicking socks
Immediate showers after sporting activity
Sandals or other footwear worn while walking on shower and locker room floors or pool decks
Thorough feet washing
Regular cleaning of shower, locker room, and pool floors
Daily application of antifungal cream to feet

Another investigator studied a swimming pool on the first day of classes and 12 days later. No dermatophytes were detectable on the pool or shower floors on the first day of classes. After 6 weeks (twice-per-week classes), the investigator found 16% positive cultures taken from the same floors (Bolanos, 1991). Given these findings, athletes must always wear sandals or other protective footwear while walking on pool decks and the floors of showers and the locker room. One study of a professional hockey team was unable to detect any dermatophytes and surmised that the code of never going barefoot in the locker room contributed greatly to the lack of tinea pedis (Mohrenschlager et al., 2001).

It is incumbent upon practitioners to ensure that the cleaning staff thoroughly cleans the floors and pool decks. A very early study revealed that, after the floors were cleaned, all cultures of the floors were negative even though they had been positive before the cleaning (Gentles, 1957). Another study showed that washing the feet radically reduces the fungal load on the foot (Gip, 1967).

Athletes with a tendency for recurrent tinea pedis should use daily prophylactic ciclopirox to the feet. One trial supports this approach, with investigators showing a statistically significant decrease in the prevalence of tinea pedis in swimmers from 21.5% to 6.9% over 3 years simply with use of antifungal powder after bathing at the pool (Gentles et al., 1974). Another unique application is the use of tolnaftate-impregnated swabs. These nonprescription swabs cost $7 (US) for 36 applicators. The approach is convenient because the athlete can store the applicator in a gym bag and use the once-only swab after sports activity.

Athletes and clinicians should remember that shoes can harbor these organisms. One study cultured fungus from 15% of shoes kept in storage for a period from 1 to 4 weeks (Ajello and Getz, 1954).

Tinea Unguium (Onychomycosis)

Epidemiology

Onychomycosis has been noted in runners and swimmers, but any athlete is at risk for developing onychomycosis (tinea unguium). One large study of 100,000 people showed that children younger than 18 years who played sports had statistically more onychomycosis than nonathletes (1.5 times more). No difference between adult athletes and nonathletes was observed (Caputo et al., 2001). Another study of 277 adult swimmers revealed that they were at least three times as likely to develop onychomycosis compared with the rest of the population (Gudnadottir et al., 1999). Thirty percent of the swimmers were culture or potassium hydroxide examination positive.

The three main genera of dermatophytes that cause nail infection are *Trichophyton*, *Epidermophyton*, and *Microsporum*. Dermatophytes of the first genus are the main cause of onychomycosis; *Trichophyton mentagrophytes* and *Trichophyton rubrum* comprise nearly all the causative species. In the normal population, in terms of onychomycosis, the ratio of *T. rubrum* to *T. mentagrophytes* is >9:1 (Kemna and Elewski, 1996). Unlike tinea pedis, the ratio of

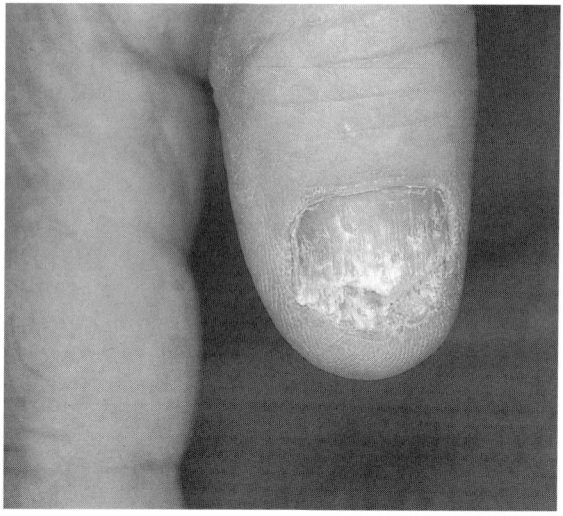

Figure 3-5. Subungual hyperkeratosis, nail thickening, and brittleness characterize onychomycosis.

organisms causing onychomycosis is the same in athletes as in nonathletes, also 9:1 (Gudnadottir et al., 1999).

Clinical Presentation

One of the most common types of onychomycosis is distal onychomycosis. It nearly always is related to concomitant tinea pedis. If the athlete has onychomycosis, the entire foot must be examined. Clinically the nail is thickened and yellow (Figure 3-5). If the onychomycosis is relatively advanced, subungual debris and onycholysis is present, and the nail becomes quite brittle. Occasionally the nail is secondarily infected with *Pseudomonas* and appears green. However, not all green nails suggest *Pseudomonas*, because primary and secondary molds also create green nails. Usually the athlete complains about the cosmetic appearance of the nail. Occasionally the patient reports pain.

Diagnosis

The diagnosis can be challenging, especially in the athlete. The differential diagnosis includes toenail changes related to sporting activity (which has been termed *tennis toe, runner's toe,* etc.), which can mimic onychomycosis clinically.

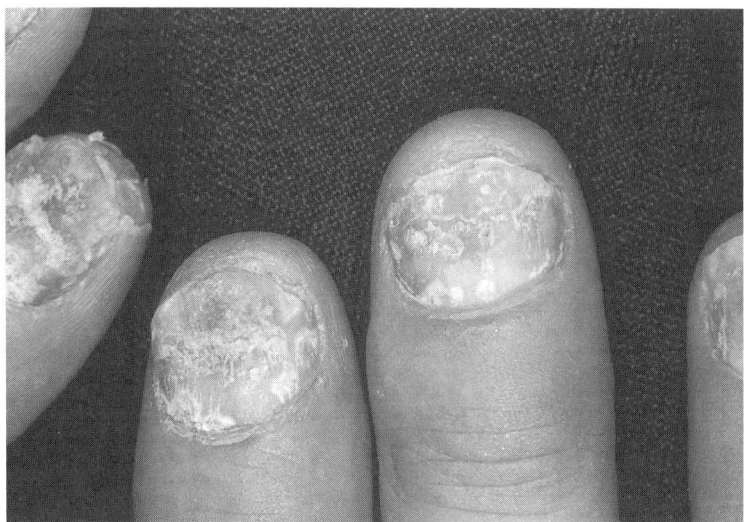

Figure 3-6. Psoriasis may resemble onychomycosis. Psoriatic nails, however, demonstrate nail pits and oil spots.

Psoriasis also must be considered, but nail pits and oil spots help differentiate psoriasis from onychomycosis (Figure 3-6).

Periodic acid–Schiff examination of the subungual debris by the histology laboratory probably is the most sensitive test to detect dermatophyte infection of the nail. The clinician also can confirm the diagnosis by using potassium hydroxide examination. The clinician should scrape an adequate amount of scale onto a glass slide for microscopic evaluation. To obtain subungual debris for potassium hydroxide examination, the clinician should use a curette. Under low-power magnification, long branching hyphae are seen traversing the cell borders (Figure 3-4). The clinician should send the scrapings for culture to confirm or speciate the microorganism.

Treatment

Oral antifungal agents are the standard therapy. Oral antifungal therapy includes itraconazole 200 mg twice per day or terbinafine 250 mg once per day for 3 months. These regimens are not particularly effective for toenail onychomycosis; a cure rate of only 25% is expected after 1 year. Therapy for onychomycosis of the fingernails must be performed for 6 weeks and has a much higher cure rate. Careful attention should be paid to the athlete's preexisting medication list. Several medications are contraindicated if the athlete is taking either oral terbinafine or itraconazole. Results of liver function tests and complete blood counts should be normal before and 1 month after therapy is started.

Athletes who cannot undergo oral therapy for a variety of reasons should be given topical therapy. Use of the fungicidal (and not the fungistatic) type of topical cream is preferred. My preference is to use ciclopirox because it has fungicidal as well as antibacterial properties. The topical antifungal preparations typically do not penetrate nails, so an athlete must attempt one of two approaches for the treatment to be effective. Application of urea 40% cream along with the topical antifungal (ciclopirox) is necessary twice per day. Ciclopirox is approved by the US Food and Drug Administration (FDA) for use as a nail lacquer. The athlete applies the lacquer like nail polish to the affected nail on a daily basis. Once per week the nail and its lacquer must be cleared using alcohol. This process takes up to 1 year.

No recommendations from the NCAA regarding onychomycosis are available. The NCAA guidelines on skin infections have some latitude, however, and college athletes with exposed feet during competition should ensure prompt therapy of their tinea pedis. The NCAA (2005) guidelines on skin infections begin by in general stating that "infectious skin conditions that cannot be adequately protected should be considered cause for medical disqualification from practice and competition."

Prevention

Clearing dermatophytes from the nail is difficult, so prevention is paramount (Table 3-1). First, athletes should wear synthetic moisture-wicking socks that keep the feet dry even as the athletes sweat profusely. Second, athletes must immediately remove these "advanced socks" and their shoes and take a shower. Showers (along with the locker room floor and pool deck) are not without their own peril. Several studies have noted a high prevalence of dermatophytes in these areas (Detandt and Nolard, 1988; English and Gibson, 1959; Gentles, 1956, 1957). Investigators cultured samples taken from a pool twice per day every other week for 1 year. Dermatophytes were cultured from the pool or locker rooms each time the areas were sampled (Detandt and Nolard, 1988). Therefore, athletes must always wear sandals or other protective footwear while walking on pool decks and on the floors of showers and the locker room.

It is incumbent upon practitioners to ensure that the cleaning staff thoroughly cleans the floors and pool decks. A very early study revealed that, after the floors were cleaned, all cultures of the floors were negative even though they had been positive before the cleaning (Gentles, 1957). Another study showed that washing the feet radically reduces the fungal load on the foot (Gip, 1967).

Athletes with a tendency for recurrent tinea pedis should use daily prophylactic ciclopirox to the feet, although no evidence has shown that this method decreases the recurrence of tinea pedis. Another unique application is the use of tolnaftate impregnated swabs. These nonprescription swabs cost $7 (US) for 36 applicators. The approach is convenient because the athlete can store the applicator in a gym bag and use the once-only swab after sports activity.

3. Fungal Skin Infections 69

Tinea Versicolor

Epidemiology

Any athlete is at risk for developing tinea versicolor. No epidemiologic study has focused on athletes. Tinea versicolor is caused by *Pityrosporum ovale* and predominates on warm moist skin.

Clinical Presentation

Tinea versicolor appears as asymptomatic, well-defined, hypopigmented or hyperpigmented, discrete, confluent macules and patches over the upper extremities, neck, and trunk (Figures 3-7 and 3-8). Scale may be apparent only after the affected area is scraped with a microscope slide or plastic table knife.

Diagnosis

The diagnosis is generally straightforward but can be easily confused with a relatively rare skin condition known as *confluent and reticulated papillomato-*

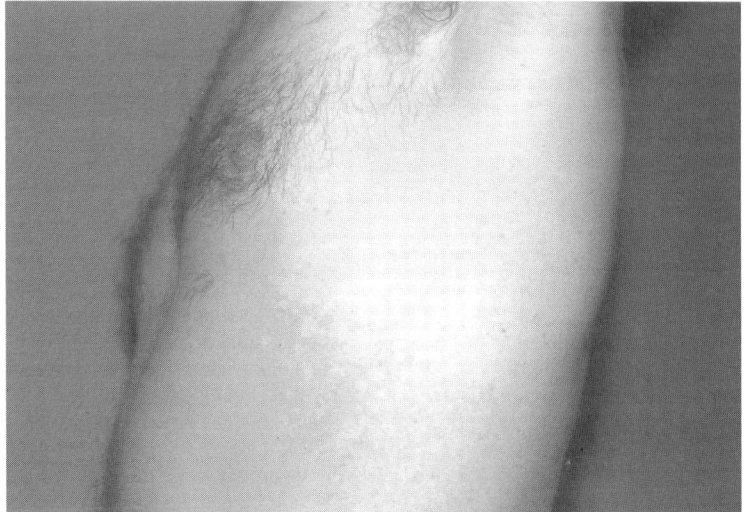

Figure 3-7. Extensive tinea versicolor on the trunk.

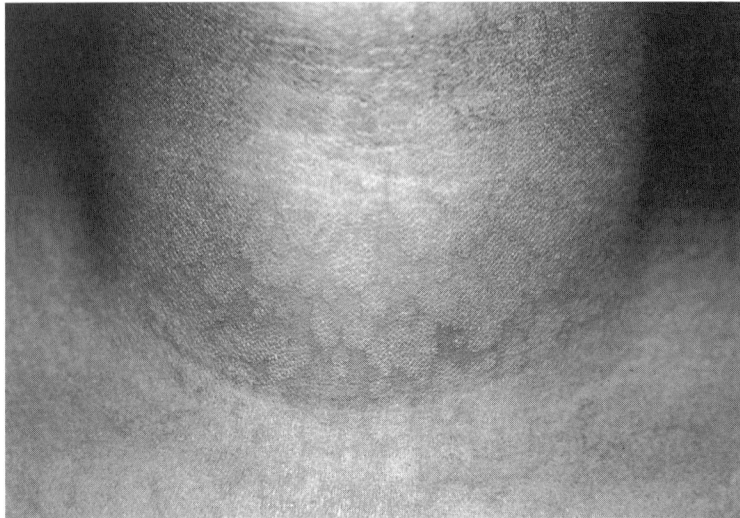

Figure 3-8. Hyperpigmented round, discrete, confluent patches and macules exemplify tinea versicolor.

sis. Potassium hydroxide examination should be performed to confirm the diagnosis. The clinician should scrape an adequate amount of scale onto a glass slide for microscopic evaluation. Another glass slide or a plastic table knife makes an ideal scraper. Spores and short hyphae (so-called *spaghetti and meatballs)* are seen under low-power magnification. Wood's lamp examination of the affected skin may reveal a yellow color.

Treatment

The standard therapy has been topical treatment with selenium sulfide 2.5% lotion applied to the affected area and washed off 15 minutes later. This treatment can be repeated once per day for 1 week. This therapy is somewhat cumbersome, and oral regimens are available. The athlete can take a single dose of two 200-mg ketoconazole tablets. The athlete then should exercise to allow the medication to concentrate in the sweat. Occasionally this regimen is repeated 1 week later.

Liver function tests are not needed during this regimen for athletes without a history of liver disease. Careful attention should be paid to the athlete's preexisting medication list. Several medications are contraindicated if the athlete is taking ketoconazole.

Remind the athlete that although the treatment very likely clears dermatophyte overgrowth, the color in the light or dark areas on the skin may not normalize for months.

Prevention

Tinea versicolor flourishes on the hot humid skin of an athlete. Athletes should wear synthetic moisture-wicking shirts that keep the athlete drier. After exercise or competition, the athlete should immediately shower to help prevent tinea versicolor. Finally, to prevent tinea versicolor, once per week athletes can apply selenium sulfide 2.5% lotion to the areas typically involved and wash the lotion off 15 minutes later.

Tinea Cruris
Epidemiology

Tinea cruris is also known as *jock itch*, but only one study has examined tinea cruris in athletes. Forty-five percent of 55 varsity college football players developed tinea cruris within 6 weeks of the start of the season (Malamatinis et al., 1968). No player on the freshman team had tinea cruris. The most common organisms that cause tinea cruris are *T. rubrum, T. mentagrophytes,* and *Candida albicans.*

Clinical Presentation

Athletes have pruritic, well-defined, erythematous, scaling plaques in the groin extending from the groin to the inner thighs (Figure 3-9). The border may be raised more than the rest of the lesion.

Diagnosis

The diagnosis of tinea cruris can be challenging. The differential diagnosis includes inverse psoriasis, seborrheic dermatitis, contact dermatitis, candidiasis, intertrigo, erythrasma, and extramammary Paget disease. Potassium hydroxide examination and/or culture should be performed to confirm the diagnosis. The clinician should scrape an adequate amount of scale onto a glass slide for micro-

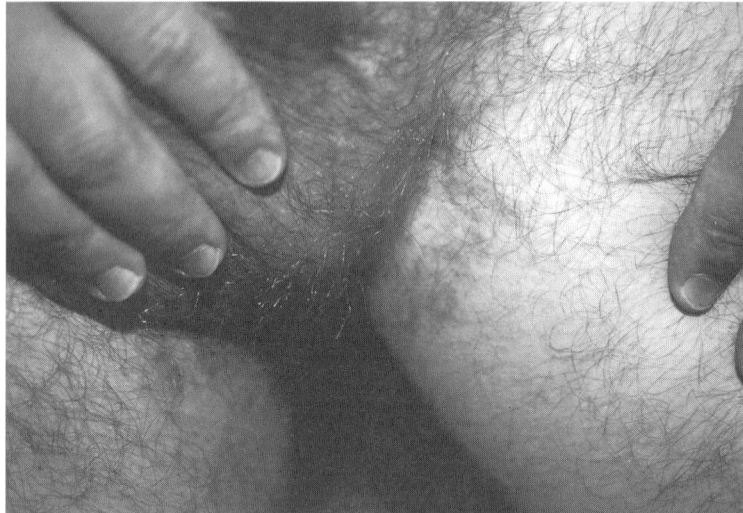

Figure 3-9. Tinea cruris occurs in the groin and manifests as a well-defined, erythematous, scaling plaque with an advancing border.

scopic evaluation. Another glass slide or a plastic table knife makes an ideal scraper. Under low-power magnification, long branching hyphae are seen traversing the cell borders (Figure 3-4). A biopsy may be required if the diagnosis is questionable, especially if extramammary Paget disease is possible.

Treatment

In most scenarios, topical therapy with an antifungal cream (either the azoles or allylamines) once or twice per day for 2 weeks should be effective. Rarely, the athlete requires oral therapy with terbinafine or one of the azoles.

Prevention

In the one reported epidemic of *Candida* intertrigo in football players, investigators cultured *Candida* from the bulk lubrication ointment bin and the tongue depressors used to obtain the ointment. It is very important to ensure that these ointment jars and the equipment placed in them are clean. The athlete should wear synthetic moisture-wicking underwear that maintains dryness. Immediately after the sporting activity, the athlete should shower and apply powder to keep the groin dry. On occasion the athlete may need to use a hair dryer to keep the groin as dry as possible and to create a microenvironment inhospitable for dermatophytes.

Tinea Corporis Gladiatorum

Epidemiology

Tinea corporis gladiatorum, also known as *trichophytosis gladiatorum* or *tinea gladiatorum,* creates epidemics every wrestling season. The prevalence ranges from 20% to 77% and vary because of different study methodologies (Adams, 2002). Professional, collegiate, and high school teams all suffer epidemics. The median prevalence, which likely best represents the actual prevalence, is 31%. One study of a high school wrestling team (without a known epidemic) and a track team discovered prevalence of 24% and 0%, respectively. Based on data from the National Collegiate Athletic injury surveillance system (NCAAISS), tinea corporis gladiatorum composed 23% of all skin infections in collegiate wrestlers between 1991 and 2003. *Trichophyton rubrum* causes tinea corporis, and *Trichophyton tonsurans* causes tinea capitis most commonly in nonwrestlers. This distribution is not replicated in wrestlers.

In most cases, infection with *T. tonsurans* causes tinea corporis gladiatorum; more than 100 cases are reported. *Trichophyton rubrum*, *Trichophyton equinum*, and *Trichophyton verrucosum* have been cultured in 45, 30, and 24 total wrestlers, respectively. Because tinea corporis gladiatorum nearly always is caused by *T. tonsurans*, wrestlers in some cases are believed to contract the infection from asymptomatic scalp carriers who act as reservoirs.

Clinical Presentation

The infected athlete demonstrates well-defined, erythematous, scaling, round papules and plaques on the head, neck, and arms (Figures 3-10 and 3-11). Thirty-eight percent of lesions develop on the arms, and 32% occur on the head and neck. Less commonly, lesions appear on the trunk (24%) and legs (6%). The typical annular configuration may not be apparent because wrestlers most often present to the clinician before the lesion has matured and become annular. The differential diagnosis includes acneiform papules, atopic dermatitis, early herpes gladiatorum, and early impetigo.

74 Sports Dermatology

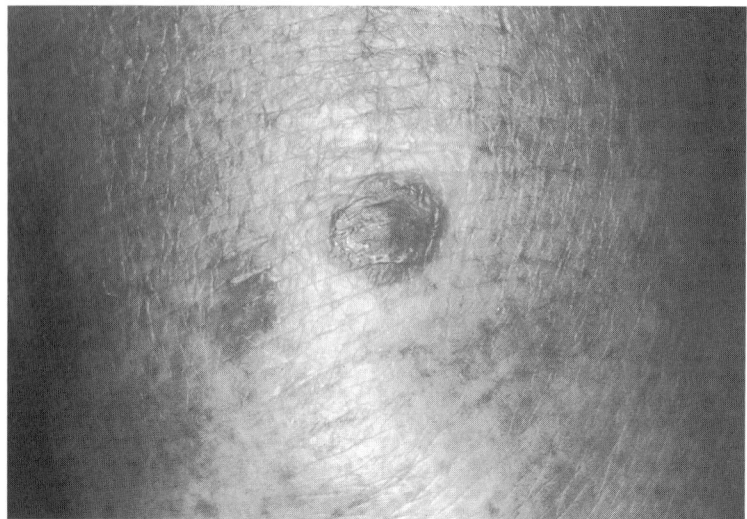

Figure 3-10. Lesions of tinea corporis gladiatorum do not often attain the annular or ring appearance typical of ringworm.

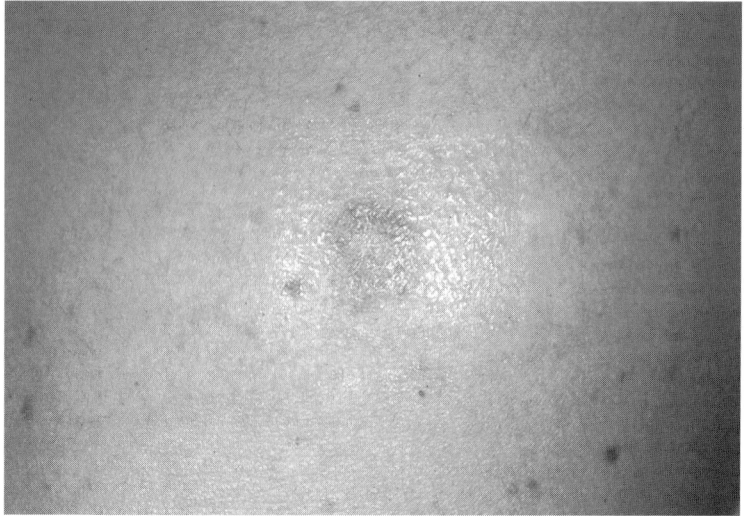

Figure 3-11. Athletes frequently attempt to conceal suspicious lesions, so tinea corporis gladiatorum may appear slightly macerated from being covered with an adhesive bandage.

Diagnosis

The diagnosis can be challenging, especially when the athlete presents early in the course of the disease. Potassium hydroxide examination should be performed to confirm the diagnosis. The clinician should scrape an adequate amount of scale onto a glass slide for microscopic evaluation. Another glass slide or plastic table knife makes an ideal scraper. Under low-power magnification, long branching hyphae are seen traversing the cell borders (Figure 3-4). Culture confirms the diagnosis and identifies the organism type.

Treatment

Two studies using a prospective open-label design examined the treatment of tinea corporis gladiatorum. Fluconazole once per week for 3 weeks results in clearance of the fungus (0% of cultures were positive at 3 weeks) (Kohl et al., 2000). Topical clotrimazole does not result in timely clearance of tinea corporis gladiatorum; after application twice per day for 3 weeks, 50% of cultures still were positive (Kohl et al., 1999). Other treatments that lack evidence-based support include ketoconazole 200 mg per day for 2 to 4 weeks and itraconazole 200 mg per day for 1 to 2 weeks.

Liver function tests are not needed during this regimen for athletes without a history of liver disease. Careful attention should be paid to the athlete's preexisting medication list. Several medications are contraindicated if the athlete is taking fluconazole, itraconazole, or ketoconazole.

No studies have examined the newer topical or oral fungicidal antifungal agents. One study showed that 67% of cultures became negative after only 1 week of topical terbinafine. In fact, the NCAA guidelines specifically require 72 hours of therapy with a fungicidal agent such as terbinafine or naftifine before a wrestler can safely participate. If lesions persist after this period of therapy, the athlete may be able to participate in competition as long as the athlete follows a series of interventions. Before the match, the lesions should be washed with ketoconazole or selenium sulfide shampoo and covered with naftifine or terbinafine cream. Subsequently the same lesion must be protected by a gas-permeable dressing such as Op-site or Bioclusive and finally Pro-Wrap and stretch tape. If scalp lesions are present, the athlete must have undergone 2 weeks of oral antifungal therapy before the infected wrestler can participate in intercollegiate competition (NCAA, 2005).

Prevention

The time-honored tradition of cleaning mats to ward off fungal infection is not supported by any scientific evidence. In fact, many studies have failed to culture any fungus from the wrestling mats. Only one study cultured *T. tonsurans* from the mats (El Fari et al., 2000). No study has definitively determined the transmissibility of the organism on equipment, but avoiding all sharing of equipment still is best practice. Most authorities also recommend immediate showers after activity and daily laundering of clothing, although a study revealed that wrestlers who followed this regimen still had a prevalence of 35% (Kohl and Lisney, 2000).

The keys to thwarting epidemics in teams and leagues are extensive surveillance coupled with rapid institution of oral therapy. Daily practices are ideal times to examine the athletes' skin. Coaches, trainers, and athletes themselves should join forces to ensure that all lesions are detected as early as possible. The ultimate control of epidemics in contact sports will come when a specifically trained clinician is assigned to each single school or, if funding is an issue, a group of schools. At present, especially on the high school level of sports activity, a medley of clinicians cares for the athletes of a team. In most states, wrestlers must present a completed evaluation and authorization form to the pre-competition official. However, the policy is not consistent, and no uniform or logical diagnostic approach or treatment and prevention plan is available. In addition, those individuals who disqualify or qualify athletes need not be clinicians with any particular expertise in the area. Early identification of lesions permits rapid institution of therapy so that athletes do not unintentionally infect team members or opponents. Identified athletes may continue to practice with bandages, but most interscholastic and intercollegiate competitions do not permit bandaging of infectious lesions.

Two studies have investigated season-long oral prophylaxis. In an open-label, prospective trial, authors decreased the incidence of tinea corporis gladiatorum from 27% to 0% with itraconazole 400 mg every other week (Hazen and Weil, 1997). Another double-blind, placebo-controlled study revealed that fluconazole 100 mg once per week significantly decreased the incidence of tinea corporis gladiatorum compared to placebo (Kohl et al., 2000).

For either of these season-long prophylaxis schedules, liver function tests should be performed before starting therapy and at mid-season. Careful attention should be paid to the athlete's preexisting medication list. Several medications are contraindicated if the athlete is taking fluconazole or itraconazole.

Tinea Corporis (Nonwrestlers)

Epidemiology

One case report noted tinea corporis occurred beneath a cast applied for broken bones.

Clinical Presentation

A 6-year-old child developed widespread tinea corporis beneath his cast after he went swimming several times per week (Marks et al., 1983). The cast never had an opportunity to dry, which provided an optimal microenvironment for fungal growth.

Diagnosis

The diagnosis can be challenging and can be confused with contact dermatitis. Potassium hydroxide examination should be performed to confirm the diagnosis.

Treatment

Topical allylamines should be used twice per day until the lesions are clear. Extensive disease may require oral antifungal agents.

Prevention

Injured athletes should not swim and should avoid wetting their casts.

Runner's Rubrum

Epidemiology

One case has been reported (Ross, 1978).

Clinical Presentation

A runner developed chronic tinea faciei on the upper lip caused by *T. rubrum*. The author believed profuse nasal discharge during every run propagated the infection.

Diagnosis

The diagnosis requires culture. Clinicians also must consider sycosis barbae, which is caused by *Staphylococcus* species.

Treatment

Topical allylamines should be used twice per day until the lesions are clear. Extensive disease may require oral antifungal agents.

Prevention

Profuse nasal discharge can be controlled by nasal spray decongestants. Care must be taken not to use these decongestants for more than 3 consecutive days. Decongestants can include substances that are banned from use during national and international competitions.

Curvularia Lunata

Epidemiology

One case is reported (Rohwedder et al., 1979).

Clinical Presentation

An immunocompetent football player suffered inoculation from *Curvularia lunata* (brown/black pigmented saprophytic soil fungus) on the football field. Multiple abscesses developed at the sites of abrasions and turf burns. Systemic dissemination occurred and affected the brain, lung, and bones.

Diagnosis

The diagnosis requires culture. Clinicians also must consider atypical mycobacterial infections, furunculosis, and deep fungal infections.

Treatment

Infected athletes require immediate treatment with surgical excision and amphotericin B.

Prevention

Infection with this rare fungus illustrates the importance of immediate and careful attention to treatment of turf burns and abrasions.

Bibliography

Adams BB. Tinea corporis gladiatorum. J Am Acad Dermatol 2002;47:286–290.

Ajello L, Getz ME. Recovery of dermatophytes from shoes and shower stalls. J Invest Dermatol 1954;22:17–24.

Attye A, Auger P, Joly J. Incidence of occult athletes foot in swimmers. Eur J Epidemiol 1990;6:244–247.

Badillet G, Puissant A, Jourdan-Lemoine M, et al. Pratique du judo et risque de contamination fongique. Ann Dermatol Venereol 1982;109:661–664.

Bakos L, Brito AC, Castro CM, et al. Open clinical study of the efficacy and safety of terbinafine cream 1% in children with tinea corporis and tinea cruris. Pediatr Infect Dis J 1997;16:545–548.

Bolanos B. Dermatophyte feet infection among students enrolled in swimming courses at a university pool. Bol Asoc Med P Rico 1991;83:181–184.

Caputo R, DeBoulle K, DelRosso J, et al. Prevalence of superficial fungal infections among sports-active individuals: results from the Achilles survey. J Eur Acad Dermatol Venereol 2001;15:312–316.

Detandt M, Nolard N. Dermatophytes and swimming pools: seasonal fluctuations. Mycoses 1988;31:495–500.

Detandt M, Nolard N. Fungal contamination of the floors of swimming pools particularly subtropical swimming paradises. Mycoses 1995;38:509–513.

El Fari M, Gräser Y, Presber W, et al. An epidemic of tinea corporis caused by *Trichophyton tonsurans* among children (wrestlers) in Germany. Mycoses 2000;43:191–196.

English MP, Gibson MD. Studies in the epidemiology of tinea pedis (dermatophytes on the floors of swimming baths). Br Med J 1959;June:1446–1448.

Gentles JC, Evans EGV, Jones GR. Control of tinea pedis in a swimming bath. Br Med J 1974;2:577–580.

Gentles JC, Evans EGV. Foot infections in swimming baths. Br Med J 1973;3:260–262.

Gentles JC, Jones GR, Roberts DT. Efficacy of miconazole in the topical treatment of tinea pedis in sportsmen. Br J Dermatol 1975;93:79–84.

Gentles JC. Athlete's foot fungi on floors of communal bathing-places. Br Med J 1957;March:746–748.

Gentles JC. The isolation of dermatophytes from the floors of communal bathing places. J Clin Pathol 1956;9:374–377.

Gip L. Estimation of incidence of dermatophytes on floor areas after barefoot walking with washed and unwashed feet. Acta Derm Venereol 1967;47:89–93.

Gudnadottir G, Hilmarsdottir I, Sigurgeirsson B. Onychomycosis in Icelandic swimmers. Acta Dermatol Venereol 1999;79:376–377.

Hazen PG, Weil ML. Itraconazole in the prevention and management of dermatophytosis in competitive wrestlers. J Am Acad Dermatol 1997;36:481–482.

Kamihama T, Kimura T, Hosokawa JI, et al. Tinea pedis outbreak in swimming pools in Japan. Pub Health 1997;111:249–253.

Kemna ME, Elewski BE. A U.S. epidemiologic survey of superficial fungal diseases. J Am Acad Dermatol 1996;35:539–542.

Kohl TD, Lisney M. Tinea Gladiatorum. Sports Med 2000;6:439–447.

Kohl TD, Martin DC, Berger MS. Comparison of topical and oral treatments for tinea gladiatorum. Clin J Sport Med 1999;9:161–166.

Kohl TD, Martin DC, Nemeth R, et al. Fluconazole for the prevention and treatment of tinea gladiatorum. Pediatr Infect Dis J 2000;19:717–722.

Lacroix C, Baspeyras M, de La Salmoniere P, et al. Tinea pedis in European marathon runners. J Eur Acad Dermatol Venereol 2002;16:139–142.

Leyden JJ, Kligman AM. Aluminum chloride in the treatment of symptomatic athlete's foot. Arch Dermatol 1975;111:1004–1010.

Mailler EA, Adams BB. The wear and tear of 26.2: dermatological injuries reported on marathon day. Br J Sports Med 2004;38:498–501.

Malamatinis JE, Mattmiller ED, Westfall JN. Cutaneous moniliasis affecting varsity athletes. J Am Coll Health Assoc 1968;16:294–295.

Marks MI, Guruswamy A, Gross RH. Ringworm resulting from swimming with a polyurethane cast. J Ped Orthop 1983;3:511–512.

Millikan LE, Galne WK, Gewirtzman GB, et al. Naftifine cream 1% versus econazole cream 1% in the treatment of tinea cruris and tinea corporis. J Am Acad Dermatol 1988;18:52–56.

Mohrenschlager M, Seidl HP, Schnopp C, et al. Professional ice hockey players: a high risk group for fungal infection of the foot? Dermatology 2001;203:271.

NCAA. Wrestling rules and interpretations. 2005;WA-15.

Rohwedder JJ, Simmons JL, Colfer H, et al. Disseminated Curvularia lunata infection in a football player. Arch Intern Med 1979;139:940–941.

Ross MS. Complication of jogging. Arch Dermatol 1978;114:1856.

van Heerden JS, Vismer HF. Tinea corporis/cruris: new treatment options. Dermatology 1997;194:14–18.

4. Atypical Mycobacterial Skin Infections

This fourth chapter in the section on sports-related skin infections discusses atypical mycobacterial infections in the athlete, specifically *Mycobacterium marinum*. This infection is unusual but has occurred in epidemic proportions.

A swimmer's skin is ideal for infection with atypical mycobacteria. First, supersaturation of the stratum corneum (the first layer of protection of the skin) as a result of water immersion permits easy passage of microorganisms through the epidermis. Second, swimmers experience abrasions and cuts from the pool deck, diving boards, and pool walls. These breaks in the epidermis allow additional entrance of atypical mycobacteria into the deeper layers of the skin.

Swimming Pool Granuloma

Epidemiology

Mycobacterium marinum, an acid-fast atypical mycobacterium, causes swimming pool granuloma. In rare cases, *Mycobacterium scrofulaceum* is the cause (Sowers, 1972). The organism typically lives in fresh water or seawater. Affected athletes include boaters, jet skiers, lifeguards, sailors, swimmers, snorkelers, scuba divers, high divers, surfers, rafters, wind surfers, water skiers, and water polo players. After injury to the skin of the aquatic athlete, the organism gains entry into the dermis. Several epidemics of swimming pool granuloma have occurred around the world. Eighty people (73 children) in England developed *M. marinum* infection from one pool. Investigators were able to culture the organism from cracks in the pool tile (Galbraith, 1980). One pool in Colorado yielded 290 cases of *M. marinum.* The pool had very rough surfaces, and inoculating traumas occurred to most of the swimmers while they were getting in and out of the pool (Philpott et al., 1963).

In Spain a retrospective review of an 8-year period detected 45 cases of *M. marinum* infection. Eighteen percent of the infections were related to swimming pools (the majority was related to fish tanks). Eighty percent of all patients had a history of local trauma (Casal et al., 2001). Three fourths of all *M. marinum* infections occur in individuals younger than 30 years.

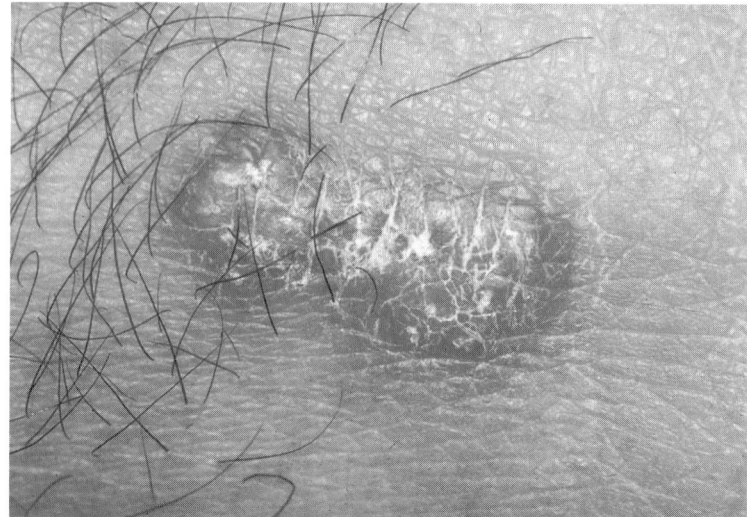

Figure 4-1. Well-defined, brown to red, minimally scaling, somewhat lobulated nodule typical of swimming pool granuloma located on an extremity.

Clinical Presentation

An erythematous papule occurs at the site of skin injury. After 1 to 2 months, the papule evolves into a verrucous nodule that may ulcerate (Figure 4-1). During epidemics, the most common locations have been the elbow (85% in many studies) and the hand (82% in some studies). The organism may migrate along the lymphatics and cause multiple linear nodules. Low-grade fevers and extension to the lungs may occur. Cutaneous complications include scarring and pigmentary changes.

Diagnosis

Biopsy reveals a granulomatous infiltrate in the mid-dermis. Cultures grow the organism in 1 to 2 weeks, most optimally at 32°C. Eighty percent of affected individuals have a positive Tb test. The differential diagnosis includes sporotrichosis (which also produces a pattern of lymphatic spread of red nodules), furunculosis, gout, leishmaniasis, sarcoidosis, and verruca vulgaris.

Verrucous squamous cell carcinoma mimics swimming pool granuloma and must be considered. This delay in diagnosis occurred in a 37-year-old scuba diver who was incorrectly diagnosed with an infectious process after receiving an injury from a coral formation (Sinnott et al., 1988).

Treatment

Warm-water soaks should be applied for 5 to 10 minutes three or four times per day. Typical useful oral antibiotic regimens include minocycline 100 mg twice per day or clarithromycin 500 mg twice per day for at least 6 weeks (most require 2–4 four months for total healing). Others have used rifampin 600 mg per day in conjunction with ethambutol 15 mg/kg per day (Fisher, 1988). Doxycycline, tetracycline, ciprofloxacin, and trimethoprim-sulfamethoxazole are other options (Johnston and Izumi, 1987). In a large retrospective study, 99% of *M. marinum* infections cleared within 2 to 4 months. Surgical excision also has been suggested. Many believe that 80% of lesions will resolve spontaneously within 3 years.

Prevention

Chlorine has little influence on *M. marinum*.

Bibliography

Casal M, del Mar Casal M. Multicenter study of incidence of Mycobacterium marinum in humans in Spain. Int J Tuberc Lung Dis 2001;5:197–199.

Fisher AA. Swimming pool granulomas due to Mycobacterium marinum: an occupational hazard of lifeguards. Cutis 1988;41:397–398.

Galbraith NS. Infections associated with swimming pools. Environ Health 1980;Feb:31–33.

Johnston JM, Izumi AK. Cutaneous Mycobacterium marinum infection. Clin Dermatol 1987;5:68–75.

Philpott JA, Woodburne AR, Philpott OS, et al. Swimming pool granuloma. Arch Dermatol 1963;83:158–162.

Sinnott JT, Trout T, Berger L. The swimming-pool granuloma that wouldn't heal. Hosp Pract 1988;23:82–84.

Sowers WF. Swimming pool granuloma due to Mycobacterium scrofulaceum. Arch Dermatol 1972;105:760–761.

5. Parasitic Skin Infections

The final chapter in the section on sports-related skin infections in athletes reviews the several parasites that infest humans. These infestations are more unusual than the infections discussed in previous chapters and rarely have long-term sequelae. Nonetheless, contracting these infections just prior to competition can severely limit an athlete's ability to participate. Scabies and lice are the two conditions that athletes contract directly from other athletes. Athletes acquire cutaneous larva migrans from the venue in which they compete.

Cutaneous Larva Migrans

Epidemiology

One case of cutaneous larva migrans in a world-class volleyball player is reported. The parasite's larva causing this condition resides in the sand and attaches to barefoot athletes (Biolcati and Alabiso, 1997). *Ancylostoma braziliense* causes cutaneous larva migrans.

Clinical Presentation

A pruritic, well-defined, linear, erythematous plaque is seen on the lower extremities (Figure 5-1).

Diagnosis

The diagnosis is made based on the clinical findings. Peripheral eosinophilia and secondary bacterial infection may be present. Migratory pulmonary infiltrates occur, so a chest radiograph is recommended.

Treatment

Topical or oral thiabendazole 400 mg twice per day for 5 days clears the infestation. The athlete should not have any pruritus after 2 days.

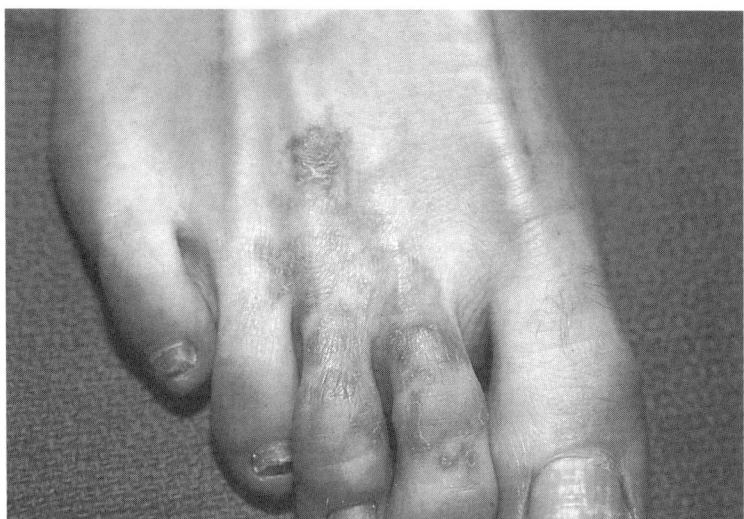

Figure 5-1. Serpiginous and erythematous plaques with cutaneous larvae migrans on the foot.

Prevention

Protective footwear should be worn when the athlete is playing in sand known to harbor the parasite. The areas where beach volleyball matches occur should be clean and clear of animal feces, which can contain eggs that produce the larva.

Cutaneous Myiasis

Epidemiology

A swimmer developed cutaneous myiasis after donning swimming trunks that had been left to dry outside in Africa (Jacobs and Orrey, 1997). The tumbu fly *(Cordylobia anthropophaga)* had deposited its eggs and larvae within the bathing suit.

Clinical Presentation

Several tender, pruritic, erythematous nodules with punctum developed on the buttocks. The swimmer complained of tender lymphadenopathy and malaise.

Diagnosis

The diagnosis is made based on the clinical findings. Biopsy reveals the larvae. Examination of the swimming trunks can reveal numerous 1-mm eggs. The differential diagnosis primarily includes furunculosis.

Treatment

Multiple therapies for cutaneous myiasis include surgical excision or application of petroleum jelly, beeswax, and mineral oil to suffocate the larvae.

Prevention

In endemic areas, swimming suits should not be left to dry in the open environment.

Pediculosis

Epidemiology

Any athlete with close skin-to-skin contact is at risk for developing scabies, but wrestling is the one sport that has dominated the literature and guideline recommendations. Based on data from the National Collegiate Athletic Association injury surveillance system (NCAAISS), 0.1% of all skin infections in collegiate wrestlers between 1991 and 2003 were caused by pediculosis.

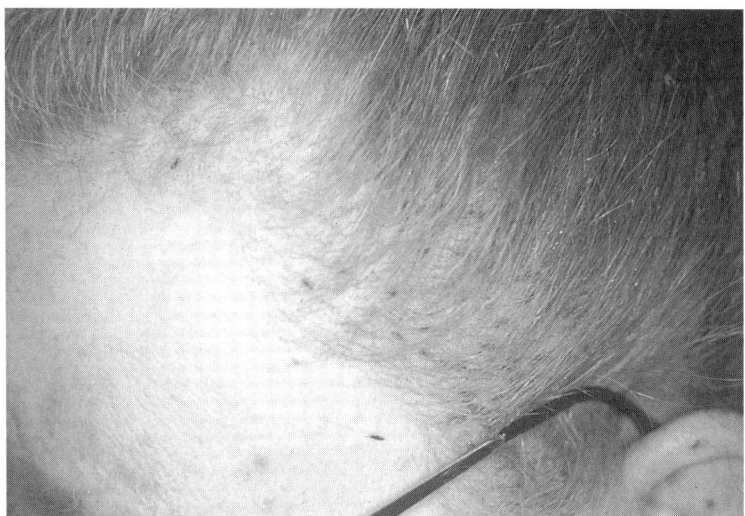

Figure 5-2. Slender moving organisms populate the hair of an athlete with pediculosis capitis.

Clinical Presentation

Pediculosis corporis (body lice), pediculosis capitis (head lice), and pediculosis pubis (genital lice) are the three types of lice that may infect the athlete (Figure 5-2). Once exposed, the athlete develops the condition in up to 10 days. Athletes complain of pruritus in the affected area.

Diagnosis

The diagnosis is made upon direct visualization of the nits or live lice. The lice can be seen on the hair or on the seams of clothes.

Treatment

Affected athletes must apply permethrin 5% cream, lindane shampoo, or petrolatum to the affected area once per day for 1 week. All clothes and equipment worn and bed sheets slept upon within 3 to 5 days prior to treatment should be laundered and dried in a hot cycle. If laundering is not possible, then at-risk material should be placed in an airtight bag for 3 to 5 days. Athletes must avoid upholstered furniture that they sat upon within the past 3 to 5 days. Intimate contacts require treatment.

Prevention

Athletes with lice should not participate in sports with plentiful skin-to-skin contact. According to NCAA rules, wrestlers must be adequately treated before competition. Athletes must be without lice. The ultimate disposition of the athlete is decided by the certified athletic trainer or physician at the time of skin check.

Scabies

Epidemiology

Any athlete with close skin-to-skin contact is at risk for developing scabies, but wrestling is the one sport that has dominated the literature and guideline recommendations. Based on data from the National Collegiate Athletic injury surveillance system (NCAAISS), 0.5% of all skin infections in collegiate wrestlers between 1991 and 2003 were caused by scabies. *Sarcoptes scabiei,* the mite that causes scabies, burrows through the epidermis and deposits its feces and eggs.

Clinical Presentation

Once exposed to another affected athlete, the competitor develops lesions within 3 to 4 weeks. Athletes develop intense pruritus that worsens in the evening. Lesions appear on the arms, hands, and groin (Figure 5-3) and progress to include the trunk (Figure 5-4) and lower extremities. Most of the lesions on the body reflect a subacute dermatitis related to the host immune system's reaction to the mite. Extremely careful examination of the volar aspects of the wrist (Figure 5-5), interdigital spaces, and elbows reveal subtle, thin, linear, scaling plaques with or without erythema. The presence of a barely visible black speck is the burrowing organism.

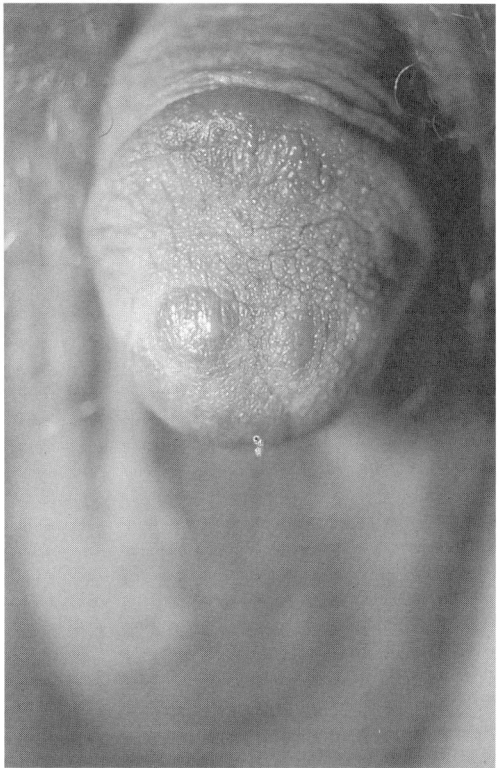

Figure 5-3. Reactive erythematous papules occur in scabies, not uncommonly in the genital region.

Diagnosis

Not uncommonly, both athletes and nonathletes with scabies are misdiagnosed. The differential diagnosis includes atopic dermatitis, contact dermatitis, and eczematous drug eruption. It is incumbent upon the clinician to perform a scabies preparation.

The best manner in which to perform a scabies preparation is as follows. The clinician dips a no. 15 blade into mineral oil and places a drop of mineral oil on a microscopic slide. The liner plaque should be scraped in one direction toward the end with the black speck. After three or four continuous scrapes, the clinician should rub the blade's contents on the microscopic slide in the area of the drop of mineral oil. This process should be repeated several times for as many burrows as can be identified on the athlete. Increasing the number of

90 Sports Dermatology

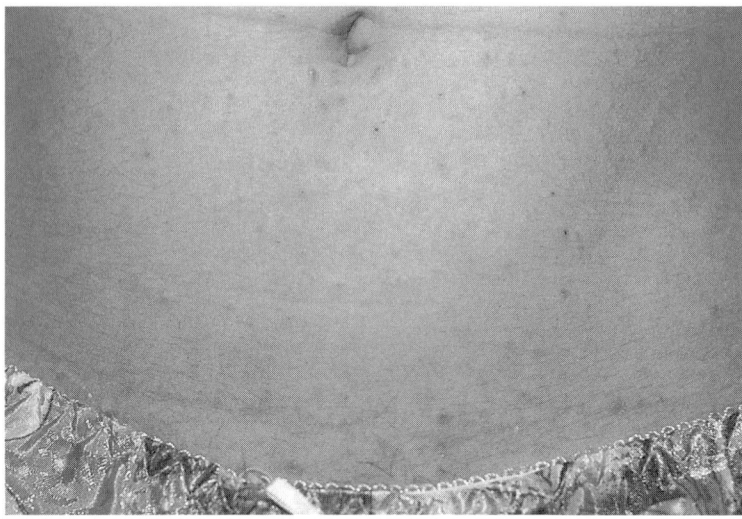

Figure 5-4. Much of the rash of scabies consists of nonspecific erythematous papules on the trunk and extremities.

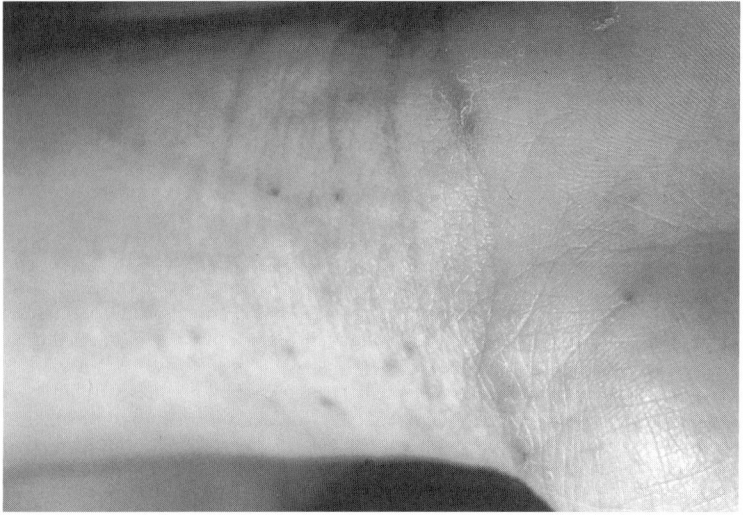

Figure 5-5. Extremely careful examination of the volar aspects of the wrist and elbows to detect burrows is critical.

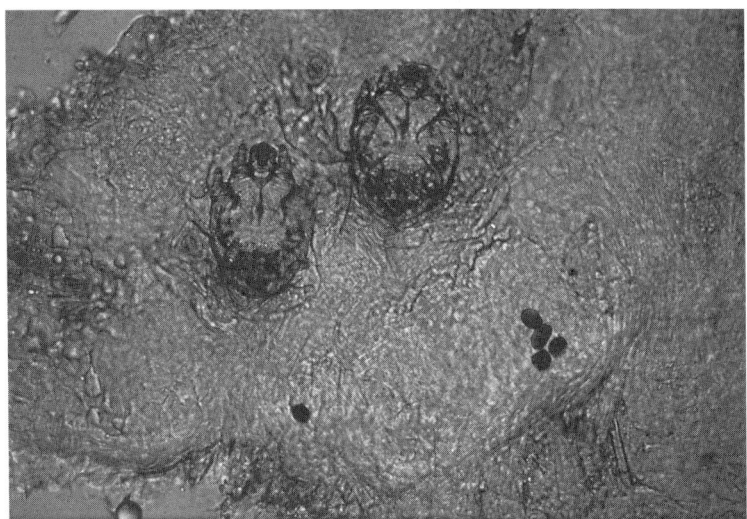

Figure 5-6. Presence of the scabies organism determined by microscopic examination confirms the diagnosis. The small brown clumps represent scybala (scabies' feces).

burrows examined increases the chance of a positive preparation. A coverslip should be placed upon the mineral oil and the slide examined under low-power magnification. A positive mineral oil preparation reveals live or dead mites. Eggs and feces (scybala) also confirm the diagnosis (Figure 5-6).

Treatment

Affected athletes must apply permethrin 5% cream applied to *all* skin surfaces from the neck to the toes at bedtime. They should not neglect the umbilicus, groin, interdigital areas or beneath the nails. The cream should be washed off in the morning. The same therapy should be repeated 1 week later. Alternatively, 200 µg/kg oral ivermectin can be taken, with a repeat dose recommended 1 to 2 weeks later. All clothes and equipment worn and bed sheets slept upon within 3 to 5 days prior to treatment should be laundered and dried in a hot cycle. If laundering is not possible, then at-risk material should be placed in an airtight bag for 3 to 5 days. Athletes must avoid upholstered furniture that they sat upon within the past 3 to 5 days. Intimate contacts require treatment.

Pruritus resolves very quickly. Unfortunately, in rare cases, pruritus persists in an athlete. The scabies organism is generally killed, but the pruritus is a persistent hypersensitivity reaction that may require topical or oral steroids.

Prevention

Athletes with scabies should not participate in sports with extensive skin-to-skin contact. According to NCAA rules, athletes must have a negative scabies preparation before competition. The ultimate disposition of the athlete is decided by the certified athletic trainer or physician at the time of skin check.

Bibliography

Biolcati G, Alabiso A. Creeping eruption of larva migrans: a case report in a beach volley athlete. Int J Sports Med 1997;18:612–613.

Jacobs P, Orrey L. Micro-abscesses in the swimming trunk area. S Afr Med J 1997; 87:1559–1560.

Section II Sports-Related Aberrant Growths

6. Athlete's Nodules

Section II of this book discusses tumors or tumorlike growths (both benign and malignant) on the skin of athletes. Compared to the immediate morbidity of many of the infections discussed in Section I, the disorders discussed in this section do not cause as much disruption to athletes, at least in the acute setting. Also, in general the incidence of tumors and tumorlike growths pale in comparison to the incidence of sports-related skin infections. Nonetheless, athletes do develop skin cancers at epidemic proportions, albeit often after they have long retired their athletic equipment. Sunburns and the eventual skin cancers should be of critical concern to athletes and the clinicians entrusted with their care. Chapter 7, the second chapter in this section, reviews melanoma and nonmelanoma skin cancers and the sun exposure leading to them as they relate to sports participation.

Chapter 6, the first chapter in Section II, concentrates on the benign growths that develop as a result of athletes' participation in sports. Controversy over the exact nomenclature of these benign growths of athletes rages on in the literature. Most believe the term *athlete's nodules* is a general term referring to all benign neoplasms that occur in areas of repeated traumas. Many different athletes are afflicted, and the exact trauma that leads to the nodule varies with the sport. Because of variations in pathogenesis, clinical presentation, and treatment, clinicians ultimately subcategorized athlete's nodules.

For example, because of their relatively common occurrence in actual athletes or perhaps just in the literature, nodules occurring after cycling and surfing have garnered their own designations and are described separately in this chapter. Furthermore, evidence suggests that the "nodules" seen in runners and hockey players have different etiologies and are discussed as a separate group. Finally, not all growths are thick enough to be classified as nodules; investigators refer to these growths as *pads* in boxers and soccer players. Thus, these two conditions are discussed as a separate group.

In summary, this chapter discusses separately athlete's nodules, surfer's nodules, cycler's nodules, pseudonodules, and knuckle pads.

Athlete's Nodules

Epidemiology

Athlete's nodules has been a general term for reactive nodules occurring in individuals who engage in sports. The specific sports discussed under this nomenclature are football and canoeing. No data on incidence exist for either sport. There is no reason to believe that any athlete whose skin rubs repeatedly on equipment could not also develop a similar condition. Chronic rubbing on the ankle from tight-fitting shoes is believed to cause athlete's nodules in foot-

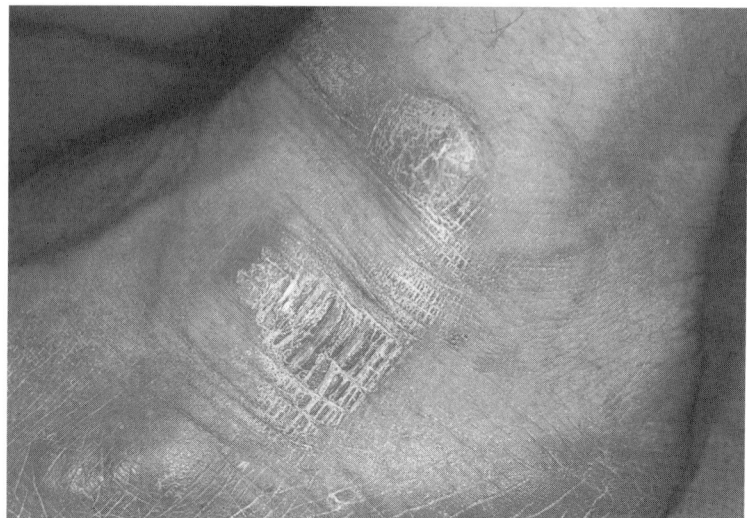

Figure 6-1. Two thick nodules occurring over the dorsal aspects of the foot after tight-fitting athletic footwear is worn for a prolonged period. Biopsy of this lesion would reveal a collagenoma.

ball players (Figure 6-1). The chronic rubbing of the canoe's floor against the canoeist's knees results in athlete's nodules.

Clinical Presentation

In the case of one football player, large (3.5-cm), well-defined, skin-colored nodules appeared on the dorsal aspect of the feet after the player wore tight-fitting sneakers several hours per day for up to 5 months per year for 6 years. The lesions enlarged even after the player stopped participating in football. Thirty-eight years later the lesions persisted (Cohen et al., 1992). Canoeists develop similar lesions on the knees.

Diagnosis

To confirm the diagnosis of athlete's nodules, the clinician most often needs to perform a punch or excisional biopsy. The differential diagnosis is vast and varies with the location of the nodule. The clinical differential diagnosis of a lesion on the foot includes ganglion cyst, granuloma annulare, rheumatoid nodule, gout, foreign body reaction, and elastoma (Adams, 2001). The differential diagnosis of lesions on the knee is the same as for the foot and includes bursitis and xanthoma (Table 6-1).

Athlete's nodules (specifically of these types) are collagenomas. Histologically, a normal or hyperkeratotic and acanthotic epidermis may be present. An increased density of normal-appearing collagen bundles is seen in the dermis. The repeated trauma to the skin may increase collagen production or decrease local degradation of collagen.

Treatment

Both medical and surgical modalities are available for treatment of athlete's Nodules. In cases with significant hyperkeratosis, topical keratolytics such as salicylic acid, urea, and lactic acid may be useful (Adams, 2001). However, this treatment does not influence the dermal component of athlete's nodules. Intralesional steroids (triamcinolone) or potent topical steroids may be useful. Surgical excision can be performed. The risks regarding keloids, severe scarring, and recurrence should be discussed with the patient, although some authors noted none of these complications (Cohen et al., 1992).

Prevention

Because the primary etiology for athlete's nodules is repeated friction between equipment and the skin, the clinician and athlete can make alterations to decrease the condition's incidence. Athletes should promptly alert their

Table 6-1. Differential Diagnosis of Athlete's Nodules Depending on Anatomic Location

Foot Lesion	Knee Lesion
Elastoma	Bursitis
Foreign body reaction	Elastoma
Ganglion cyst	Foreign body reaction
Gout	Ganglion cyst
Granuloma annulare	Gout
Keloid	Granuloma annulare
Rheumatoid nodule	Keloid
Scar	Rheumatoid nodule
	Scar
	Xanthoma

athletic trainer or sports clinician if they have such ill-fitting shoes and nodules are developing. Properly fitted footwear does not create the physical forces necessary to create athlete's nodules. Protective padding can be worn to decrease friction. The football player would wear this protection on the foot, and the canoeist would wear it on the knees.

Surfer's Nodules

Epidemiology

Surfer's nodules also are termed *surfer's knots* and *surfer's ulcers*. This condition apparently is so common among surfers the nodules are readily apparent even in cartoons of surfers. These nodules only rarely are brought to the attention of clinicians; in fact, some surfers express pride in having them.

Clinical Presentation

There are at least five different clinical presentations of surfer's nodules. The etiology may differ among the various subtypes. Most lesions present on the pretibial portions of the leg, the dorsal aspect of the foot, and the knee. Most akin to the athlete's nodules of football players and canoers, surfers develop collagenomas on the pretibial region below the knee or over the metatarsophalangeal joints with an increased amount of collagen (Cohen et al., 1990, 1992; Swift, 1965). One author noted another type of skin change (Gelfand, 1966). He found that four of the eight surfers with foot nodules (he termed them *surfer's knots*) examined had radiographic evidence of chipping or spurring of an underlying bone. These nodules on the dorsal aspect of the feet are soft tissue swellings that evolve based on the duration of surfing. Initially the lesions are soft, painful, erythematous, and fluctuant and have discharge. Over 1 to 2 years of regular surfing, the lesions become firm, fibrous, and less painful. If surfing is discontinued during the fluctuant period of the nodule's evolution, the nodules may disappear. Once surfer's nodules become firm, they persist even after months out of the water.

A third type of skin change seen in surfer's nodules is a ganglionlike cyst over the proximal dorsal aspect of the foot. It is a soft swelling that varies in size and grows rapidly. A gelatinous material exudes if the cyst ruptures. This lesion is essentially a bursa forming in the synovial sheath of the extensor digitorum longus tendon (Cohen et al., 1992; Swift, 1965). A fourth type of surfer's nodule is a subcutaneous infrapatellar bursal cyst that surfers note as nodules just beneath the knee (Cragg, 1973). Finally, surfer's nodules can be knee nodules that ulcerate (hence their name *surfer's ulcers*). The histology of this type of

Table 6-2. Classification of Clinical/Histologic Types of Surfer's Nodules

Type	Location	Pathology
A	Pretibial or metatarsophalangeal joints	Collagenoma
B early	Dorsal aspects of the feet	Soft tissue swellings
B late	Dorsal aspects of the feet	Fibrous nodules with chipping and spurring of underlying bone
C	Proximal dorsal aspect of the feet	Ganglionlike cyst
D	Infrapatellar region	Bursal cyst
E	Knee	Granulomatous infiltrate with pseudoepitheliomatous hyperplasia

surfer's nodule shows pseudoepitheliomatous hyperplasia and hyperkeratosis. A granulomatous infiltrate of neutrophils seen in the dermis (Cohen et al., 1992) may be a foreign body response to grains of sand obtained by friction with sand embedded in the paraffin wax on the surfboard (Table 6-2) (Pharis et al., 1997).

Diagnosis

To confirm the diagnosis of surfer's nodules, the clinician most often must perform a punch or excisional biopsy. The differential diagnosis includes not only many non-sports–related skin diseases but also the various types of surfer's nodules. The clinical differential diagnosis of lesions on the foot includes ganglion cyst, granuloma annulare, rheumatoid nodule, gout, foreign body reaction, and elastoma (Adams, 2001). The differential diagnosis of lesions on the knee is the same as for the foot and includes bursitis and xanthoma (Table 6-1). Histologic examination helps the clinician determine if the nodules are related to surfing. In the case of surfer's nodules, the biopsy also allows the clinician to determine the mechanism of lesion origin.

Treatment

Most of the lesions do not require treatment, and many surfers do not present to the clinician for treatment (Swift, 1965). However, the lesions can be quite painful, and surfers may call upon the sports clinician for therapy. In fact, surfer's nodules can be so painful that some surfers dangle their affected legs into the cold water to anesthetize them before putting them firmly on the board (Gelfand, 1966). Other surfer's nodules become secondarily infected and develop cellulitis.

Both medical and surgical treatments are available for treatment of athlete's nodules. In cases of significant hyperkeratosis, topical keratolytics such as salicylic acid, urea, and lactic acid may be useful (Adams, 2001). However, this treatment does not influence the dermal component of athlete's nodules. Intralesional steroids (triamcinolone) or potent topical steroids may be useful. Surgical excision can be performed. The risks regarding keloids, severe scarring, and recurrence should be discussed with the patient, although some authors noted none of these complications (Cohen et al., 1990, 1992).

Prevention

Many cases of surfer's nodules occur in Californian and British surfers, who paddle out to catch the waves in relatively cold water (55°F–60°F). They kneel and rest all their body weight on the board between just the knees and feet. Surfers in Hawaii, where the water is warmer, seem to have fewer surfers' nodules. These warm-water surfers, who lie prone on the seaward journey to the waves, distribute their body's weight more equally and do not develop surfer's nodules. If cold-water surfers use wet suits to keep them warm, they too can lie prone on the surfboard as they paddle out to the waves. Use of protective padding on their knees and ankles seems to decrease the development of surfer's nodules (Adams, 2001; Cohen et al., 1990).

Cycler's Nodules

Epidemiology

No epidemiologic study has examined the incidence of nodules in cyclists; however, nodules resembling either collagenoma or cysts are reported in multiple series. The collagenoma-like lesion can occur in the area of the ischial tuberosities or the sacrococcygeal region. At least seven Japanese males with the collagenoma-like nodules in the sacrococcygeal region were reported (Kawaura et al., 2000; Nakamura et al., 1995). The mean age was 16 years (range 13–19 years). The onset of disease was between 4 and 13 years, and the nodules were present for between 1 and 14 years. Family members did not have similar lesions.

The cysts have occurred in the perineum of racers and other intense cyclists (Mellion, 1991).

Clinical Presentation

Some authors believe cycler's nodules that resemble collagenoma are caused by mechanical irritation between the skin and the bicycle saddle. Individuals with a sharply angulated sacrococcygeal joint seem at particular risk. Thirty percent of the normal Japanese population has sharply angulated sacrococcygeal joints, which may explain the high incidence of cycler's nodules in Japanese cyclists (Kawaura et al., 2000). The nodules seen in Japanese bike riders are well-defined, skin-colored, oval, hard, 2- to 7-cm nodules in the sacrococcygeal area. Similar nodules may appear over the ischial tuberosities in cyclists. These nodules likely are caused by constant pressure and trauma (Mellion, 1991).

The cysticlike nodules in the perineum that cyclers can develop are related to pressure and trauma. Clinically these cycler's nodules are a bit different from the nodules in the sacrococcygeal area. Because of the location and somewhat pendulous appearance of these particular cycler's nodules, some authors note their resemblance to "accessory testicles."

Diagnosis

Although cycler's nodules may be suspected, especially if an astute clinician inquires about cycling and observes the nodules in the perineum region or over the ischial tuberosities or sacrococcygeal area, a biopsy is necessary to confirm the diagnosis. The differential diagnosis includes teratoma, epidermoid cyst, dermoid cyst, and coccygeal cyst.

On histopathologic examination, the cycler's nodules over the ischial tuberosities or sacrococcygeal area reveal hyperkeratosis, acanthosis, and an increased amount of collagen in the dermis and into the subcutaneous fat. Magnetic resonance imaging of the sacrococcygeal joint likely will reveal a sharp angle (Kawaura et al., 2000; Nakamura et al., 1995). The other diagnoses in the clinical differential will be easily excluded.

The histopathology of the cycler's nodules in the perineum is different. No significant epidermal change is noted, but necrosis and pseudocysts involving connective tissue are observed in the superficial fascia. This pathology allows the clinician to differentiate among the other clinical diagnoses.

Treatment

Cycler's nodules of the collagenoma type have been excised without recurrence, and excision should be performed if the nodules affect the athlete's daily life or cycling. Some authors have noted that nonsurgical approaches can be attempted first (Mellion, 1991). Rest, oral antiinflammatory agents, warm-water soaks (several times per day for several minutes each time), and use of protective padding on the bicycle seat should assuage early lesions of cycler's nodules.

Prevention

For cyclists who spend a great deal of time on the saddle, trauma and pressure are part of the game. Attention to proper padding of the seat and extra padding in their shorts may help to decrease the incidence of cycler's nodules. Athletes should be aware that certain anatomic variations might make them more at risk for developing cycler's nodules.

Pseudonodules

Epidemiology

The incidence of pseudonodules in athletes is unknown. These lesions have been termed *Nike nodules* in runners and *skate bite* in hockey players, although theoretically they can occur in athletes participating in any sport requiring footwear. Both Nike nodules and skate bites are caused by chronic pressure and friction in tight-fitting shoes or hockey skates, respectively (Basler and Jacobs, 1991).

Clinical Presentation

Nike nodules and skate bite occur on the dorsal aspects of both feet where the ill-fitted shoes exert the greatest pressure.

Diagnosis

The diagnosis should be straightforward and is confirmed by rapid resolution of the pseudonodules upon obtaining properly fitted shoes or hockey skates. Although pseudonodules have not often been biopsied, they likely represent a type of pseudobursa because the pseudonodules rapidly resolve upon discontinuation of the offending footwear.

Treatment

Pseudonodules rapidly clear once the athlete starts wearing proper-fitting footwear.

Prevention

Athletes of all types, especially those whose footwear is so integral to their sport (e.g., runners), should acquire shoes or skates only from specialized stores. Specialty running stores can be found in most major cities and are staffed by extremely knowledgeable assistants whose goal is to find the best fitting shoes based upon a person's height, weight, foot shape, and running style. These or similar professionals can educate the athlete about different lacing techniques that will distribute the pressure more equally. Protective padding may be helpful but should not be necessary with proper athletic footwear and lacing.

Knuckle or Sports-Related Pads

Epidemiology

No studies have examined the incidence of knuckle pads in athletes. Although lesions do not always occur exactly on the knuckles, the literature still refers to these lesions as *knuckle pads.* Boxers and soccer players with the condition are reported (Dickens et al., 2002; Kanerva, 1998).

Clinical Presentation

Knuckle or sports-related pads tend to be plaques, whereas athlete's nodules are dome-shaped nodules representing a deeper dermatologic process. Boxers traumatize their hands during their sport and develop well-defined, hyperpigmented plaques over their knuckles (Kanerva, 1998). A female soccer player developed thick, rough, scaling, 2-cm plaques over both anterior ankles after wearing skin guards while playing soccer and softball for 2 years (Figure 6-2). The lesions persisted even 2 years after she stopped playing, although the lesion size decreased (Dickens et al., 2002).

Diagnosis

The diagnosis is made clinically. Biopsy is rarely needed or desired but is helpful to confirm the diagnosis. The differential diagnosis includes foreign body reactions, granuloma annulare, warts, xanthomas, and sports-related callosities. This last condition may be difficult to distinguish from sports-related pads, but callosities related to sports typically resolve more quickly after the athlete stops the activity (Dickens et al., 2002).

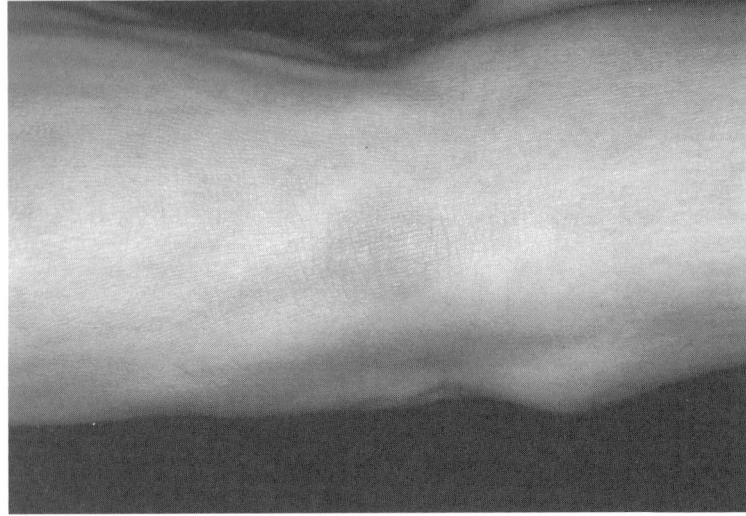

Figure 6-2. Shin guards may cause sufficient friction and pressure to create sports-related pads on the athlete.

Treatment

Knuckle or sports-related pads resolve slowly after the activity that caused them is discontinued. Keratolytic agents such as lactic acid or urea cream may be helpful. Topical or intralesional steroids can be tried. The surgical approach that is often needed for the nodules of athletes is not required as frequently for sports-related pads.

Prevention

Boxers can wear protective padding during sparring to decrease the production of knuckle pads. Soccer, baseball, and softball players may require additional padding under their shin guards if they notice increased friction and pressure.

Bibliography

Adams BB. Sports dermatology. Adolesc Clin 2001;12:305–322.
Basler RSW, Jacobs SI. Athlete's nodules [letter]. J Am Acad Dermatol 1991;24:318.

Cohen PR, Eliezri YD, Silvers DN. Athlete's nodules. Cutis 1992;50:131–135.
Cohen PR, Eliezri YD, Silvers DN. Athlete's nodules. Sports Med 1990;10:198–203.
Cragg J. Surfers' nodules. Br J Clin Pract 1973;11:418–419.
Dickens R, Adams BB, Mutasim DF. Sports-related pads. Int J Dermatol 2002;41:291–293.
Gelfand DW. Surfer's knots. JAMA 1966;197:189–190.
Kanerva L. Knuckle pads from boxing. Eur J Dermatol 1998;8:359–361.
Kawaura K, Yano K, Takama H, et al. Nodular lesion on the sacrococcygeal area in a bicycle rider. Br J Dermatol 2000;143:1097–1131.
Mellion MB. Common cycling injuries. Sports Med 1991;11:52–70.
Nakamura A, Inoue Y, Ishihara T, et al. Acquired coccygeal nodule due to repeated stimulation by a bicycle saddle. J Dermatol 1995;22:365–369.
Pharis DB, Teller C, Wolf JE. Cutaneous manifestations of sports participation. J Am Acad Dermatol 1997;36:448–459.
Swift S. Surfers' "knots." JAMA 1965;192:123–124.

7. Sunburns and Skin Cancer

Chapter 6 outlined the myriad benign neoplasms that occur in athletes. Unfortunately, not all neoplasms acquired by sports participants are benign. Malignant growths have become a concern for many different athletes.

Outdoor athletes probably compose one of the most at-risk groups in terms of exposure to ultraviolet radiation. Although any outdoor athlete in general is at increased risk, this chapter elucidates why some winter and aquatic athletes may assume more risk. Athletes are at increased risk for developing side effects from the sun, not only because of their prolonged exposure to the sun but also because of other intrinsic factors related to sports and sports' equipment.

Once athletes are exposed to ultraviolet radiation, both acute and chronic consequences occur. Acutely, athletes may endure painful sunburns that prevent practice or competition. Chronically exposed athletes likely may experience skin cancer, which includes melanoma, squamous cell carcinoma, and basal cell carcinoma. Both cumulative and intermittent extensive exposures to the sun increase the risk of squamous cell carcinoma, basal cell carcinoma, and melanoma.

This chapter specifically reviews the therapeutic and preventative modalities not only for the acute ultraviolet toxicity but also for the chronic skin changes that lead to skin cancer.

Sunburn

Epidemiology

Almost every outdoor athlete has experienced an overdose of ultraviolet irradiation. Several studies have examined sunburns and sunscreen use in athletes. Athletes' risk for sunburns relate to the environments in which their sport occurs, the equipment they wear, and intrinsic factors related to exercise (Table 7-1).

Many sports place athletes particularly at risk for sunburn because of the environment in which the athletes participate. Some athletes have little to no chance at receiving shade cover. For example, studies have shown that triathletes, cyclists, skiers, and swimmers experience an exceptional amount of ultraviolet exposure during competitions. One study quantified that the mean personal ultraviolet exposure of participants at the Ironman Triathlete World Championships in Hawaii was more than eight times the minimal erythema dose (MED) required to induce pink skin. All athletes were sunburned after their 8- to 9-hour competition even though they all wore water-resistant, sun protection factor (SPF) 25+ on exposed skin (Moehrle et al., 2001).

A study also quantified the ultraviolet exposure of professional cyclists during the eight stages of the Tour de Suisse. Cyclists received the lowest

Table 7-1. Sports for Which Studies Have Specifically Illustrated Reasons for Increased Ultraviolet Damage

Sport	Reason for Increased Ultraviolet Damage
Triathlon, cycling, baseball, softball, golf	Gross exposure to severe level of ultraviolet rays
Skiing, soccer, running	Failure to apply sunscreen
Outdoor athletics	High wind
Outdoor athletics	High temperatures
Outdoor athletics	Sweating
Skiing, snowboarding, swimming	Reflectance of ultraviolet rays

exposure during the prologue of the race (0.2 MED), but received more than 17 times their MED during the mountain surge. The mean daily exposure for the cyclists was, as for triathletes, more than eight times the MED. This exposure is more than 30 times the international exposure limits (Moehrle et al., 2000a).

Other athletes whose environments place them at increased risk include winter and aquatic athletes. Water reflects much of the ultraviolet rays, concentrating them on the swimmer. Outdoor winter athletes experience the same concentration of ultraviolet rays from reflection off the snow. This reflection may be as great as 85% to 95% when the snow is fresh. Furthermore, winter athletes whose sport takes them to the higher mountain elevations must endure more intense rays. At higher elevations, less ultraviolet light is scattered or absorbed. One study revealed that skiers at noon in Vail, Colorado, experience nearly the same ultraviolet B intensity as those standing at sea level in Orlando, Florida, at the same time. The study also determined that an average unprotected skier at an elevation of 11,000 feet at noon would receive enough ultraviolet B radiation to make them pink (reach their MED) in only 6 minutes (Rigel et al., 1999). The same authors also studied 10 professional skiers for 1 month to assess the actual dose of ultraviolet rays. Individuals with type II skin experienced 0.5 to 7.6 times their MED total while skiing during the day. Ten percent of the skiers received more than one MED per hour at peak ultraviolet times (Rigel et al., 2003).

Despite these obvious risk factors for skiers, one study exposed the lack of knowledge and understanding among skiers. Only about half of the skiers and snowboarders surveyed were wearing sunscreen (mean SPF 23) while they were on the resort slopes (Buller et al., 1998). Of those wearing sunscreen, nearly all had it on their face, but only half of the sunscreen wearers applied any sunscreen to their neck (half wore neck covers) or ears (most wore hats that covered their ears). Only 64% of all skiers used lip balm with sunscreen. Seventy percent had burned while skiing or snowboarding, and 27% had burned that winter. Of the burns, 25% resulted in skin blistering and 29% resulted in lip blistering.

Of the variables tested, only female gender correlated positively with a skier's or snowboarder's use of lip balm with SPF. This study also examined the variables associated with the SPF level used on the body. Skiers and snowboarders used higher SPFs when they hit the slopes later in the day, when the temperature rose or the wind was less, or if they had been burnt in the past. Skiers were much more likely than snowboarders to use higher SPF.

Other outdoor athletes experience increased exposure to the sun. Using personal electronic ultraviolet radiation dosimeters, researchers showed that golfers received an inordinate amount of ultraviolet radiation (Thieden et al., 2004). Another study showed that baseball players received an excess of ultraviolet radiation. Their arms received the most radiation and the forehead the least, likely related to use of brimmed hats (Melville et al., 1991).

Outdoor environments provide increased risk through unique factors. Interesting information from rat research shows that wind exposure (Owens et al., 1974) and hotter temperatures (Freeman and Knox, 1964) increase damage to skin after ultraviolet irradiation.

Finally, intrinsic athlete factors play a role. Participants sweat during most athletic activities. One study discovered that the sweat itself increased the chance of sunburn. An athlete's MED is decreased by more than 40% after only 15 minutes of sweating during jogging (Moehrle et al., 2000b).

Clinical Presentation

Most clinicians do not experience difficulty in identifying sunburn. Less than 1 day after sun exposure, patients are diffusely red with very sharp lines of demarcation corresponding to areas covered by clothing. Sunburns may show signs of blisters. Occasionally, severe sunburns are associated with systemic signs of fever, malaise, nausea, and chills.

Diagnosis

The diagnosis of sunburn is obvious. The effect of systemic medications that the athlete may be taking also must be considered. For example, antibiotics taken for acne are classic photosensitizing medications (Figure 7-1). Many other medications also can make the athlete more sensitive to the sun.

Treatment

The long-term changes caused by the sun cannot be reversed. The acute changes caused by the sun can be treated with cool water or Burrow's compresses. Topical petroleum jelly, Sarna lotion, steroids, and oral nonsteroidal antiinflammatory drugs such as aspirin and indomethacin can be soothing.

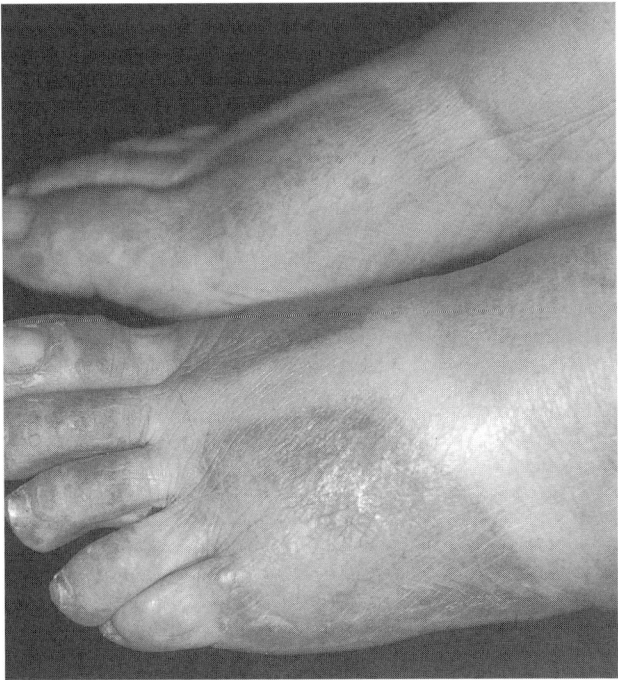

Figure 7-1. Athletes taking photosensitizing medication (e.g., doxycycline) may develop an intense sunburn on their feet after wearing sandals without sunscreen.

A number of studies have examined the evidence for such treatments in patients with sunburns. Most studies agree that nonsteroidal agents decrease erythema after ultraviolet B irradiation, but they must be taken immediately after sun exposure. Use of emollients improves the symptoms associated with sunburn but does not decrease recovery time. Antihistamines offer no benefit. The only double-blind, placebo-controlled study showed that oral corticosteroids were no better than placebo in the acute management of sunburn (Han and Maibach, 2004).

Prevention

The keys to sunburn prevention include sun avoidance, use of sunscreen, and photoprotective clothing. Obviously, prevention from sunburn resides in avoiding the sun, especially during the peak hours of ultraviolet radiation between

10 AM and 3 PM (Table 7-2). Unfortunately, many practices and competitions are scheduled during this period. Some very competitive national teams creatively schedule practices in the late afternoon or early morning to avoid these peak hours.

Athletes must wear broadband-blocking sunscreen, preferably with an SPF of at least 30. Despite the importance of sunscreen use for athletes, many athletes do not routinely apply it. One study of 186 collegiate soccer players and cross-country runners revealed that 85% had not worn any sunscreen in the past 7 days and only 6% of them reported using sunscreen at least 3 of the past 7 days (Hamant and Adams, 2005). Studies of skiers and snowboarders also document the scarcity of sunscreen use.

Coaches and instructors must be advocates for sunscreen use. Skiers note that less than one fourth of ski instructors provided warnings regarding the increased risk of sunburn while skiing. Less than half of the skiers recalled seeing any sign or brochure regarding sun safety at the ski resorts. A study of more than 1000 youth soccer players showed that using coaches as advocates for sunscreen use significantly increased its use from the beginning to the end of the season (Adams, unpublished data).

Athletes do not regularly apply sunscreen for many reasons. In a study of collegiate soccer players and cross-country runners, the investigators discovered that the main reasons why collegiate athletes did not wear sunscreen during their outdoor exposure related to access to sunscreen in 46% and misinformation about sunscreen use in 33%. For example, many people, including athletes, have the misconception that a "base" tan provides adequate protection from ultraviolet radiation. A "base" tan for the average skin-type athlete provides the equivalent of only SPF 2 sunscreen (Kaidbey and Kilgman, 1978). By providing education and sunscreen in accessible locations to outdoor athletes, organizers of youth, collegiate, and professional sports likely will overcome some of the most common barriers to sunscreen use.

Athletes regularly sweat or frequently are in the water. Both of these activities decrease the effectiveness of sunscreen, and reapplication is mandatory. Swimmers who wear sunscreen are more likely to sunburn than are nonswimming sunscreen users (Wright et al., 2001). Use of sunscreen is not without controversy. Some investigators have linked sunscreen use to a higher incidence of skin cancer. Clinicians should be aware of some data suggesting that use of sunscreen while exercising at low humidity retards sweat evaporation (Wells et al., 1984).

Finally, athletes' equipment should protect them not only from physical contact during sports activity but also from ultraviolet radiation. Hats should be

Table 7-2. Smart Sun Safety Tips for Athletes

Avoid the sun between 10 AM and 3 PM, if possible
Apply SPF 30 sunscreen 30 minutes before participating in outdoor sports
Reapply sunscreen often while sweating or swimming
Wear hats
Wear sun-protective clothing

Table 7-3. Factors Influencing the Protection Factor of an Athlete's Clothing

Fabric Variable	Effect on Protection Factor
Nylon, wool, silk	Relatively increases
Cotton, rayon, linen	Relatively decreases
Dark color	Increases
Ultraviolet absorbers added	Increases
Increasing wetness	Decreases
Increasing numbers of washes	Increases

worn whenever reasonable. Baseball players who wear hats receive significantly less ultraviolet exposure to their foreheads compared to their cheeks and arms. A great deal of research involves evaluation of the ultraviolet protection provided by clothing (Table 7-3). Most summer clothing does not provide sufficient ultraviolet protection. One study found that one English soccer shirt provided an ultraviolet protection factor of only 5 to 10 (Wright et al., 2001). Dyeing fabrics or adding an ultraviolet-absorbing material during laundering increases the clothing's protection. Blue dye increases the SPF by 544%, whereas yellow dye increases the SPF by only 212%. Simply laundering with soap and water increases the SPF of clothing (through fabric shrinkage). Fabric material and the wetness of clothing also influence the protection factor. Nylon, wool, and silk have higher protection factors than other fabrics. Wetness of cotton fabric decreases the protection factor (Table 7-3).

Melanoma

Epidemiology

Extensive epidemiologic studies regarding melanoma in athletes in the United States are not available. Many epidemiologic studies have been performed in Denmark, Italy, and Australia. One Italian study linked outdoor sports with melanoma, with outdoor athletic men 4.1 times more likely to develop melanoma (Zanetti et al., 1988). An Argentinean study also showed that participation in sports was linked to melanoma (Loria and Matos, 2001). Athletes who had spent considerable time practicing outdoors (mostly playing soccer) had a risk 3.2 times that of nonathletes. However, at least one study in the United States did not find any association between land sports (e.g., winter sports and hiking) with melanoma (Herzfeld et al., 1993).

More consistently positive results on the association of sports with melanoma were found when water sports were studied. The same study in the United States found that athletes participating in water sports were 2.67 times more likely to develop melanoma than were nonparticipants. A study in the

Netherlands found that sun-sensitive athletes participating in water sports (excluding swimming) were 22.7 times more likely to develop melanoma than were nonathletes (Nelemans et al., 1993). Several studies of hundreds of patients demonstrated an association of melanoma with intermittent sun exposure (Basler et al., 2000). Swimming in these studies was not associated with increased risk of melanoma. However, one interesting study determined that swimming was partly related to melanoma. Danish researchers studied subjects with or without melanoma and compared those who swam in "polluted" water (defined as rivers or chlorinated water) to those who swam in unpolluted water (defined as lakes and Dutch Fens) or those who did not swim at all. Persons who swam in "polluted" water were at significantly greater risk to develop melanoma compared with those who did not swim in "polluted" water. More extensive epidemiologic research is needed to determine the influence of swimming on melanoma development.

Unlike the sports discussed above, no large epidemiologic studies have focused on cyclists. However, one British group reported five cyclists who were diagnosed with melanoma within 1 year (Williams et al., 1989). Four of the cyclists were women. All but one of the lesions were located on the posterior calf; one was located on the anterior thigh of a female. Interestingly, these particular anatomic locations are the areas of maximal irradiation when the cyclist assumes the flexed cycling position. As illustrated by the irradiation studies of professional cyclists, intermittent intense sun exposure is par for the course. Furthermore, because the cyclists travel at great speeds and experience the cooling effect of the wind, they do not experience the warming signs foreboding a sunburn.

Clinical Presentation

Unlike squamous and basal cell carcinoma, melanoma is more associated with intermittent, intense ultraviolet exposure. Melanomas can be found anywhere on the body, but clinicians should be particularly careful to screen areas that have received intense intermittent exposure. Melanomas typically are irregularly shaped, irregularly colored macules, patches, papules, or plaques (Figure 7-2). Often, yet not universally, several different colors (blue, black, brown) are seen within the lesion. In rare instances, the color of a melanoma is not very impressive (so-called *amelanotic melanoma).* Lesions that are changing rapidly should be examined carefully.

Diagnosis

The differential diagnosis of melanoma is vast and most often consists of dysplastic nevi, pigmented seborrheic keratoses, pigmented basal cell carcinomas, and blue nevi. All suspicious lesions must be biopsied by an expert in skin diseases. Superficial biopsies must be avoided because inadequate tissue may

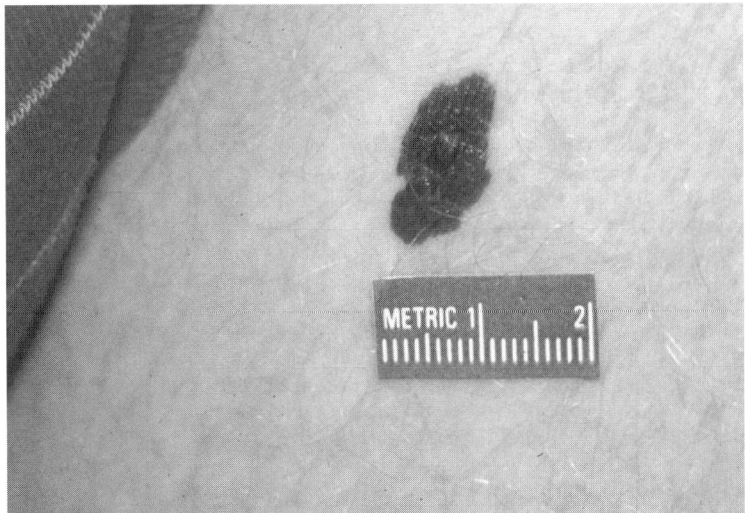

Figure 7-2. Typical irregularly shaped, irregularly colored, black plaque characteristic of melanoma.

lead to an incorrect diagnosis or misleading depth of invasion. The specimen should be read by a dermatopathologist known to the clinician who is sending the biopsy.

Treatment

Trained surgeons should excise melanoma. Surgical margins differ based on the depth and presence of cutaneous ulceration or lack thereof. Long-term survival is best correlated with the depth of lesion and the presence of ulceration. Sentinel lymph node biopsy should be considered for lesions more than 1 mm deep. Patients then should be followed-up closely by a dermatologist for an indefinite period.

Prevention

Athletes are at risk for developing skin cancers because of their intense and frequent exposure to ultraviolet radiation during peak ultraviolet times of the day. Reflectance of ultraviolet rays by the snow and water enhances the exposure of athletes whose venues include those elements. Sweating increases the chances of sunburn, not only by making the athlete more sun-sensitive but also by diluting the effect of applied sunscreen.

The keys to sunburn prevention include sun avoidance, use of sunscreen, and photoprotective clothing. Obviously, prevention of sunburn resides in avoiding the sun, especially during the peak hours of ultraviolet radiation between 10 AM and 3 PM (Table 7-2). Unfortunately, many practices and competitions are scheduled during this period. Some very competitive national teams creatively schedule practices in the late afternoon or early morning to avoid these peak hours.

Athletes must wear broadband-blocking sunscreen, preferably with an SPF of at least 30. Despite the importance of sunscreen use for athletes, many athletes do not routinely apply it. One study of 186 collegiate soccer players and cross-country runners revealed that 85% had not worn any sunscreen in the past 7 days, and only 6% of them reported using sunscreen at least 3 of the past 7 days (Hamant and Adams, 2005). Studies of skiers and snowboarders also document the scarcity of sunscreen use.

Coaches and instructors must be advocates for sunscreen use. Skiers note that less than one fourth of ski instructors had provided warnings regarding the increased risk of sunburn while skiing. Less than half of the skiers recalled seeing any sign or brochure regarding sun safety at the ski resorts. A study of more than 1000 youth soccer players showed that using coaches as advocates for sunscreen use significantly increased its use from the beginning to the end of the season (Adams, unpublished study).

Athletes do not regularly apply sunscreen for many reasons. In the study of collegiate soccer players and cross-country runners, the investigators discovered that the main reasons why collegiate athletes did not wear sunscreen during their outdoor exposure related to access to sunscreen in 46% and misinformation about sunscreen use in 33%. For example, many people, including athletes, have the misconception that a "base" tan provides adequate protection from ultraviolet radiation. A "base" tan for the average skin-type athlete provides the equivalent of only SPF 2 sunscreen (Kaidbey and Kilgman, 1978). By providing education and sunscreen in accessible locations to outdoor athletes, organizers of youth, collegiate, and professional sports likely will overcome some of the most common barriers to sunscreen use.

Athletes regularly sweat or frequently are in the water. Both of these activities decrease the effectiveness of sunscreen, and reapplication is mandatory. Swimmers who wear sunscreen are more likely to sunburn than are nonswimming sunscreen users (Wright et al., 2001). Use of sunscreen is not without controversy. Some investigators have linked its use to a higher incidence of skin cancer. Clinicians should be aware of some data suggesting that use of sunscreen while exercising at low humidity retards sweat evaporation (Wells et al., 1984).

Finally, athletes' equipment should protect them not only from physical contact during sports activity but also from ultraviolet radiation. Hats should be worn whenever reasonable. Baseball players who wear hats receive significantly reduced ultraviolet exposure to their foreheads compared to their cheeks and arms. A great deal of research involves evaluation of the ultraviolet protection provided by clothing (Table 7-3). Most summer clothing does not provide sufficient ultraviolet protection. One study found that one English soccer shirt provided an ultraviolet protection factor of only 5 to 10 (Wright et al., 2001). Dyeing fabrics or adding an ultraviolet-absorbing material during laundering increases the clothing's protection. Blue dye increases the SPF by 544%, whereas yellow dye increases the SPF by only 212%. Simply laundering with soap and water increases the SPF of clothing (through fabric shrinkage) (Wang et al., 2001). Fabric material and the wetness of the clothing also influence the protection factor. Nylon, wool, and silk have higher protection factors than other fabrics. Wetness of cotton fabric decreases the protection factor (Table 7-3).

Basal Cell Carcinoma
Epidemiology

Few studies on basal cell carcinoma and outdoor sports are available, and the results are mixed. One study showed no association with basal cell carcinoma when all outdoor sports were examined together (Rosso et al., 1996). However, restricting analysis to only water sports (e.g., swimming, boating, surfing, and sailing) revealed an association with basal cell carcinoma. Another smaller study of Swiss athletes showed a weak association between outdoor athletes and basal cell carcinoma (Rosso et al., 1999). Examined separately, water sports enthusiasts were no more likely to develop basal cell carcinoma.

Although no epidemiologic study has investigated the incidence of nonmelanoma skin cancers in golfers, an interesting study from Japan suggests that a golfer's exposed skin shows characteristics of chronic and severe sun damage (Kikuchi-Numagami et al., 2000). Researchers in this study took advantage of the fact that golfers had one hand chronically exposed to the sun and one hand chronically protected by a golfing glove. Morphologic and functional changes were observed in the exposed hand compared to the glove-protected hand. Exposed hands were darker and had more freckles and wrinkles.

Clinical Presentation

Basal cell carcinomas have several clinical morphologies. The classic basal cell carcinoma is a well-defined pearly papule with tiny blood vessels running through it (Figure 7-3). It may ulcerate and bleed easily. Another more unusual variant of basal cell carcinoma is an irregularly shaped, scaling, erythematous patch or plaque.

116 Sports Dermatology

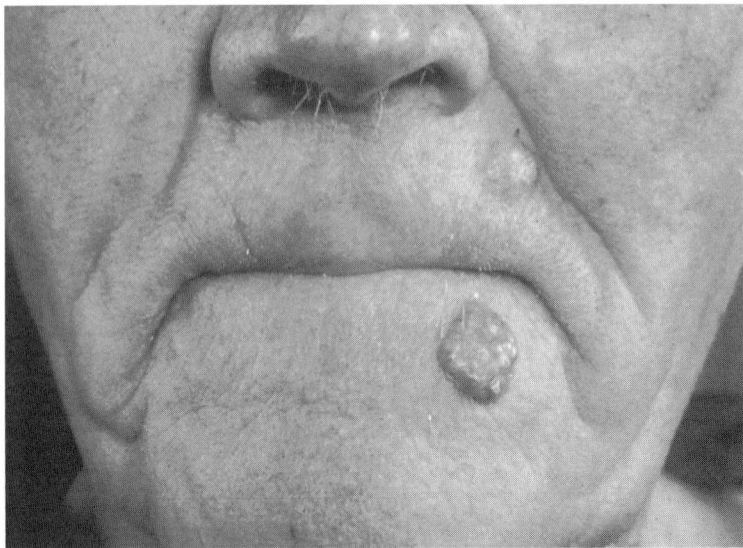

Figure 7-3. Classic basal cell carcinoma with a pearly color and telangiectasias coursing through it.

Diagnosis

The diagnosis of basal cell carcinoma requires a shave biopsy. The classic lesion may be confused with acne papules or tiny cysts. The superficial variant most often may be confused with psoriasis or dermatitis.

Treatment

Basal cell carcinomas should be destroyed by curettage or surgical excision. The surgical approach depends on several patient variables. An experienced physician should perform all surgical procedures. Close, at least yearly, follow-up with a dermatologist is essential. In very special circumstances, topical agents (e.g., imiquimod) may be beneficial to the athlete instead of surgical therapy. Close interaction with a dermatologist is essential.

Prevention

Athletes are at risk for developing skin cancers because of their intense and frequent exposure to ultraviolet radiation during peak ultraviolet times of the day. Reflectance of ultraviolet rays by the snow and water enhances the exposure for athletes whose venues include those elements. Sweating increases the chances of sunburn, not only by making the athlete more sun sensitive but also by diluting the effect of applied sunscreen.

The keys to sunburn prevention include sun avoidance, use of sunscreen, and photoprotective clothing. Obviously, prevention of sunburn resides in avoiding the sun, especially during the peak hours of ultraviolet radiation between 10 AM and 3 PM (Table 7-2). Unfortunately, many practices and competitions are scheduled during this period. Some very competitive national teams creatively schedule practices in the late afternoon or early morning to avoid these peak hours.

Athletes must wear broadband-blocking sunscreen, preferably with an SPF of at least 30. Despite the importance of sunscreen use for athletes, many athletes do not routinely apply it. One study of 186 collegiate soccer players and cross-country runners revealed that 85% had not worn any sunscreen in the past 7 days, and only 6% of them reported using sunscreen at least 3 of the past 7 days (Hamant and Adams, 2005). Studies of skiers and snowboarders also document the scarcity of sunscreen use.

Coaches and instructors must be advocates for sunscreen use. Skiers note that less than one fourth of ski instructors provided warnings regarding the increased risk of sunburn while skiing. Less than half of the skiers recalled seeing any sign or brochure regarding sun safety at the ski resorts. A study of more than 1000 youth soccer players showed that using coaches as advocates for sunscreen use significantly increased its use from the beginning to the end of the season (Adams, unpublished data).

Athletes do not regularly apply sunscreen for many reasons. In the study of collegiate soccer players and cross-country runners, the investigators discovered that the main reasons why collegiate athletes did not wear sunscreen during their outdoor exposure related to access to sunscreen in 46% and misinformation about sunscreen use in 33%. For example, many people, including athletes, have the misconception that a "base" tan provides adequate protection from ultraviolet radiation. A "base" tan for the average skin-type athlete provides the equivalent of only SPF 2 sunscreen (Kaidbey and Kilgman, 1978). Providing education and sunscreen in accessible locations to outdoor athletes, organizers of youth, collegiate, and professional sports likely will overcome some of the most common barriers to sunscreen use.

Athletes regularly sweat or frequently are in the water. Both of these activities decrease the effectiveness of sunscreen, and reapplication is mandatory. Swimmers who wear sunscreen are more likely to sunburn than are nonswimming sunscreen users (Wright et al., 2001). Use of sunscreen is not without controversy. Some investigators have linked its use to a higher incidence of skin cancer. Clinicians should be aware of some data suggesting that use of sunscreen while exercising at low humidity retards sweat evaporation (Wells et al., 1984).

Finally, athletes' equipment should protect them not only from physical contact during sports activity but also from ultraviolet radiation. Hats should be worn whenever reasonable. Baseball players who wear hats receive significantly reduced ultraviolet exposure to their foreheads compared to their cheeks and arms. A great deal of research involves evaluation of the ultraviolet protection provided by clothing (Table 7-3). Most summer clothing does not provide sufficient ultraviolet protection. One study found that one English soccer shirt provided an ultraviolet protection factor of only 5 to 10 (Wright et al., 2001). Dyeing fabrics or adding an ultraviolet-absorbing material during laundering increases the clothing's protection. Blue dye increases the SPF by 544%, whereas yellow dye increases the SPF by only 212%. Simply laundering with soap and water increases the SPF of clothing (through fabric shrinkage) (Wang et al., 2001). Fabric material and the wetness of the clothing also influence the protection factor. Nylon, wool and silk have higher protection factors than other fabrics. Wetness of cotton fabric decreases the protection factor (Table 7-3).

Squamous Cell Carcinoma

Epidemiology

Few studies on squamous cell carcinoma and outdoor sports are available, and the results are mixed. One study showed a negative association with squamous cell carcinoma when all outdoor sports were examined together (Rosso et al., 1996). Athletes who practiced outdoor sports for more than 1000 hours during a lifetime developed squamous cell carcinoma 1/2 as many times as nonathletes. However, restricting analysis to only water sports (e.g., swimming boating, surfing, and sailing) did not reveal any relationship with squamous cell carcinoma. Another smaller study showed that neither outdoor sports nor water sports alone were associated with squamous cell carcinoma (Rosso et al., 1999).

Clinical Presentation

Precancers (otherwise known as *actinic keratoses)* present as erythematous, somewhat ill-defined, rough, scaling papules (Figures 7-4 and 7-5). Squamous cell carcinomas typically are characterized by well-defined, rough, thick, scaling papules and plaques (Figure 7-6). These lesions may be painful and occasionally bleed.

Diagnosis

The diagnosis of actinic keratoses is made clinically. Hypertrophic actinic keratoses may be difficult to distinguish from squamous cell carcinoma, and biopsy is required. The diagnosis of squamous cell carcinoma requires a shave biopsy. The classic lesion may be confused with seborrheic keratoses especially those which are inflamed.

7. Sunburns and Skin Cancer 119

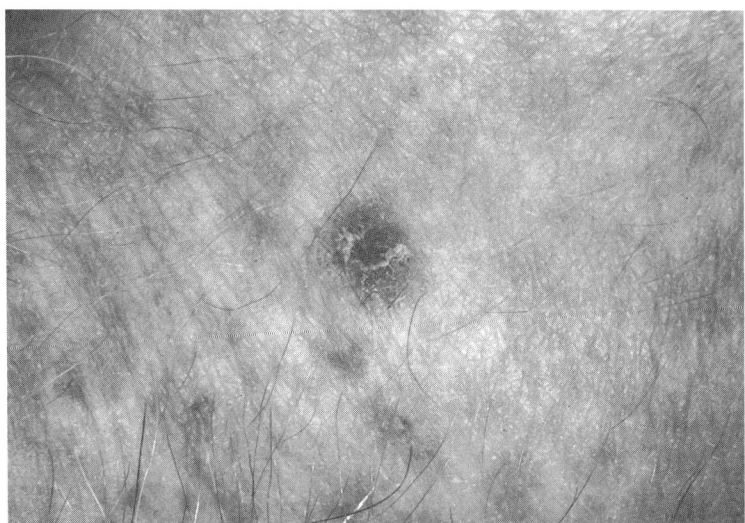

Figure 7-4. Chronically exposed skin of athletes demonstrates not only sun damage freckles but also a rough (sandpaperlike) and scaling papule typical of actinic keratosis. These lesions often are unimpressive visually but are not mistakable after palpation.

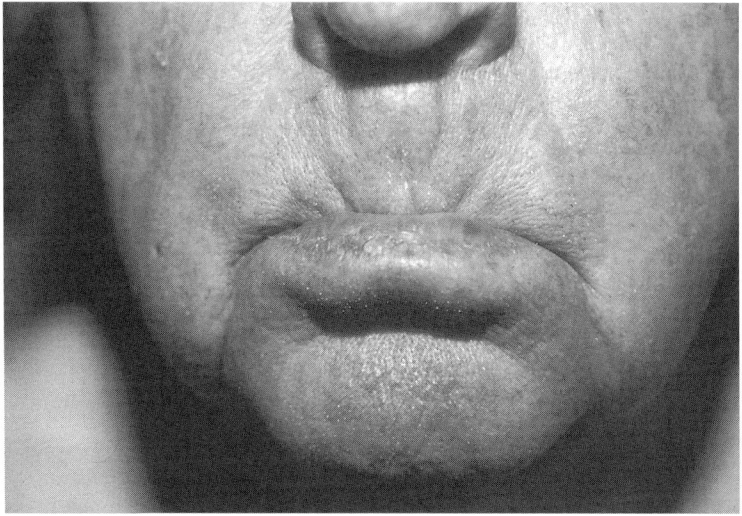

Figure 7-5. Athletes often neglect using sunscreen on their lips and are at risk for developing actinic cheilitis, which is extensive precancer of the lips.

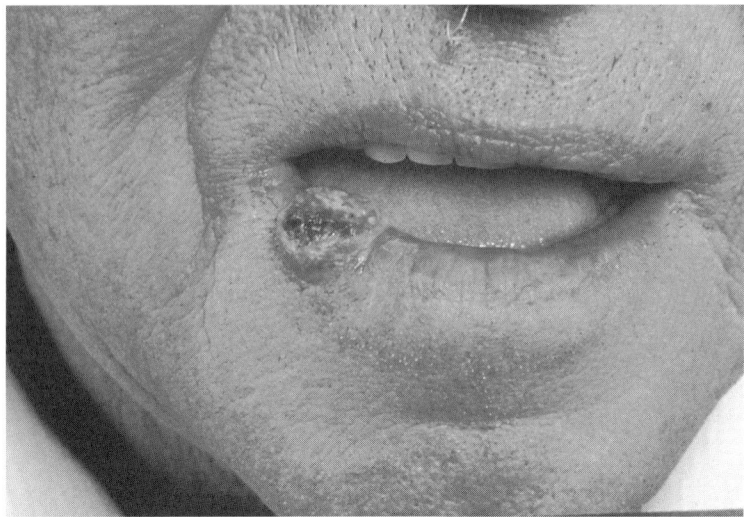

Figure 7-6. Thick, scaling, erythematous, well-defined, centrally necrotic papulonodule illustrates squamous cell carcinoma.

Treatment

Treatment of actinic keratoses includes destructive methods such as liquid nitrogen. Topical creams such as 5-fluorouracil and imiquimod effectively eradicate actinic keratoses. Squamous cell carcinomas should be destroyed by curettage or surgical excision. The surgical approach depends on several patient variables. An experienced physician should perform all surgical procedures. Close, at least yearly, follow-up with a dermatologist is essential. In very special circumstances, topical agents (e.g., 5-fluorouracil) may be beneficial to the athlete instead of surgical therapy. Close interaction with a dermatologist is essential.

Prevention

Although some authors found that nonwater outdoor sports provide a "protective effect" against the development of squamous cell carcinoma, protection from sun exposure still seems prudent. Athletes are at risk for developing skin cancers because of their intense and frequent exposure to ultraviolet radiation during peak ultraviolet times of the day. Reflectance of ultraviolet rays by the snow and water enhances the exposure for athletes whose venues include those elements. Sweating increases the chances of sunburn, not only by making the athlete more-sun sensitive but also by diluting the effect of applied sunscreen.

The keys to sunburn prevention include sun avoidance, use of sunscreen, and photoprotective clothing. Obviously, prevention of sunburn resides in avoiding the sun, especially during the peak hours of ultraviolet radiation that are between 10 AM and 3 PM (Table 7-2). Unfortunately, many practices and competitions are scheduled during this period. Some very competitive national teams creatively schedule practices in the late afternoon or early morning to avoid these peak hours.

Athletes must wear broadband-blocking sunscreen, preferably with an SPF of at least 30. Despite the importance of sunscreen use for athletes, many athletes do not routinely apply it. One study of 186 collegiate soccer players and cross-country runners revealed that 85% had not worn any sunscreen in the past 7 days, and only 6% of them reported using sunscreen at least 3 of the past 7 days (Hamant and Adams, 2005). Studies of skiers and snowboarders also document the scarcity of sunscreen use.

Coaches and instructors must be advocates for sunscreen use. Skiers note that less than one fourth of ski instructors provided warnings regarding the increased risk of sunburn while skiing. Less than half of the skiers recalled seeing any sign or brochure regarding sun safety at the ski resorts. A study of more than 1000 youth soccer players showed that using coaches as advocates for sunscreen use significantly increased its use from the beginning to the end of the season (Adams, unpublished data).

Athletes do not regularly apply sunscreen for many reasons. In the study of collegiate soccer players and cross-country runners, the investigators discovered that the main reasons why collegiate athletes did not wear sunscreen during their outdoor exposure related to access to sunscreen in 46% and misinformation about sunscreen use in 33%. For example, many people, including athletes, have the misconception that a "base" tan provides adequate protection from ultraviolet radiation. A "base" tan for the average skin type athlete provides the equivalent of only SPF 2 sunscreen (Kaidbey and Kilgman, 1978). By providing education and sunscreen in accessible locations to outdoor athletes, organizers of youth, collegiate, and professional sports likely will overcome some of the most common barriers to sunscreen use.

Athletes regularly sweat or frequently are in the water. Both of these activities decrease the effectiveness of sunscreen, and reapplication is mandatory. Swimmers who wear sunscreen are more likely to sunburn than are nonswimming sunscreen users (Wright et al., 2001). Use of sunscreen is not without controversy. Some investigators have linked its use to a higher incidence of skin cancer. Clinicians should be aware of some data suggesting that use of sunscreen while exercising at low humidity retards sweat evaporation (Wells et al., 1984).

Finally, athletes' equipment should protect them not only from physical contact during sports activity but also from ultraviolet radiation. Hats should be worn whenever reasonable. Baseball players who wear hats receive significantly reduced ultraviolet exposure to their foreheads compared to their cheeks and arms.

A great deal of research involves evaluation of the ultraviolet protection provided by clothing (Table 7-3). Most summer clothing does not provide sufficient ultraviolet protection. One study found that one English soccer shirt only provided an ultraviolet protection factor of 5–10 (Wright et al., 2001). Dyeing fabrics or adding an ultraviolet-absorbing material during laundering increases the clothing's protection. Blue dye increases the SPF by 544%, whereas yellow dye increases the SPF by only 212%. Simply laundering with soap and water increases the SPF of clothing (through fabric shrinkage) (Wang et al., 2001). Fabric material and the wetness of the clothing also influence the protection factor. Nylon, wool, and silk have higher protection factors than other fabrics. Wetness of cotton fabric decreases the protection factor (Table 7-3).

Bibliography

Basler RS, Basler GC, Palmer AH, et al. Special skin symptoms in swimmers. J Am Acad Dermatol 2000;43:299–305.

Buller DB, Andersen PA, Walkosz B. Sun safety behaviours of alpine skiers and snowboarders. Can Prev Control 1998;2:133–139.

Freeman RG, Knox JM. Influence of temperature on ultraviolet injury. Arch Dermatol 1964;89:858–864.

Hamant E, Adams BB. Sunscreen use among collegiate athletes. J Am Acad Dematol 2005;53:237–241.

Han A, Maibach HI. Management of acute sunburn. Am J Clin Dermatol 2004;5:39–47.

Herzfeld PM, Fitzgerald EF, Hwang SA, et al. A case-control study of malignant melanoma of the trunk among white males in upstate New York. Cancer Detect Prevent 1993;17:601–608.

Kaidbey KH, Kilgman AM. Sunburn protection by longwave ultraviolet-induce pigmentation. Arch Dermatol 1978;114:46–48.

Kikuchi-Numagami K, Suetake T, Yanai M, et al. Functional and morphological studies of photodamaged skin on the hands of middle-aged Japanese golfers. Eur J Dermatol 2000;10:277–281.

Loria D, Matos E. Risk factors for cutaneous melanoma: a case-control study in Argentina. Int J Dermatol 2001;40:108–114.

Melville SK, Rosenthal FS, Luckmann R, et al. Quantitative skin exposure in children during selected outdoor activities. Photodermatol Photoimmunol Photomed 1991;8:99–104.

Moehrle M, Heinrich L, Schmid A, et al. Extreme UV exposure of professional cyclists. Dermatology 2000a;201:44–45.

Moehrle M, Koehle W, Dietz, et al. Reduction of minimal erythema dose by sweating. Photodermatol Photoimmunol Photomed 2000b;16:260–262.

Moehrle M. Ultraviolet exposure in the Ironman triathlon. Med Sci Sport Exer 2001;33:1385–1386.

Nelemans PJ, Groenendal H, Kiemeney LALM, et al. Effect of intermittent exposure to sunlight on melanoma risk among indoor workers and sun-sensitive individuals. Env Health Perspect 1993;101:252–255.

Owens DW, Knox JM, Hudson HT et al. Influence of wind on ultraviolet injury. Arch Dermatol 1974;109:200–201.

Rigel DS, Rigel EG, Rigel AC. Effects of altitude and latitude on ambient UVB radiation. J Am Acad Dermatol 1999;40:114–116.

Rigel EG, Lebwohl MG, Rigel et al. Ultraviolet radiation in alpine skiing. Arch Dermatol 2003;139:60–62.

Rosso S, Zanetti R, Martinez C, et al. The multicentre south European study "Helios" II: different sun exposure patterns in the aetiology of basal cell and squamous cell carcinomas of the skin. Br J Cancer 1996;73:1447–1454.

Rosso S, Joris F, Zanetti R. Risk of basal and squamous cell carcinomas of the skin in Sion, Switzerland: a case-control study. Tumori 1999;85:435–442.

Thieden E, Philipsen PA, Heydenreich J, et al. UV radiation exposure related to age, sex, occupation, and sun behavior based on time-stamped personal dosimeter readings. Arch Dermatol 2004;140:197–203.

Wang SQ, Kopf AW, Marx J, et al. Reeducation of ultraviolet transmission through cotton T-shirt fabrics with low ultraviolet protection by various laundering methods and dyeing: clinical implications. J Am Acad Dermatol 2001;44:767–774.

Wells TD, Jessup GT, Langlotz KS. Effects of sunscreen use during exercise in the heat. Phys Sportsmed 1984;12:132–144.

Williams H, Brett J, Vivier A. Cyclist's melanoma. J R Coll Physicians Lond 1989;23:114–115.

Wright MW, Wright ST, Wagner RF. Mechanisms of sunscreen failure. J Am Acad Dermatol 2001;44:781–784.

Zanetti R, Rosso S, Faggiano F, et al. Etude cas-temoins sur le melanome de la peau dans la provinve de Torino, Italie. Rev Epidemiol Sante Publique 1988;36:309–317.

Section III Sports-Related Inflammatory Reactions

8. Allergic Contact Dermatitis

Section III of this book examines the inflammatory reactions that occur in the skin as a result of sports participation. The scope of disorders in this section is vast. Cutaneous conditions in this section range from very common disorders such as poison ivy to very rare conditions such as aquagenic urticaria. The severity of lesions ranges from inconvenient, focal, slightly itchy skin rashes to life-threatening diffuse skin conditions (exercise-induced anaphylaxis).

Urticaria is not an uncommon disorder in the normal population. Unfortunately, it may occur at a greater frequency in athletes and poses unique problems. Chapter 10 of this section discusses the several types of physical urticaria that afflict athletes. Chapter 11 examines the athletes who develop hivelike reactions but also have potential severe systemic complications (exercise-induced anaphylaxis).

Chapters 8 and 9 of this section focus on the dermatitis that occurs when the athlete reacts to the physical components of their sport. Chapter 9 reviews the uncommon incidence of irritant contact dermatitis that results from direct skin toxicity with the sport's environment. Chapter 8 reviews the more ubiquitous occurrence of allergic contact dermatitis in athletes. In this type of dermatitis, the athlete's skin is exposed to a foreign antigen. The athlete's immune system reacts to this antigen, resulting in the clinical manifestation of dermatitis. The antigens that cause problems for athletes are found in sports equipment, clothing, topical medications, and objects in the environment of the athletic venue. Because generic dermatitis (eczema) is so common in the normal population, clinicians may forget the role of the athlete's surroundings in creating dermatitis.

Equipment

Water-Related

Swim Goggles

Epidemiology

One of the most commonly reported types of allergic contact dermatitis is a reaction to swimming goggles. The incidence among all swimmers has not been demonstrated in a rigorous manner. One study examined 43 athletes who developed contact dermatitis. A control group of 38 students who did not play sports demonstrated a low incidence of contact dermatitis. Of the 43 athletes, 23.3% and 21% of the contact dermatitis cases were related to thiurams and mercaptobenzothiazole, respectively. This study did not specify which athletes were sensitive to which antigen, although it was clear from the data that swimmers were allergic to those two most common sensitizers (Ventura et al., 2001).

All the reported cases of allergic contact dermatitis identified the rubber or neoprene cushion as the culprit. Several ingredients in goggles are implicated as causing allergic contact dermatitis. These chemicals include benzoyl peroxide, phenol-formaldehyde resin, diethylthiourea, ethylbutylthiourea, dibutylthiourea, IPPD (N-Isopropyl-N'-phenyl-p-phenylenediamine), CPPD (N-Phenyl-N'-cyclohexyl-p-phenylenediamine), DPPD (N N-Diphenyl-p-phenylenediamine). These substances are used in the production of rubber (Alomar and Vilaltella, 1985; Azurdia and King, 1998; Romaguera et al., 1988; Vaswani et al., 2003).

Clinical Presentation

Swimmers present with pruritic, erythematous (occasionally vesicular, if acute), edematous, scaling, well-defined plaques periorbitally (Figure 8-1). Yellow exudates may be present if the condition is severe. The conjunctiva may be affected.

Although not technically an allergic reaction, a highly unusual hypopigmentation resulting from goggle use was noted in at least 13 swimmers (Goette,

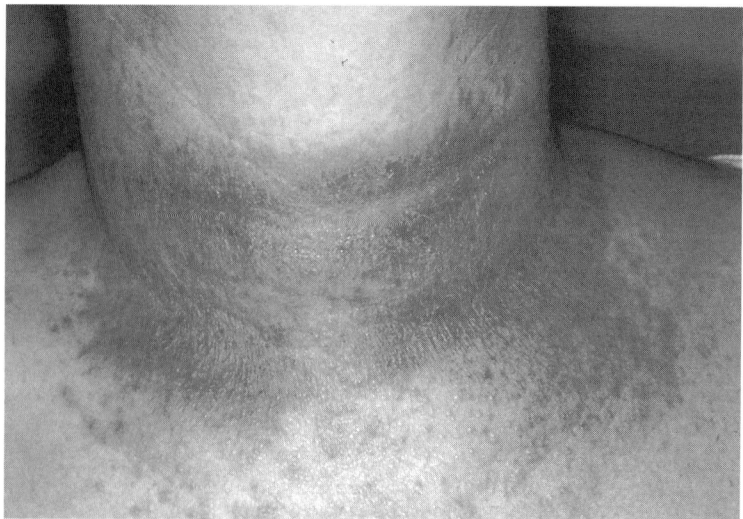

Figure 8-1. Allergic contact dermatitis to protective equipment (or any athletic equipment) produces a sharply demarcated, erythematous, vesicular, scaling eruption.

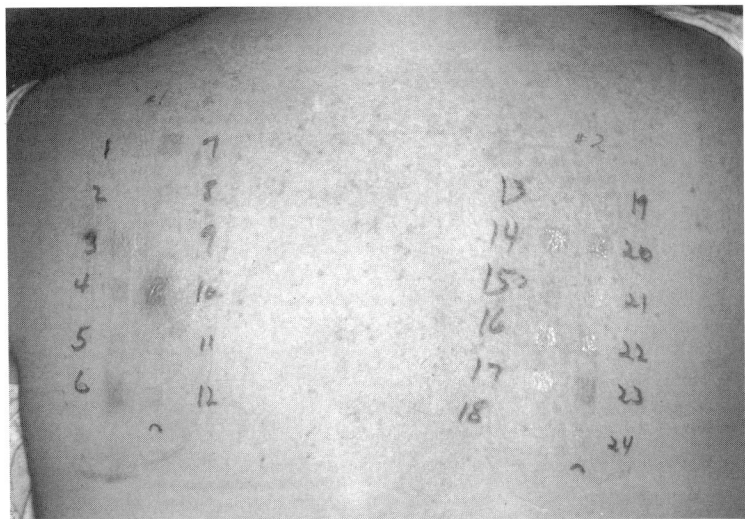

Figure 8-2. A typical patch test that evaluates two dozen of the most common allergens.

1984). This disorder has been termed *raccoonlike periorbital leukoderma*. The author proposed that leakage of breakdown products in the neoprene rubber or glue of the goggles caused a toxic reaction rather than an allergic reaction. The leached chemicals allegedly inhibited melanin production. The swimmer was able to reuse the goggles later because the chemicals eventually had completely leached out of the goggles.

Diagnosis

The clinical diagnosis is not difficult, although it is important to identify the culprit ingredient in the goggles that is causing the dermatitis. Patch testing of suspected chemicals is necessary (Figure 8-2). It is critical not to confuse the severe exudates of the dermatitis that may become yellow and crusted for secondary impetigo.

Treatment

The treatment of choice includes medium-potency (class III–IV) topical steroids used for a brief period. A rapid burst of oral steroids may be necessary for severe outbreaks. Topical immunomodulators (e.g., pimecrolimus) can be used for milder or chronic conditions.

Prevention

It is incumbent upon the clinician to determine the ingredient causing the dermatitis. A call to the manufacturer should reveal alternative goggles that do not contain the offending agent. Speedo makes two alternatives to the black neoprene rubber padding goggles that seem to create dermatitis. One type of swimming goggle uses a polyvinyl chloride pad to protect the eyes ("freestyle antifog model 750127) (Fisher, 1999). The other type is a padded goggle with air-blown neoprene that does not require rubber accelerators (Fisher, 1987). Competitive swimmers like to use foamless goggles that do not leak, are comfortable, and do not cause dermatitis. Obviously the dermatitis will improve quickly if the swimmer does not use the goggles, but this alternative is unacceptable for intent swimmers.

Wet Suits

Epidemiology

No epidemiologic study has reported the incidence of allergic contact dermatitis to wet suits. A variety of athletes might use wet suits in their pursuits, including kayakers, surfers, snorkelers, scuba divers, swimmers, water and jet skiers, and wind surfers. The reported sensitizers reported in wet suits include diethylthiourea, dibutylthiourea, diphenylthiourea, ethylbutylthiourea, nickel, and para-tertiary-butylphenol-formaldehyde resin (Adams, 1982; Balestrero et al., 1999; Boehnckee et al., 1997; Corazza and Virgili, 1998; Nagashima et al., 2003; Reid et al., 1993). The inciting chemical usually is one of the agents used as the rubber accelerator or the glue. Leached nickel from metal on the suit also causes dermatitis. Use of Tego 103G disinfectant to clean a wet suit is also a reported sensitizer (Munro et al., 1989).

Clinical Presentation

Athletes with contact dermatitis to wet suits present with a diffuse, pruritic, erythematous, scaling, vesicular eruption several hours after exposure to the wet suit if they have been sensitized by a prior exposure to the offending agent. Sometimes the eruption is so severe that it requires hospitalization (Adams, 1982).

Diagnosis

The history and distribution of the eruption should clue the clinician to the diagnosis of contact dermatitis. It is important to identify the culprit ingredient in the wet suit that is causing the dermatitis. Patch testing suspected chemicals is necessary. The differential diagnosis includes pressure urticaria and noncontact dermatitis. It is critical not to confuse the severe exudates of the dermatitis that may become yellow and crusted for secondary impetigo.

Treatment

The treatment of choice includes medium- to high-potency (class I–II) topical steroids. A rapid burst of oral steroids or an intramuscular injection of triamcinolone may be necessary for severe or diffuse outbreaks.

Prevention

It is important to find alternatives for athletes who are allergic to rubber or neoprene suits. Wet suits without thiourea accelerators are available (Adams, 1982). Material R-5012-A made by Rubatex uses ethylene vinyl acetate as material for suit-sensitive divers. The same company also makes material G231-N, which is an ethylbutylthiourea-free diving suit material as an alternative (Fisher, 1999).

Swim Fins

Epidemiology

No epidemiologic studies of swim fin dermatitis are available (Foussereau et al., 1990). This type of contact dermatitis affects scuba divers and snorkelers. The reputed ingredients causing swim fin dermatitis are dibutylthiourea, diethylthiourea, and IPPD.

Clinical Presentation

Athletes with contact dermatitis to fins present with a focal, pruritic, erythematous, scaling, vesicular eruption on their feet several hours after exposure to the fins, if they have been sensitized by a prior exposure to the offending agent.

Diagnosis

The diagnosis should be evident, but patch testing suspected chemicals is necessary. The differential diagnosis includes pressure urticaria and noncontact dermatitis. It is critical not to confuse the severe exudates of the dermatitis that may become yellow and crusted for secondary impetigo.

Treatment

The treatment of choice includes medium- to high-potency (class I–II) topical steroids. A rapid burst of oral steroids or an intramuscular injection of triamcinolone may be necessary for severe outbreaks.

Prevention

Athletes may need to obtain fins without the sensitizer or wear protective clothing on their feet to protect them from the fins.

Underwater Masks

Epidemiology

Although mini-epidemics are reported in the literature, no epidemiologic studies of underwater mask dermatitis are available (Maibach, 1975). This type of contact dermatitis affects scuba divers and snorkelers. Most underwater enthusiasts notice erythema on the face, termed *mask burn*, when they remove their mask. In sensitive individuals, the dermatitis can be much more severe. The suspected agent causing diving mask dermatitis is the rubber antioxidant IPPD (Maibach, 1975; Tuyp and Mitchell, 1983).

Clinical Presentation

This type of dermatitis occurs as early as 10 minutes after mask exposure or as long as 48 hours after exposure. The rash in areas where the mask touched the skin consists of well-defined, erythematous, scaling, vesicular plaques.

Diagnosis

The diagnosis should be evident given the characteristic distribution on the face, but patch testing suspected chemicals is necessary. The differential diagnosis includes pressure urticaria and noncontact dermatitis. It is critical not to confuse the severe exudates of the dermatitis that may become yellow and crusted for secondary impetigo.

Treatment

The treatment of choice includes low- to medium-potency (class III–IV) topical steroids. A rapid burst of oral steroids or an intramuscular injection of triamcinolone may be necessary for severe outbreaks. Topical immunomodulators (e.g., pimecrolimus) can be used for milder or chronic conditions.

Prevention

Affected athletes have been able to prevent this eruption by using silicone masks (Fisher, 1999).

Swimming Caps

Epidemiology

No epidemiologic studies of swim cap dermatitis are available (Cronin, 1980). This type of contact dermatitis affects swimmers who react to mercaptobenzothiazole in the swim cap.

Clinical Presentation

Well-defined, erythematous, scaling plaques occur in the same distribution as the swimming cap. Vesicles may be present.

Diagnosis

The diagnosis should be evident given the characteristic distribution on the scalp extending onto the forehead, but patch testing suspected chemicals is necessary. The differential diagnosis includes pressure urticaria and noncontact dermatitis. It is critical not to confuse the severe exudates of the dermatitis that may become yellow and crusted for secondary impetigo.

Treatment

The treatment of choice includes low- to medium-potency (class III–IV) topical steroids for a brief period. A rapid burst of oral steroids or an intramuscular injection of triamcinolone may be necessary for severe outbreaks. Topical immunomodulators (e.g., pimecrolimus) can be used for milder or chronic conditions.

Prevention

Companies such as Speedo make a silicone swim cap that sensitive swimmers can use without problem (Fisher, 1999).

Nose Clips and Earplugs

Epidemiology

No epidemiologic studies of these pieces of swimming equipment are available (Fisher, 1999). This type of contact dermatitis affects swimmers who are allergic to the rubber accelerators used to make the equipment.

Clinical Presentation

Affected swimmers have well-defined, erythematous, scaling plaques on the nose or ears, depending on the type of equipment used.

Diagnosis

The diagnosis should be evident given the characteristic distribution on the nose or ears, but patch testing suspected chemicals is necessary. The differential diagnosis includes pressure urticaria and noncontact dermatitis. It is critical not to confuse the severe exudates of the dermatitis that may become yellow and crusted for secondary impetigo.

Treatment

The treatment of choice includes low- to medium-potency (class III–IV) topical steroids for a brief period. A rapid burst of oral steroids or an intramuscular injection of triamcinolone may be necessary for severe outbreaks. Topical immunomodulators (e.g., pimecrolimus) can be used for milder or chronic conditions.

Prevention

Nonsensitizing nose and earplugs are commercially available (Fisher, 1999).

Land Footwear

Athletic Shoes

Epidemiology

Any athlete theoretically is at risk for developing dermatitis from their athletic footwear. However, runners and tennis players have been the main targets in the literature. Mini-epidemics are noted in runners (Roberts and Hanifin, 1979). Several components of athletic shoes can cause allergic contact dermatitis. These include not only the typical rubber accelerators (ethylbutylthiourea, mercaptobenzothiazole, and dibenzothiazyl disulfide) but also dyes (paraphenylenediamine) (Roberts and Hanifin, 1979; Jung et al., 1988; Romaguera et al., 1988).

Clinical Presentation

Athletes note the development of a pruritic eruption on the plantar aspects of the feet 2 weeks to several months after wearing new athletic shoes. Clinically, diffuse erythematous, fissured, vesicular plaques are observed on the sole of feet.

Diagnosis

Contact dermatitis of the foot is not a simple diagnosis in any patient, especially athletes. Several other skin conditions can closely mimic contact dermatitis. The clinician should perform a potassium hydroxide examination or refer the patient to a specialist who can rule out dermatophyte infection. Psoriasis and foot dermatitis (noncontact related) also can be challenging to differentiate. It is critical not to confuse the severe exudates of the dermatitis that may become yellow and crusted for secondary impetigo. Biopsies may be helpful. Patch testing suspected chemicals is necessary.

Although not necessary on a case-by-case basis, investigators have mixed synthetic solvents to mimic human sweat. By combining this mixture with shoe material, investigators have shown that the sensitizers diethylthiourea, ethylbutylthiourea, and dibutylthiourea all leach from shoe materials at high levels (Emmett et al., 1994).

Treatment

The treatment of choice includes medium- to high-potency (class I–II) topical steroids. A rapid burst of oral steroids or an intramuscular injection of triamcinolone may be necessary for severe outbreaks. In the mini-epidemic of athletic shoe dermatitis, topical steroids were not helpful, and the eruption resolved only when new nonallergenic innersoles were developed (Roberts and Hanifin, 1979).

Prevention

Through collaborative efforts in the mid-1970s, several companies have manufactured innersoles for running shoes that do not contain ethylbutylthiourea (Roberts and Hanifin, 1979). Tennis shoes that contain polyurethane are available for those who are sensitive, for example, the "Wimbledon Player" by Nike, Inc. (Fisher, 1999).

Protective Equipment

Shin and Knee Guards

Epidemiology

Two specific sports were singled out when two athletes developed contact dermatitis. A young soccer player was allergic to his shin guards, whereas a female basketball player was allergic to her knee guard (Sommer et al., 1999; Vincenzi et al., 1992). There is no reason to suspect that other athletes who use similar implements are not also at risk. Urea-formaldehyde resin was the cause of the reported shin guard dermatitis (Sommer et al., 1999). Para-tertiary-butylphenol-formaldehyde resin has caused contact dermatitis in athletes, and this compound was a component of the glue used in the knee guard manufacturing (Vincenzi et al., 1992).

Clinical Presentation

Shin guards can cause a pruritic, erythematous, scaling, well-defined, occasionally vesicular eruption on both anterior shins where they protect the lower leg from other players' kicks. Knee guards can cause a similar eruption on the knee.

Diagnosis

The diagnosis should be evident given the characteristic distribution beneath the protective equipment. Patch testing suspected chemicals confirms the diagnosis. The differential diagnosis includes pressure urticaria and noncontact dermatitis. It is critical not to confuse the severe exudates of the dermatitis that may become yellow and crusted for secondary impetigo.

Treatment

The treatment of choice includes medium- to high-potency (class I–II) topical steroids for a brief period. A rapid burst of oral steroids or an intramuscular injection of triamcinolone may be necessary for severe outbreaks. Topical immunomodulators (e.g., pimecrolimus) can be used for milder or chronic conditions.

Prevention

Affected athletes can apply tape or another barrier (e.g., Coban wrap, liquid adhesive, or petroleum jelly) to the skin before donning the guards. Alternatively, athletes can obtain guards that lack the sensitizers to which they react.

Helmets and Face Masks

Epidemiology

No epidemiologic studies of helmet or face mask dermatitis are available. This type of contact dermatitis affects any athlete who wears this protective gear (e.g., baseball, football, hockey, lacrosse, and softball players). Athletes are allergic to the epoxy resins used to make the equipment.

Clinical Presentation

Well-defined, erythematous, scaling papules and plaques are observed on the face, especially the chin and lateral aspects of the head.

Diagnosis

The diagnosis should be evident given the characteristic distribution on the face, but patch testing suspected chemicals is necessary. The differential diagnosis includes pressure urticaria and noncontact dermatitis. It is critical not to confuse the severe exudates of the dermatitis that may become yellow and crusted for secondary impetigo.

Treatment

The treatment of choice includes low- to medium-potency (class III–IV) topical steroids for a brief period. A rapid burst of oral steroids or an intramuscular injection of triamcinolone may be necessary for severe outbreaks. Topical immunomodulators (e.g., pimecrolimus) can be used for milder or chronic conditions.

Prevention

Silicone adhesives should be used if the athlete is allergic to epoxy resins.

Manual Implements

Bowls Grip

Epidemiology

No epidemiologic studies of lawn bowlers and their grips are available; however, many serious bowlers are exposed to chemicals to which they may become sensitive. Most lawn bowlers grip the bowl with their bare hand, but some like to polish the bowl with mixtures (bowls grip). Millions of containers of bowls grip are sold each year. Bowls grip can contain colophony, perfume mix, and balsam of Peru.

Clinical Presentation

Affected bowlers develop an erythematous and scaling eruption on the palms (Blair, 1982; Paterson et al., 1993).

Diagnosis

Contact dermatitis of the palm is not a simple diagnosis in any patient, especially athletes. Several other skin conditions can closely mimic contact dermatitis. The clinician should perform a potassium hydroxide examination or refer the patient to a specialist who can to rule out dermatophyte infection. Psoriasis and hand dermatitis (noncontact related) also can be challenging to differentiate. It is critical not to confuse the severe exudates of the dermatitis that may become yellow and crusted for secondary impetigo. Biopsies may be helpful. Patch testing suspected chemicals is necessary. Obtaining the bowls grip and noting its ingredients are important.

Treatment

The treatment of choice includes medium- to high-potency (class I–II) topical steroids. A rapid burst of oral steroids or an intramuscular injection of triamcinolone may be necessary for severe outbreaks.

Prevention

If the bowler must use a bowls grip, several commercial brands are available. The bowler should use one that does not contain the substance to which they are sensitive.

Handles

Wishbone

Epidemiology

Two cases of wind surfers allergic to the wishbone, which is the handle (often made of black rubber) by which the sailor guides the sail through the water, are reported (Tennstedt et al., 1978).

Clinical Presentation

The wishbone contains CPPD, IPPD, and DPPD, which cause a well-defined, scaling, fissured, erythematous, severely pruritic eruption of both palms.

Diagnosis

Without obtaining a history from the athlete and making the link between sailing and the eruption, the differential diagnosis may be difficult. Psoriasis, hand dermatitis (unrelated to a contactant), and tinea manuum must be considered. Potassium hydroxide examination and/or biopsies are indicated. Patch tests confirm the diagnosis.

Treatment

Potent topical steroids (class I–II) should be tried; however, the reported cases were somewhat resistant to topical steroids. Topical immunomodulators (e.g., pimecrolimus) can be used for milder or chronic conditions.

Prevention

Because therapy is less than effective, sailors should be encouraged to exchange a wishbone made of black rubber for one made of aluminum.

Tennis Racquet

Epidemiology

No studies have examined the incidence of tennis racquet dermatitis. Tennis players may react to isophorone diamine or epoxy resin found in the tennis racquet (Lachapelle et al., 1978). Other racquet sport athletes (e.g., squash, racquetball, and badminton players) also may develop this type of contact dermatitis.

Clinical Presentation

Sensitive players develop a well-defined, scaling, fissured, erythematous, severely pruritic eruption mainly of the dominant hand. If the tennis player uses two hands (i.e., on backhand shots), the nondominant hand also can be affected but often to a lesser degree.

Diagnosis

Without obtaining a history from the athlete and making the link between tennis and the eruption, the differential diagnosis may be difficult. Psoriasis, hand dermatitis (unrelated to a contactant), and tinea manuum must be considered. Psoriasis and hand dermatitis are less likely diagnoses because these diseases most often affect both hands. Potassium hydroxide examination and/or biopsies are indicated. Patch tests confirm the diagnosis.

Treatment

Potent topical steroids (class I–II) should be tried. Oral or intramuscular steroids should be used in severe cases. Topical immunomodulators (e.g., pimecrolimus) can be used for milder or chronic conditions.

Prevention

Tennis players can find handles for their racquets that do not contain the sensitizer that causes their hand dermatitis.

Fishing Rods

Epidemiology

No epidemiologic studies of fishers with allergies to rods are available. In one reported case, IPPD from the fishing rod caused the dermatitis (Minciullo et al., 2004).

Clinical Presentation

Unilateral, erythematous, scaling plaques on the hands are observed in sensitive fishers.

Diagnosis

Without obtaining a history from the athlete and making the link between fishing and the eruption, the differential diagnosis may be difficult. Tinea manuum must be considered. Potassium hydroxide examination and/or biopsies are indicated. Psoriasis and hand dermatitis (unrelated to a contactant) are less likely diagnoses because these diseases most often affect both hands. Patch tests confirm the diagnosis.

Treatment

Potent topical steroids (class I–II) should be tried. Topical immunomodulators (e.g., pimecrolimus) can be used for milder or chronic conditions.

Prevention

The reported fisher was able to fish without hand rashes when he covered the handle with insulating tape.

Balls

Basketball

Epidemiology

One case of basketball contact dermatitis is reported.

Clinical Presentation

Athletes allergic to thiuram and mercaptobenzothiazole (rubber accelerators) in rubber basketballs present with symmetrical erythematous, fissured, scaling plaques on the palms, especially on the fingers and thenar eminence (Rodriguez-Serna et al., 2002).

Diagnosis

Without obtaining a history from the athlete and making the link between basketball and the eruption, the differential diagnosis may be difficult. Psoriasis, hand dermatitis (unrelated to a contactant), and tinea manuum must be considered. Potassium hydroxide examination and/or biopsies are indicated. Patch tests confirm the diagnosis.

Treatment

Potent topical steroids (class I–II) should be tried. Topical immunomodulators (e.g., pimecrolimus) can be used for milder or chronic conditions.

Prevention

Affected basketball players should be cautioned to only use leather balls. Avoiding rubber balls should clear the eruption.

Squash

Epidemiology

There is no reason to believe that squash is the only sport in which players react to the rubber ball, but to date it is the only sport for which the ball has been reported to cause reactions (Cronin, 1980). In the one reported case, patch testing revealed that IPPD in the rubber caused the eruption.

Clinical Presentation

The athlete develops a pruritic, erythematous, scaling eruption on the hand that holds the ball before service.

Diagnosis

Without obtaining a history from the athlete and making the link between the squash ball and the eruption, the differential diagnosis may be difficult. Psoriasis, hand dermatitis (unrelated to a contactant), and tinea manuum must be considered. Potassium hydroxide examination and/or biopsies are indicated. Patch tests confirm the diagnosis.

Treatment

Potent topical steroids (class I–II) should be tried. Topical immunomodulators (e.g., pimecrolimus) can be used for milder or chronic conditions.

Prevention

To my knowledge, a hypoallergenic squash ball is not available. The unfortunate squash player may attempt to use synthetic skin to coat the area of the most affected hand.

Accessories

Metal Weights and Chalk

Epidemiology

No epidemiologic studies exist regarding allergic contact dermatitis and athletes who lift weights. Any athlete whose training program includes weight training is potentially at risk. Two case reports relate contact sensitivity to metal weights and chalk (Guerra et al., 1988; Scott et al., 1992). One weightlifter presented with an allergic contact dermatitis to pallidium.

Clinical Presentation

The weightlifter had an erythematous and vesicular eruption on the neck, forearms, and legs (Guerra et al., 1988). Whether pallidium was found in the weights used by this athlete is not known. Other weightlifters have developed contact sensitivity to chalk that was liberally applied to the hands before weightlifting (Scott et al., 1992).

Diagnosis

Clinicians must consider the athlete's activity or they may risk missing the diagnosis of allergy related to weightlifting tools. Patch testing the metal found in the weights will be positive if the weights are causing the dermatitis.

Treatment

Potent topical steroids (class I–II) should be tried. Topical immunomodulators (e.g., pimecrolimus) can be used for milder or chronic conditions.

Prevention

Athletes who are sensitive to the metal in weights should ensure that clothes or petroleum jelly covers the contact points during weightlifting.

Billiard Cue

Epidemiology

Only one case report exists regarding billiard cue contact dermatitis (Goncalo et al., 1992). Patch testing revealed that he was allergic to the epoxy resin in the varnish of the cue.

Clinical Presentation

An older man presented with pruritic, hyperkeratotic, fissured, erythematous plaques on the palms extending to the first interdigital web space.

Diagnosis

Without obtaining a history from the athlete and making the link between billiards and the eruption, the differential diagnosis may be difficult. Psoriasis, hand dermatitis (unrelated to a contactant), and tinea manuum must be considered. Potassium hydroxide examination and/or biopsies are indicated. Patch tests confirm the diagnosis.

Treatment

Potent topical steroids (class I–II) should be tried. Topical immunomodulators (e.g., pimecrolimus) can be used for milder or chronic conditions.

Prevention

The affected patient removed the varnish from his cue completely and protected it only with petrolatum. He did not experience recurrences of his dermatitis.

Fishing Bait

Epidemiology

Several cases of fishers developing contact dermatitis are reported (Virgili et al., 2001; Warren and Marren, 1997). Prick test and radioallergosorbent test

(RAST) reveal that fishers can become allergic to *Calliphora vomitoria* (flesh fly maggots), midge larvae, and the azo compounds used to dye some live bait.

Clinical Presentation

Fishers may develop pruritic, well-defined, erythematous, hyperkeratotic, vesicular plaques on their palms, thumb, and first finger (corresponding to the location of primary bait handling).

Diagnosis

Without obtaining a history from the athlete and making the link between fish bait and the eruption, the differential diagnosis may be difficult. Psoriasis, hand dermatitis (unrelated to a contactant), and tinea manuum must be considered. Potassium hydroxide examination and/or biopsies are indicated. Patch testing, prick test, and RAST confirm the diagnosis.

Treatment

Potent topical steroids (class I–II) should be tried. Topical immunomodulators (e.g., pimecrolimus) can be used for milder or chronic conditions.

Prevention

Sensitive fishers should wear gloves and avoid dyed bait.

Medical Supplies for the Injured Athlete

Athletic Tape

Epidemiology

Almost any athlete who has been injured or is trying to prevent injury using athletic tape may develop a contact allergy. Basketball players and track and field athletes are reported in the literature. Para-tertiary-butylphenol-formaldehyde resin is used in adhesives, and all athletes in the one case series were patch test, positive for this compound.

Clinical Presentation

Beneath the tape, the athlete develops erythematous, well-defined, scaling, occasionally vesicular plaques.

Diagnosis

The diagnosis should be evident given the characteristic distribution beneath the tape. Patch testing suspected chemicals confirms the diagnosis. The differential diagnosis includes pressure urticaria and noncontact dermatitis. It is critical not to confuse the severe exudates of the dermatitis that may become yellow and crusted for secondary impetigo.

Treatment

The treatment of choice includes medium- to high-potency (class I–II) topical steroids for a brief period. A rapid burst of oral steroids or an intramuscular injection of triamcinolone may be necessary for severe outbreaks. Topical immunomodulators (e.g., pimecrolimus) can be used for milder or chronic conditions.

Prevention

Tapes without the offending compound are available, such as acrylate tape called Micropore. Alternatively, the athlete can apply a barrier between the skin and the adhesive tape.

Topical Creams/Analgesics/Anesthetics/Antibiotics

Jogging Cream

Epidemiology

One case report of contact dermatitis to jogging cream exists (de Leeuw and den Hollander, 1987). Patch testing revealed that she was allergic to several of the 31 ingredients in the cream, which included lipacide, palmitoyl hydrolyzed milk protein, palmitoyl collagen amino acids, and arnica.

Clinical Presentation

A runner who was using jogging cream to prevent blisters during her activity developed dermatitis on her face, hands, and feet.

Diagnosis

Without obtaining a history from the athlete and making the link between the jogging blister cream and the eruption, the differential diagnosis may be difficult. Psoriasis, atopic dermatitis, and dermatophyte infection must be considered. Potassium hydroxide examination and biopsies are indicated. Patch tests confirm the diagnosis.

Treatment

Potent topical steroids (class I–II) should be tried. Topical immunomodulators (e.g., pimecrolimus) can be used for milder, facial, or chronic conditions.

Prevention

Runners, especially those who are allergic, need not use these creams because petroleum jelly and synthetic socks by themselves should solve the blister problem.

Topical Antiinflammatory Agents

Epidemiology

A few case reports of contact dermatitis to topical analgesics exist (Camarasa, 1990; Vilaplana and Romaguera, 2000). A professional athlete developed dermatitis from eucalyptus in an antiinflammatory cream (Vilaplana and Romaguera, 2000). Analgesic salicylate sprays also cause pruritic and bullous dermatitis (Camarasa, 1990). Menthol or methyl salicylate (oil of wintergreen) may be culprits.

Clinical Presentation

Athletes develop the reaction on the skin where they applied the cream or spray. Unfortunately, sensitive individuals also can become exposed via the aerosol route when they use sprays. With this method, systemic symptoms (e.g., angioedema and respiratory symptoms) have occurred, so athletes must be cautioned.

Diagnosis

Without obtaining a history from the athlete and making the link between the analgesic and the eruption, the differential diagnosis may be difficult. The differential diagnosis mainly consists of acute vesicular dermatitis of various non–sports-related causes. Patch tests confirm the diagnosis.

Treatment

Potent topical steroids (class I–II) should be tried. Topical immunomodulators (e.g., pimecrolimus) can be used for milder, facial, or chronic conditions. Oral steroids are necessary for severe conditions, especially with systemic symptoms. Although respiratory symptoms are rare, careful attention to the respiratory status of the athlete is important.

Prevention

Sensitive individuals should avoid topical salicylate analgesics. Other topical analgesics are commercially available.

Topical Anesthetics

Epidemiology

A few case reports of contact dermatitis to topical anesthetics exist (Aberer and Zonzits, 1989; Kriechbaumer et al., 1998; Ventura et al., 2001). Ethyl chloride is a halogenated hydrocarbon used as an aerosolized cooling agent (−3°C). In one study of only athletes, investigators found that 9.3% had positive patch tests results to the topical anesthetic benzocaine. The athletes who developed reactions to benzocaine were runners, cyclists, and football players (Ventura et al., 2001).

Clinical Presentation

A handball player developed a vesicular eruption after using ethyl chloride on injured areas (Kriechbaumer et al., 1998). Any sprayed surface is susceptible. Those athletes sensitive to benzocaine develop a dermatitis on exposed skin.

Diagnosis

Without obtaining a history from the athlete and making the link between topical anesthetics and the eruption, the differential diagnosis may be difficult. The differential diagnosis includes frostbite related to the cold nature of the spray (in the case of ethyl chloride), contact dermatitis to adhesive bandages, and acute vesicular dermatitis not related to sports-related contactants. Patch tests confirm the diagnosis.

Treatment

Potent topical steroids (class I–II) should be tried. Topical immunomodulators (e.g., pimecrolimus) can be used for milder, facial, or chronic conditions.

Prevention

Sensitive athletes should avoid ethyl chloride and benzocaine.

Neosporin (Topical Antibiotic)

Epidemiology

Up to 10% of the normal population may be allergic to Neosporin. Any injured athlete using this topical antibiotic risks contact dermatitis.

Clinical Presentation

Injured athletes develop intensely pruritic, well-defined, erythematous, frequently vesicular plaques, often in geographic patterns correlating to the manner in which the antibiotics were applied to the skin (Figure 8-3).

152 Sports Dermatology

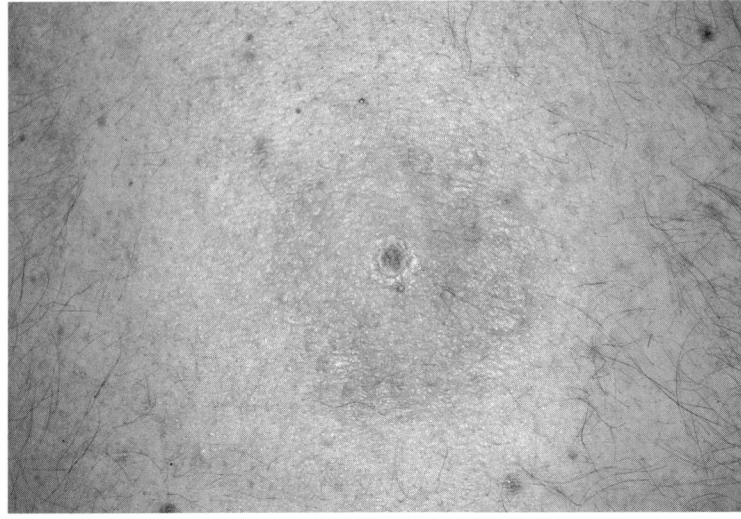

Figure 8-3. Topical Neosporin creates an allergic contact dermatitis around the wound on which the antibiotic was applied. Note the well-defined, erythematous, vesicular papules coalescing into a plaque.

Diagnosis

Without obtaining a history from the athlete and making the link between Neosporin and the eruption, the differential diagnosis may be difficult. The differential includes contact allergy to the adhesive in bandages and impetigo. Patch tests confirm the diagnosis.

Treatment

Potent topical steroids (class I–II) should be tried.

Prevention

Injured athletes should use petroleum jelly alone for cuts and abrasions.

Knee and Ankle Braces, Elbow Splints

Epidemiology

One report noted contact dermatitis to an elbow splint (Diphenylthiourea, found in a neoprene) used by a tennis player (Thomson et al., 1998). Thiourea, found in neoprene, can cause allergic contact dermatitis when sensitized individuals wear ankle or knee supports (Blum and Gerd, 1997; Haapasaari and Niinimaki, 2000).

Clinical Presentation

Injured athletes develop intensely pruritic, well-defined, erythematous, frequently vesicular plaques, often in geographic patterns correlating to the manner in which the braces or splints touched the skin.

Diagnosis

The diagnosis should be evident given the characteristic distribution beneath the protective equipment. Patch testing suspected chemicals confirms the diagnosis. The differential diagnosis includes pressure urticaria and noncontact dermatitis. It is critical not to confuse the severe exudates of the dermatitis that may become yellow and crusted for secondary impetigo.

Treatment

The treatment of choice includes medium- to high-potency (class I–II) topical steroids for a brief period. A rapid burst of oral steroids or an intramuscular injection of triamcinolone may be necessary for severe outbreaks. Topical immunomodulators (e.g., pimecrolimus) can be used for milder or chronic conditions.

Prevention

Affected athletes can apply tape or another barrier (such as Coban wrap, liquid adhesive, or petroleum jelly) to the skin before donning braces or splints. Alternatively, athletes can obtain braces or splints that lack the sensitizers to which they react.

Dermatitic "Obstacles" in the Environment

Rhus (Plants)

Epidemiology

Any outdoor athletes whose activity brings them to the woods or the woods' edge can develop rhus dermatitis. I have seen poison ivy in cross-country runners and golfers (who had been searching for errant balls). Urushiol is the hearty oil that causes poison ivy.

Clinical Presentation

If urushiol is not washed off after being on the skin for 1 hour, a sensitized athlete likely will develop contact dermatitis. Athletes also commonly, yet unwittingly, spread the causative protein to other parts of the body. Therefore, the distribution of poison ivy is not limited to the exposed areas. The clinician should search for even small areas of linear, erythematous, vesicular papules and plaques. The linear nature is highly characteristic of an external insult (Figure 8-4).

Diagnosis

The diagnosis typically is made given the pattern and morphology of the eruption. In extensive cases, the differential diagnosis must also include atopic dermatitis, eczematous drug eruption, and viral exanthems. It is critical not to confuse the severe exudates of the dermatitis that may become yellow and crusted for secondary impetigo. Patch testing and biopsy may be necessary to confirm the diagnosis.

Treatment

The treatment of choice includes medium- to high-potency (class I–II) topical steroids for a brief period. A rapid burst of oral steroids or an intramuscular injection of triamcinolone may be necessary for severe outbreaks. Topical

8. Allergic Contact Dermatitis   155

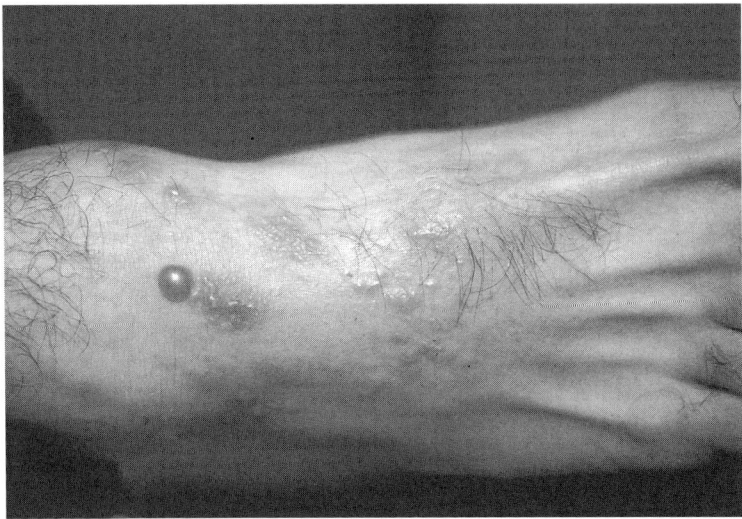

Figure 8-4. Classic linear erythematous plaques appear after exposure to poison ivy (rhus dermatitis). Note the large bullae and nonlinear nature of some red lesions.

immunomodulators (e.g., pimecrolimus) can be used for milder, facial, or chronic conditions.

Prevention

IvyBlock, which protects the athlete from poison ivy, poison oak, and poison sumac, contains the active ingredient bentoquatam. This lotion should be applied 15 minutes before outdoor exposure and reapplied every 4 hours.

Plants and Sun

Epidemiology

One small case series alleged that three professional soccer players developed dermatitis after they fell (Balabanova et al., 1993). Three professional soccer players developed a photolichenoid dermatitis from contact with plants on the playing field. It is theorized that these players came in contact with some unidentified plant in the grassy stadium after they tumbled. The fall coupled with ultraviolet irradiation caused the photolichenoid dermatitis (histology was highly suggestive of this clinical diagnosis).

Clinical Presentation

On physical examination, the players had moderately pruritic, erythematous, scaling, discrete, confluent papules and plaques on the lower legs, buttocks, and trunk (Figure 8-5). The eruption lasted up to 2 months.

Diagnosis

The diagnosis of photolichenoid contact dermatitis was tentatively made based on the characteristic histopathologic findings. The agent to which the soccer players were photoallergic is unknown. Patch testing was negative.

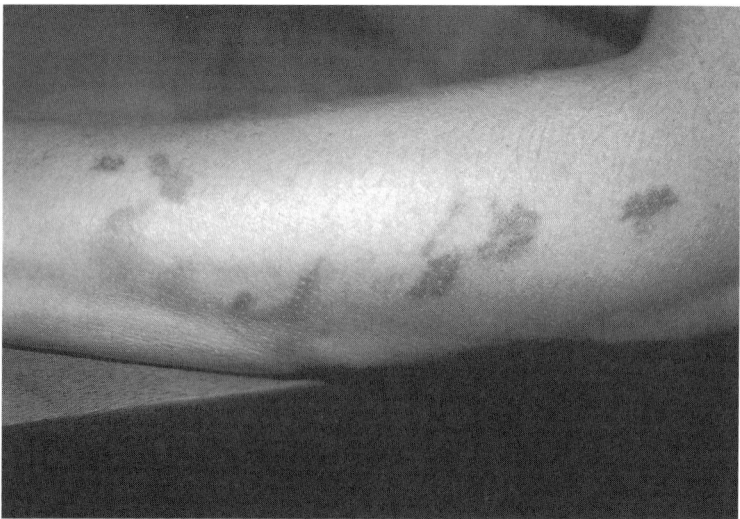

Figure 8-5. Phytophoto contact dermatitis occurs when a sensitive athlete brushes or falls on plant material that subsequently reacts upon exposure to sunlight. Well-defined, erythematous plaques occur on the extremities.

In extensive cases, the differential diagnosis must also include atopic dermatitis, eczematous drug eruption, and viral exanthems. It is critical not to confuse the severe exudates of the dermatitis that may become yellow and crusted for secondary impetigo. Biopsy may be necessary to confirm the diagnosis.

Treatment

Several therapeutic modalities were tried for these players. Topical steroids and ultraviolet therapy were used with moderate success.

Prevention

Prevention is difficult given the unknown etiology.

Sea Water

Epidemiology

Strict contact dermatitis to elements in sea water is not common. Mini-epidemics have been reported in swimmers in Hawaii who reacted to a type of seaweed (Izumi and Moore, 1987). Another incident occurred in the Red Sea when a group of swimmers developed contact dermatitis to yellow coral (Addy, 1991). Other at-risk sports include boating, kayaking, surfing, snorkeling, scuba diving, wind surfing, water tubing, waterskiing, and jet skiing.

Clinical Presentation

Swimmers who develop allergic contact dermatitis to an outside allergen can demonstrate unusual and geometric shapes such as lines and whirls. The lesions are well-defined, erythematous, scaling, potentially vesicular plaques. Covered parts of the body should not be affected. Some of the swimmers' contact dermatitis related to the yellow coral did not resolve for more than 3 months.

Diagnosis

Obtaining a history of exposure to sea water is critical. Careful attention to the pattern and distribution (particularly the areas of sparing) are key measures to determining the correct diagnosis.

In extensive cases, the differential diagnosis must also include atopic dermatitis, eczematous drug eruption, and viral exanthems. It is critical not to confuse the severe exudates of the dermatitis that may become yellow and crusted for secondary impetigo. Biopsy may be necessary to confirm the diagnosis.

Treatment

The treatment of choice includes medium- to high-potency (class I–II) topical steroids. A rapid burst of oral steroids or an intramuscular injection of triamcinolone may be necessary for severe outbreaks.

Prevention

Swimmers should avoid coral and vegetation in the sea.

Pool Water

Epidemiology

One study examined 385 swimmers at three different types of swimming pools in Australia. "Red rashes" developed on the skin within 24 hours in 4% of the swimmers in the bromine/ozone pool and in 8% of the swimmers in the chlorine and chlorine/ozone pools. The odds of a swimmer developing a red skin rash in the bromine pools were half as much compared to the chlorine pools, but this value was not statistically significant (Kelsall and Sim, 2001).

Another study reported that more than 60% of a collegiate swimming team developed what they termed *bleached swimmer syndrome* during the first few days after the pool had been cleaned and refilled. The affected swimmers developed xerosis and an erythematous macular eruption on the inner thighs and the area where the arms and chest came into contact during strokes. Additionally the swimmers noted a bleaching of dark hair and loss of hair, and they reported a few blue swimming suits had turned white (Strauss et al., 1986). Some authors believe that contact dermatitis to bromine or chlorine in pools is very rare (Fisher, 1987). Contact dermatitis to sodium hypochloride (which is used as a swimming pool disinfectant) has been reported (Fisher, 1987). Other at-risk athletes include divers, synchronized swimmers, water park enthusiasts, and water polo players.

Clinical Presentation

The chlorinated and brominated compounds can cause allergic contact dermatitis in swimmers. Affected athletes present with diffuse erythematous, scaling, pruritic plaques. Swimmers may note that the skin covered by the bathing suit is not affected (Fitzgerald et al., 1995; Sasseville et al., 1999).

Diagnosis

The clinician must specifically inquire about the relationship of the eruption to pool activities. This history coupled with sparing of clothing-covered areas should alert the clinician to the correct diagnosis. The differential diagnosis must also include atopic dermatitis, eczematous drug eruption, and viral exanthems. It is critical to distinguish the severe exudates of the dermatitis that may become yellow and crusted from secondary impetigo. Patch testing and biopsy may be necessary to confirm the diagnosis.

Treatment

The treatment of choice includes medium- to high-potency (class I–II) topical steroids. The diffuse nature of the eruption may hinder the use of topical steroids. A rapid burst of oral steroids or an intramuscular injection of triamcinolone may be necessary for diffuse or severe outbreaks.

Prevention

If possible, swimmers allergic to bromine or chlorine should partake of their aquatic activities in a nonhalogenated water supply (natural water). Swimmers who must use halogenated pools can attempt to locate a local pool that contains the halogen to which they are not allergic. Brominated pools are not common and are often found at major universities.

Judo Carpet

Epidemiology

One case report alleged that attendance at a judo club caused allergic contact dermatitis.

Clinical Presentation

A judo participant with a known allergy to red dye developed a diffuse dermatitis after attending a club with a red plastic carpet.

Diagnosis

The diagnosis would need to be confirmed with a patch test, but the red carpet in the reported case was unavailable for patch test.

Treatment

The reported individual required nearly 2 weeks of oral corticosteroids, after which the eruption cleared.

Prevention

Sensitive athletes should avoid dyed carpets.

Bibliography

Aberer W, Zonzits E. Allergy to ethyl chloride does occur, and might frequently be misdiagnosed. Contact Dermatitis 1989;21:352–353.

Adams RM. Contact allergic dermatitis due to diethylthiourea in a wetsuit. Contact Dermatitis 1982;8:277–278.

Addy JH. Red sea coral contact dermatitis. Int J Dermatol 1991;30:271–273.

Alomar A, Vilaltella I. Contact dermatitis to dibutylthiourea in swimming goggles. Contact Dermatitis 1985;13:348–349.

8. Allergic Contact Dermatitis 161

Azurdia RM, King CM. Allergic contact dermatitis due to phenol-formaldehyde resin and benzoyl peroxide in swimming goggles. Contact Dermatitis 1998;38:234–235.

Balabanova M, Kasandgieva J, Popov Y. Lichenoid dermatitis in 3 professional footballers. Contact Dermatitis 1993;28:166–168.

Balestrero S, Cozzani E, Ghigliotti G, et al. Allergic contact dermatitis from a wet suit. J Eur Acad Dermatol Venereol 1999;13:228–229.

Blair C. The dermatological hazards of bowling: contact dermatitis to resin in a bowls grip. Contact Derm 1982;8:138–139.

Blum A, Gerd L. Allergic contact dermatitis from mono-, di- and triethanolamine. Contact Dermatitis 1997;36:166.

Boehncke WH, Wessmann D, Zollner TM, et al. Allergic contact dermatitis from diphenylthiourea in a wet suit. Contact Dermatitis 1997;36:271.

Camarasa JG. Analgesic spray contact dermatitis. Dermatol Clin 1990;8:137–138.

Corazza M, Virgili A. Allergic contact dermatitis due to nickel in a neoprene wetsuit. Contact Dermatitis 1998;39:257.

Cronin E. Rubber. In: Cronin E, editor. Contact dermatitis. New York: Churchill Livingstone; 1980, p. 714.

de Leeuw J, den Hollander P. A patient with a contact allergy to jogging cream. Contact Dermatitis 1987;17:260–261.

Emmett EA, Risby TH, Taylor J, et al. Skin elicitation threshold of ethylbutyl thiourea and mercaptobenzothiazole with relative leaching from sensitizing products. Contact Dermatitis 1994;30:85–90.

Fisher AA. Contact dermatitis to diving equipment, swimming pool chemicals, and other aquatic denizens. Clin Dermatol 1987;5:36–40.

Fisher AA. Sports-related cutaneous reactions. Cutis 1999;63:202–204.

Fitzgerald DA, Wilkinson SM, Bhaggoe R, et al. Spa pool dermatitis. Contact Dermatitis 1995;33:53.

Foussereau J, Tomb R, Cavelier C. Allergic contact dermatitis from safety clothes and individual protective devices. Dermatol Clin 1990;8:127–132.

Goette DK. Raccoon-like periorbital leukoderma from contact with swim goggles. Contact Dermatitis 1984;10:129–131.

Goncalo S, Goncalo M, Matos J, et al. Contact dermatitis from a billiard cue. Contact Dermatitis 1992;26:263.

Guerra L, Misciali C, Borrello P, et al. Sensitization to palladium. Contact Dermatitis 1988;19:306–307.

Haapasaari KM, Niinimaki A. Vesicular palmar eczema from the neoprene tongue of an ankle support. Contact Dermatitis 2000;42:248.

Izumi AK, Moore RE. Seaweed (Lyngbya majuscula) dermatitis. Clin Dermatol 1987;5:92–100.

Jung JH, McLaughlin JL, Stannard J, et al. Isolation, via activity-directed fractionation, of mercaptobenzothiazole and dibenzothiazyl disulfide as 2 allergens responsible for tennis shoe dermatitis. Contact Dermatitis 1988;19:254–259.

Kelsall HL, Sim MR. Skin irritation in users of brominated pools. Int J Environ Health Res 2001;11:29–40.

Kriechbaumer N, Hemmer W, Focke M, et al. Sensitization to ethyl chloride in a handball player. Contact Dermatitis 1998;38:227–228.

Lachapelle JM, Tennstedt D, Dumont-Fruytier M. Occupational allergic contact dermatitis to isophorone diamine (IPD) used as an epoxy resin hardener. Contact Dermatitis 1978;4:109–112.

Maibach H. Scuba diver facial dermatitis: allergic contact dermatitis to N-isopropyl-N-phenylpara-phenylenediamine. Contact Dermatitis 1975;1:330.

Minciullo PL, Patafi M, Ferlazzo B, et al. Contact dermatitis from a fishing rod. Contact Dermatitis 2004;50:322.

Munro CS, Shields TG, Lawrence CM. Contact allergy to Tego 103G disinfectant in a deep-sea diver. Contact Dermatitis 1989;21:278–279.

Nagashima C, Tomitaka-Yagami A, Matsunaga K. Contact dermatitis due to para-tertiary-butylphenol-formaldehyde resin in a wetsuit. Contact Dermatitis 2003;49:267–268.

Paterson BC, White MI, Cowen PS. Further observations on adverse reactions to a bowler's grip. Contact Dermatitis 1993;29:278.

Reid CM, van Grutten M, Rycroft RJ. Allergic contact dermatitis from ethylbutylthiourea in neoprene. Contact Dermatitis 1993;28:193.

Roberts JL, Hanifin JM. Athletic shoe dermatitis. Contact allergy to ethyl butyl thiourea. JAMA 1979;241:275–276.

Rodriguez-Serna M, Molinero J, Febrer I, et al. Persistent hand eczema in a child. Am J Contact Dermatitis 2002;13:35–36.

Romaguera C, Grimalt F, Vilaplana J. Contact dermatitis from swimming goggles. Contact Dermatitis 1988;18:178–179.

Sasseville D, Geoffrion G, Lowry RN. Allergic contact dermatitis from chlorinated swimming pool water. Contact Dermatitis 1999;41:347–348.

Scott MJ, Scott, NI, Scott LM. Dermatologic stigmata in sports: weightlifting. Cutis 1992;50:141–145.

Sommer S, Wilkinson SM, Dodman B. Contact dermatitis due to urea-formaldehyde resin in shin-pads. Contact Dermatitis 1999;40:159–160.

Strauss RH, Lanesc RR, Leizman DJ. Illness and absence among wrestlers, swimmers, and gymnasts at a large university. Am J Sport Med 1986;16:653–655.

Tennstedt D, Lachapelle JM. Windsurfer dermatitis from black rubber components. Contact Dermatitis 1981;7:160–161.

Thomson KF, Wilkinson SM, Chalmers RJ, et al. Allergic contact dermatitis from a neoprene elbow splint. Contact Dermatitis 1998;38:179.

Tuyp E, Mitchell JC. Scuba diver facial dermatitis. Contact Dermatitis 1983;9:334–335.

Vaswani SK, Collins DD, Pass CJ. Severe allergic contact eyelid dermatitis caused by swimming goggles. Ann Allergy Asthma Immunol 2003;90:672–673.

Ventura MT, Dagnello M, Matino MG, et al. Contact dermatitis in students practicing sports: incidence of rubber sensitisation. Br J Sports Med 2001;35:100–102.

Vilaplana J, Romaguera C. Allergic contact dermatitis due to eucalyptol in an anti-inflammatory cream. Contact Dermatitis 2000;43:118.

Vincenzi C, Guerra L, Peluso AM, et al. Allergic contact dermatitis due to phenol-formaldehyde resins in a knee-guard. Contact Dermatitis 1992;27:54.

Virgili A, Ligrone L, Bacilieri S, et al. Protein contact dermatitis in a fisherman using maggots of a flesh fly as bait. Contact Dermatitis 2001;44:262–263.

Warren LJ, Marren P. Textile dermatitis and dyed maggot exposure. Contact Dermatitis 1997;36:106.

9. Irritant Contact Dermatitis

The first chapter in the section on sports-related inflammatory reactions discussed the aspects of sports participation that lead to allergic contact dermatitis. Intrinsic to this type of dermatitis is the idea of sensitivity. Not all athletes develop contact allergy; only those whose immune system is sensitive to the exposed allergen react. Chapter 9 reviews irritant contact dermatitis, which, unlike its allergic counterpart, can occur in any athlete if the concentration or duration of exposure of the irritant is sufficient. The athlete's immune system is irrelevant in irritant contact dermatitis. In addition, this type of dermatitis develops rapidly after exposure.

Athletes come into contact with substances that cause skin irritation through their use of equipment and the playing field. Chapter 9 is divided into three main sections based on the origin of the contact dermatitis: (1) the playing field, (2) the athletes' implements, and (3) the athletes themselves (Table 9-1). It is critical for clinicians to recognize the occurrence of irritant contact dermatitis so that they can prevent other team members from developing similar reactions.

Playing Field

Canyoning Hands

Epidemiology

There has been one case report of canyoning hands in individuals who race through ice-cold rapids, scale over rocks, and port their transportation (Descamps and Puechal, 2002).

Clinical Presentation

Athletes with canyoning hands develop painful, erythematous erosions on the palms and fingertips. The eruption results from the irritation of the cold water, sharp rocks, and rapid wet/dry cycles experienced.

Diagnosis

The diagnosis may be difficult if the clinician does not inquire into the individual's athletic activity. The differential diagnosis mainly consists of subacute to chronic hand dermatitis of various non–sports-related causes and

Table 9-1. Etiologies of the Various Sports-Related Types of Irritant Contact Dermatitis

Category	Sport	Designation	Irritant
Playing field	Mountaineering	Canyoning hands	Forces of nature (rocks, water, wind)
	Soccer	Cement burns	Calcium oxide
	Swimming	Pool dermatitis	Halogenated compounds in pool water
Athletes' implements	Basketball	Basketball pebble fingers	Pebbled nicked ball
	Hockey	Hockey dermatitis	Fiberglass
	Injured athletes	Pack dermatitis	Ammonium nitrate
	Board surfers	Surf rider's dermatitis	Mixed (board, salt, sand)
Athletes themselves	Baseball	Baseball pitcher's friction dermatitis	Questionable coarse clothing
	Swimming	Swimmer's shoulder	Hair stubble

tinea manuum. Results of potassium hydroxide examination and patch tests are negative.

Treatment

Open wounds should be covered with petroleum jelly. Topical antibiotics may be necessary. To decrease pain and healing time, the lesions should be kept moist and covered with bandages. Oral antibiotics may be necessary in case of superinfection.

Prevention

Waterproof gloves, if worn by the enthusiast, prevent canyoning hands.

Cement Burns

Epidemiology

There have been several case reports of irritant contact dermatitis to the line markers found on the soccer field. Authors have termed this type of dermatitis

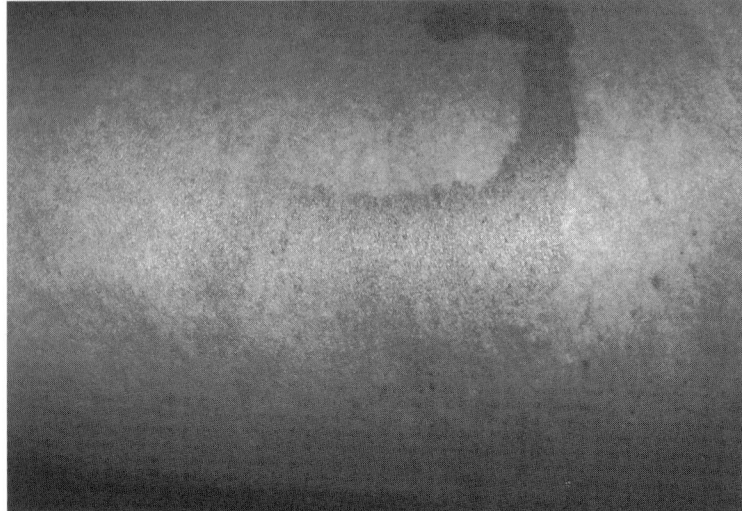

Figure 9-1 Clinical presentation of acute irritant contact dermatitis with sharply demarcated, erythematous, dusky plaques.

cement burns (Gelmetti and Cecca, 1992; Mastrolonardo et al., 1997). Calcium oxide, a white substance, has been used to mark rugby and soccer boundaries. The process consists of marking the field with chalk and then fixing the marks with wet calcium oxide.

Clinical Presentation

Soccer players with cement burns reveal well-defined, erythematous, vesicular, bullous, eroded, crusted plaques on the upper thighs (Figure 9-1). The soccer player usually complains of pruritus and burning within hours after coming in contact with the calcium oxide line markings. Some athletes even have difficulty walking after receiving the lesions. Typically the players come in contact with the line markings as they slide for the ball before it goes out of bounds, corresponding to the most common location of the rash. Taking a shower after the game worsens the lesions. The lesions heal with scarring.

Diagnosis

The diagnosis should not be difficult to make; the clinical presentation is quite distinct. The differential diagnosis mainly consists of acute vesicular dermatitis of various non–sports-related causes. Results of patch tests are negative.

Treatment

Topical antibiotics are necessary. To decrease pain and healing time, the lesions should be kept moist and covered with bandages. Oral antibiotics may be necessary in case of superinfection.

Prevention

Calcium oxide should not be used for line markings. Athletes who come into contact with the calcium oxide line markings should quickly be benched so that they can wash off the area of contact.

Pool Dermatitis

Epidemiology

Mini-epidemics of irritant contact dermatitis are reported (Rycroft and Penny, 1983). Unfortunately, the denominator of total number of swimmers was not available to make any assessment regarding prevalence among swimmers. As a result of visits to 19 brominated pools and a questionnaire sent to swimmers in those pools, the same authors discovered 65 swimmers who developed irritant contact dermatitis from swimming.

Clinical Presentation

Swimmers who develop irritant contact dermatitis to Di-halo (brominated compound in pools) usually develop a patchy, erythematous eruption in a generalized distribution. Ninety percent of swimmers develop the eruption within 12 hours of swimming. Those who spend more time in the pools seem more likely to be affected.

Diagnosis

Without obtaining a history from the athlete and making the link between the pool water and the eruption, the differential diagnosis may be quite difficult.

The differential diagnosis mainly consists of subacute dermatitis of various non–sports-related causes and worsening swimmer's xerosis. The differential diagnosis must also include atopic dermatitis, eczematous drug eruption, and viral exanthems. It is critical to distinguish the severe exudates of the dermatitis that may become yellow and crusted from secondary impetigo. Patch testing and biopsy may be necessary to confirm the diagnosis. Results of patch and prick tests with Di-halo are negative.

Treatment

Medium-potency topical steroids (class II–III) should be tried. Topical immunomodulators, such as pimecrolimus, can be used for milder, facial, or chronic conditions. Oral steroids are necessary for severe conditions, especially with systemic symptoms.

Prevention

Further studies are needed to confirm the irritancy potential of certain brominated compounds in swimming pools compared to other halogenated agents (i.e., chlorine). If swimmers have noted particular difficulty with a specific pool, then they should shower immediately after swimming in that pool.

Red Tide Dermatitis (Sea Water)

Epidemiology

There have been no epidemiologic studies regarding red tide dermatitis, but sports such as boating, scuba diving, jet skiing, kayaking, snorkeling, surfing, sailing, swimming, windsurfing, and waterskiing place athletes at risk. Under certain optimal growing conditions, unicellular phytoplankton (e.g., *Ptychodiscus brevis*) flourishes and creates huge areas of red tides in the ocean.

Clinical Presentation

The toxins from these organisms produce erythematous, urticarial eruptions on the exposed skin. Aquatic enthusiasts may develop conjunctivitis and pulmonary symptoms.

Diagnosis

The diagnosis is based on the clinical and historical findings.

Treatment

Medium-potency topical steroids (class II–III) should be tried. Topical immunomodulators, such as pimecrolimus, can be used for milder or facial conditions. Oral steroids are necessary for severe conditions, especially with systemic symptoms.

Prevention

Aquatic athletes should avoid sea water when red tides predominate.

Seaweed Dermatitis (Sea Water)

Epidemiology

There have been multiple reported skin epidemics with a type of seaweed (*Lyngbya majuscula*) affecting 86 to 242 swimmers at different beaches in Hawaii (Izumi and Moore, 1987). This organism is a blue-green alga located in the Caribbean, Pacific, and Indian Oceans, from the intertidal zones to depths of 100 feet, particularly during the summer. The organism produces two skin toxins called *debromoaplysiatoxin* and *lyngbyatoxin A* that induce an irritant contact dermatitis. It is not uncommon for the seaweed to become shredded in the surf. Small pieces eventually become lodged in the suits of unsuspecting boaters, kayakers, scuba divers, jet skiers, snorkelers, swimmers, surfers, windsurfers, water tubers, and waterskiers.

Clinical Presentation

After only a few minutes to 1 day, swimmers develop erythematous, necrotic plaques in areas covered by the bathing suit, such as the scrotum and perineal region.

Diagnosis

Without obtaining a history from the athlete and making the link between the seaweed and the eruption, the differential diagnosis may be quite difficult. The differential diagnosis mainly consists of seabather's eruption and swimmer's itch. Like seabather's eruption, the eruption of seaweed dermatitis is beneath the bathing suit.

Treatment

Experiments have shown that washing with soap and water within 1 hour of exposure can prevent or reduce the irritant contact dermatitis. Medium-potency topical steroids (class II–III) should be tried. Topical immunomodulators, such as pimecrolimus, can be used for milder or facial conditions. Oral steroids or antihistamines may be necessary.

Prevention

Swimmers should avoid ocean activities immediately after storms because the seaweed will have been pulverized and bits of the very irritating plant will abound.

Sponge Dermatitis (Sea Water)

Epidemiology

There have been no epidemiologic studies of sponge dermatitis. Affected athletes include boaters, scuba divers, jet skiers, kayakers, snorkelers, surfers, swimmers, water tubers, windsurfers, and waterskiers.

Clinical Presentation

Many sponges can create irritation when the aquatic enthusiast brushes against the colorful attractive marine life. The fine glass-like slivers on the sponge surfaces produce immediate burning pain, erythema, and blisters.

Diagnosis

The history and clinical presentation are typical.

Treatment

Some authors have used warm vinegar soaks several times per day. Medium-potency topical steroids (class II–III) may be helpful. Topical immunomodulators, such as pimecrolimus, can be used for milder or facial conditions.

Prevention

Divers, swimmers, and other athletes should not touch these attractive sponges without protective wear.

Athletes' Implements

Basketballs

Epidemiology

A review of basketball pebble fingers notes that this finding is more common than suggested by the literature. They also note that weightlifters can develop a similar reaction (Bischof and Markham, 1994).

Clinical Presentation

Repetitive contact between the fingers and fingertips with the basketball results in painful abrasions and petechiae. The area may become glazed in appearance. It appears that long periods of play, microtrauma from the ball's pebbled surface, and nicks in the surface of the ball contribute to the development of this skin condition. Playing basketball outdoors may lead to rougher ball surfaces and hence worse basketball pebble fingers.

Diagnosis

Without obtaining a history from the athlete and making the link between the basketball and the eruption, the differential diagnosis may be quite difficult. The differential diagnosis mainly consists of chronic hand dermatitis of various non–sports-related causes and tinea manuum. Results of potassium hydroxide examination and patch tests are negative.

Treatment

Basketball players who develop this condition can apply a small amount of topical antibiotics or petroleum jelly onto their fingertips.

Prevention

Basketball players can reduce their risk for this condition by playing indoors and limiting the amount of time practicing. Some have been able to assuage symptoms by applying a small amount of petroleum jelly to the fingers before play.

Hockey Sticks

Epidemiology

Contact dermatitis to hockey sticks in professional hockey players is reported (Levine, 1980). Professional hockey players have developed a contact dermatitis to fiberglass found in hockey sticks.

Clinical Presentation

The condition is characterized by fairly well-defined, erythematous, scaling plaques over the arms and areas touched by the hockey stick.

Diagnosis

Without obtaining a history from the athlete and making the link between the hockey stick and the eruption, the differential diagnosis may be quite difficult. The differential diagnosis mainly consists of subacute dermatitis of various non–sports-related causes. Results of patch tests are negative.

Treatment

Potent topical steroids (class I–II) should be tried. Topical immunomodulators, such as pimecrolimus, can be used for milder, facial, or chronic conditions.

Prevention

Hockey sticks should be repaired or replaced if the fiberglass is frayed.

Ice Packs

Epidemiology

No epidemiology of ice pack dermatitis exists. An injured athlete can use a cold pack that works by using the endothermic reaction principle. Water and solid crystals (ammonium nitrate) are kept in different compartments within the pack and are mixed once the trainer or athlete manipulates the pack. Too vigorous hand motions or smashing the pack against the other hand may result in extrusion of the ammonium nitrate crystals on the skin. The Material Safety and Data Sheet (MSDS) describes ammonium nitrate as a strong oxidizer. It is rated a 3 (severe) on the reactivity scale.

Clinical Presentation

Affected skin displays erythematous, well-defined, vesicular, or eroded plaques.

Diagnosis

The diagnosis is quite evident and occurs soon after exposure to the broken cold pack.

Treatment

The area should be washed immediately with lukewarm water and soap. Topical antibiotics or petroleum jelly should be applied. To decrease pain and healing time, the lesions should be kept moist and covered with bandages. Oral antibiotics may be necessary in case of superinfection.

Prevention

It is important to exert just enough force to combine the two inner linings of water and crystals. Excessive blunt forces risk cold pack rupture onto the skin.

Rafts and Boogie Boards

Epidemiology

One case series of surf rider's dermatitis is reported (Bischof, 1995). Women are less affected. This condition also could be described in the traumatic forces chapter of this book but is discussed here based on its term *dermatitis*.

Swimmers lie prone on rafts and boards to ride the surf. Multiple forces create surf rider's dermatitis, which results from a combination of irritant, mechanical, and allergic factors. Friction occurs between the coarse fiber surface of the rafts and the surfer's nipples. There is increased friction as a result of salabrasion (which occurs as the wind helps to evaporate water, leaving salt on the surfer's body). Finally, sand comes in contact between the skin and the board or raft. In addition to these frictional forces, the surfer's nipples experience repeated shearing forces, occlusion, and pressure. Rarely, individuals are allergic to the surfboard wax, the plasticizers, or polymers found in the raft or board.

Clinical Presentation

Clinically the board surfer complains of painful, erythematous, crusted, edematous, fissured, or eroded papules on the nipples and areolas.

Diagnosis

Without obtaining a history from the athlete and making the link between the raft or boogie board and the eruption, the differential diagnosis may be quite difficult. The differential diagnosis mainly consists of allergic contact dermatitis and acute vesicular dermatitis of various non–sports-related causes. Results of patch tests are negative.

Treatment

Lesions heal without therapy. Pain can be alleviated if the surfer applies topical antibiotic ointment or petroleum jelly to the area of irritant dermatitis. Oral analgesics, bandages, and soft clothing are helpful.

Prevention

Women seem to derive protection from bathing suits that cover their nipples. Men who wish to participate in this activity should wear shirts or apply commercially available nipple guards or petroleum jelly before surfing with boogie boards or rafts.

Shotguns

Epidemiology

One case report of trapshooter's stigma is reported (Exum and Scott, 1992).

Clinical Presentation

Trapshooters can hold their guns in several ways. Some lock their shoulders tightly, while others let their shoulders hang loose. This latter group often experiences friction between the gun and the cheek as the gun recoils abruptly during firing. The reported trapshooter held his shoulders loosely, and he also used baby powder on his cheek where the gun rubbed during recoil. Once his sweat mixed with the powder, it hardened and felt like sandpaper. A severe abrasion occurred on his cheek where the gun recoiled. Ultimately the area became lichenified, and a 1-cm scar resulted.

Incidentally, although no case reports exist, the wood or the various finishes applied to the wood is noted to possibly result in allergic contact dermatitis in areas of skin contact.

Diagnosis

Without obtaining a history from the athlete and making the link between the shotgun and the eruption, the differential diagnosis may be quite difficult. The differential diagnosis might consist of a subacute to chronic dermatitis of an allergic or noncontact type. Old lesions may resemble a basal carcinoma. Results of patch tests are negative.

Treatment

Lesions heal without therapy. Pain can be alleviated if the shooter applies topical antibiotics or petroleum jelly to the irritant dermatitis. Topical steriods may also be useful. Oral analgesics and bandages are helpful.

Prevention

If shooters experience friction dermatitis as a result of the gun's recoil, they should use petroleum jelly on the skin that is at risk for friction. Baby powder should not be used.

Hand Chalk

Epidemiology

Several cases of irritant contact dermatitis to chalk in gymnasts are reported (Strauss et al., 1988).

Clinical Presentation

The skin condition is characterized by fairly well-defined, erythematous, scaling plaques on areas of contact between the chalk on the equipment and the skin.

Diagnosis

Without obtaining a history from the athlete and making the link between gymnastics and the eruption, the differential diagnosis may be quite difficult.

The differential diagnosis mainly consists of subacute dermatitis of various non–sports-related causes and tinea manuum. Results of patch tests are negative.

Treatment

Potent topical steroids (class I–II) should be tried. Topical immunomodulators, such as pimecrolimus, may be used for milder, facial, or chronic conditions.

Prevention

There is no known alternative.

Within the Athlete

Baseball Pitcher's Friction Dermatitis

Epidemiology

One case report of irritant contact dermatitis in a baseball player exists (Inui et al., 2002).

Clinical Presentation

In the course of his pitching delivery motion, a professional baseball player developed erythematous, pruritic papules over the medial ankle and knee from friction between his coarse clothing and his skin.

Diagnosis

Without obtaining a history from the athlete and making the link between the delivery motion and the eruption, the differential diagnosis may be quite difficult. The differential diagnosis mainly consists of allergic contact dermatitis, subacute dermatitis of various non–sports-related causes, and tinea corporis. Results of patch tests are negative.

Treatment

Potent topical steroids (class I–II) can be tried; however, the reported case used oral steroids. Topical immunomodulators, such as pimecrolimus, can be used for milder, facial, or chronic conditions. Protective bandages with topical antibiotics or petroleum jelly soothe the pain and speed healing.

Prevention

No attempts should be made to change the pitcher's throwing motion because the change can lead to other biomechanical problems and alterations in accuracy. Protective dressings or petroleum jelly made be applied under the uniform to add a barrier of protection. The reported pitcher was able to continue pitching using daily topical steroids and additional stockings over the area that developed the dermatitis.

Swimmer's Shoulder

Epidemiology

Irritant contact dermatitis to unshaven hair in a swimmer is reported (Koehn, 1991).

Clinical Presentation

Males with an unshaven face may develop a well-defined, erythematous, rarely eroded plaque on the shoulders. The hair stubble is quite abrasive, and during a long workout of laps, the friction between this stubble and the skin of the shoulder produces swimmer's shoulder.

Diagnosis

Without obtaining a history from the athlete and making the link between swimming (and lack of shaving) and the eruption, the differential diagnosis may be quite difficult. The differential diagnosis mainly consists of acute to subacute dermatitis of various non–sports-related causes. Results of patch tests are negative.

Treatment

Lesions heal without therapy. Pain can be alleviated if the swimmer applies topical antibiotics or petroleum jelly to the irritant dermatitis. Oral analgesics, bandages, and soft clothing are helpful.

Prevention

Swimmers can prevent this annoying eruption by shaving before practice.

Bibliography

Bischof RO. Surf rider's dermatitis. Contact Dermatitis 1995;32:247.
Bischof RO, Markham FW. Basketball pebble fingers. J Fam Pract 1994;39:506.
Descamps V, Puechal X. "Canyoning hand": a new recreational hand dermatitis. Contact Dermatitis 2002;47:363–364.
Exum WF, Scott MJ. Trapshooter's stigma. Cutis 1992;50:110.
Gelmetti C, Cecca E. Caustic ulcers caused by calcium hydroxide in 2 adolescent football players. Contact Dermatitis 1992;27:265–266.
Inui S, Yamamoto S, Ikegami R, et al. Baseball pitcher's friction dermatitis. Contact Dermatitis 2002;47:176–177.
Izumi AK, Moore RE. Seaweed (Lyngbya majuscula) dermatitis. Clin Dermatol 1987;5:92–100.
Koehn GG. Skin injuries in sports medicine. J Am Acad Dermatol 1991;24:152.
Levine N. Dermatologic aspects of sports medicine. J Am Acad Dermatol 1980;3: 415–424.
Mastrolonardo M, Cassano N, Vena GA. Cement burns in 2 football players. Contact Dermatitis 1997;37:183–184.
Rycroft RJ, Penny PT. Dermatoses associated with brominated swimming pools. Br Med J (Clin Res Ed) 1983;287:462.
Strauss RH, Lanese RR, Leizman DJ. Illness and absence among wrestlers, swimmers, and gymnasts at a large university. Am J Sports Med 1988;16:653–655.

10. Pruritus and Urticaria

In Chapters 8 and 9, we discussed the reactions that can occur primarily in the epidermis (i.e., contact dermatitis) as a result of athletic participation. Chapters 10 and 11 switch gears and examine the sports-related allergic reactions that affect mainly the dermis. These conditions are of particular concern because of possible associated systemic findings. Susceptible athletes can develop urticaria or hives as result of genetic predisposition.

Both internal and external stimuli are important in the origin of urticaria. The rise in internal body temperature can cause hives, as can the warm or cold environment of the athletic venue. The sun and water themselves in rare cases can complicate an athlete's activity with hives. It is vital that clinicians make the appropriate diagnosis of the allergic reaction, identify the offending stimuli, and help prevent future exacerbations.

This chapter discusses first pruritus without skin lesions and then focuses on different types of urticaria. Most of the dermatologic conditions discussed in this book can be associated with pruritus to varying degrees. The urticarial reactions discussed in this chapter most characteristically have associated pruritus. Athletes, particularly those who use water as their venue, may have intense pruritus even without obvious skin lesions.

Pruritus

Epidemiology

No studies have systematically analyzed the incidence of pruritus in athletes. One study showed that swimmers were statistically more likely to develop pruritus than were nonswimmers (Momas et al., 1993). Often the pruritus of swimmers is related to xerosis (dry skin); however, a unique condition called *aquagenic pruritus* was first described in 1970 (Steinman, 1987). To date, more males than females with this unusual condition are reported. The mean age at onset is 43 years (range 8–78 years). The condition is seen most in athletes participating in water sports, such as diving, synchronized swimming, swimming, and water polo.

Clinical Presentation

Many conditions discussed in this book have associated pruritus but I am now focusing on the complaint of itching in athletes without obvious skin lesions. One of the most itchy conditions seen in a dermatology clinic is xerosis.

Swimmers may frequently get dry skin that is not clinically obvious. This propensity for dry skin originates from the paradoxical dehydration effect caused by an osmotic gradient coupled with dilution of the natural oils of the skin. This biophysical result is exacerbated by athletes' propensity to shower in very warm water with harsh soaps.

Aquagenic pruritus, which many believe is a distinct entity, is characterized by intense pruritus, burning, or stinging that develops within minutes of contact with water but with absolutely no skin changes. No hives of any sort are present, and the itching may persist up to 2 hours after water exposure. The legs seem particularly affected by aquagenic pruritus, but the face, palms, and soles are spared.

Diagnosis

The diagnosis of pruritus related to xerosis must include a careful examination of the back and flanks for any subtle signs of stratum corneum perturbation. Many authors trust that aquagenic pruritus is a distinct disorder. The diagnosis is based both on its characteristic presentation and the exclusion of urticaria, xerosis, and systemic disorders causing secondary pruritus such as polycythemia rubra vera (Table 10-1).

Treatment

Pruritus related to xerosis and swimming consistently improves with emollients and careful dry skin care. Several therapies have been attempted for aquagenic pruritus (Steinman, 1987). Standardized ultraviolet therapy seems to be the most effective. Antihistamines and topical moisturizers offer partial relief.

Table 10-1. Tests for Distinguishing the Physical Urticarias in Athletes

	Rapid Warming in Sauna	**Ice Cube Test**	**Focal Warm-Water Compress**	**Phototesting**
Aquagenic pruritus	Negative	Negative	Negative	Negative
Cholinergic urticaria	Positive	Negative	Negative	Negative
Cold urticaria	Negative	Positive	Negative	Negative
Aquagenic urticaria	Negative	Negative	Positive	Negative
Solar urticaria	Negative	Negative	Negative	Positive

Prevention

Pruritus can best be prevented by careful attention to keeping the skin moist. Thick ointments such as petroleum jelly are excellent barriers to prevent excess water evaporation from the skin while athletes are actively participating in water sports. Once out of the water, athletes should take a cool shower and use a very mild soap such as Cetaphil. Several novel in-shower moisturizers such as Olay's Moisturinse In Shower Body Lotion are available. The moisturizer is applied during the shower and improves skin hydration. Athletes should pat dry and apply additional moisturizer if needed to particularly dry areas.

Cholinergic Urticaria

Epidemiology

In the population at large, physical urticaria composes a rather small proportion (2.4%) of all types of hives; however, in athletes, physical urticaria accounts for approximately 15% of all hives (Mikhailov et al., 1977). By far the most common type of hives in athletes is cholinergic urticaria. However, one study of 30 athletes with urticaria discovered that only one fourth of the athlete population had cholinergic urticaria. The most common type of urticaria in athletes in this study was cold urticaria (50%). This unusual finding may be the result of selection bias. Prospective large epidemiologic studies likely would reveal that cholinergic urticaria is the most common type of physical urticaria in athletes.

Another study that examined 35 subjects with cholinergic urticaria used a slightly different approach (Hirschmann et al., 1987). The onset of cholinergic urticaria typically occurs between 10 and 30 years of age (mean age of onset 18 years). Nearly 90% of the subjects developed lesions after exercise, and the duration and severity correlated with the intensity of athletic activity. Nearly half of the affected subjects reported that their cholinergic urticaria was so severe that it limited their athletic activity; several stopped running, cycling, and playing football. These sports are specifically mentioned in epidemiologic studies, but in reality any sport whose activity increases the core body temperature can place the athlete at risk. The cause of cholinergic urticaria is not exactly understood. Clearly a rapid rise in core body temperature can result in cholinergic urticaria. Histamine release is widely believed to be the cause of the symptoms and signs, but the cause of mast cell degranulation is debatable. Immunoglobulin E, acetylcholine, and proteases all may play a role.

Clinical Presentation

The typical athlete with cholinergic urticaria notices symptoms before the onset of obvious skin lesions. Itching, burning, warmth, and irritation have all

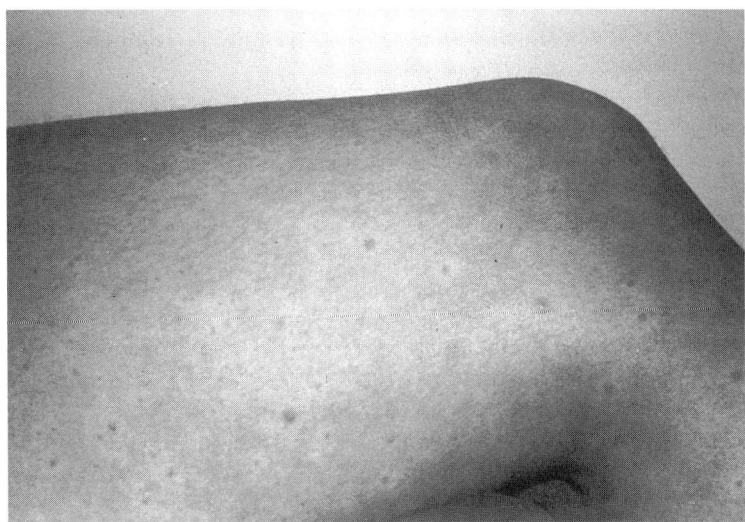

Figure 10-1. Small, well-defined, erythematous, edematous papules represent cholinergic urticaria.

been reported before the outbreak of hives. The characteristic morphology is well-defined, erythematous, edematous, discrete (and frequently confluent when severe), small (1- to 5-mm) papules (Figure 10-1). These lesions can appear anywhere on the body, but they congregate on the trunk and extremities. The median duration of hives is 30 minutes, but some patients' hives take much longer to resolve. Lesions that last longer than 24 hours are not urticaria and require expert dermatologic evaluation.

Systemic findings may be associated with cholinergic urticaria but are unusual (Hirschmann et al., 1987). Pulmonary findings include end-expiratory wheezing; syncope and nausea are possible but rare.

Diagnosis

There is no serologic test for cholinergic urticaria; rather, its diagnosis is based on a constellation of clinical signs and symptoms. The distinct small wheals are diagnostic. When the hives coalesce, the clinician may confuse cholinergic urticaria with exercise-induced anaphylaxis (discussed in Chapter 11). To confirm the diagnosis, the clinician can have the athlete sit in a sauna, where passive warming causes lesions of cholinergic urticaria to appear (Table 10-1).

Treatment

Because most athletes do not wish to abandon their sport to avoid hives, pharmacologic means for controlling cholinergic urticaria must be considered. Antihistamines, specifically hydroxyzine, may be helpful (Briner, 1993; Hirschmann et al., 1987; Pharis et al., 1997). Others have used protease inhibitors with success (Mikhailov et al., 1977). In fact, 62% of subjects believe that antihistamines improve their condition (Hirschmann et al., 1987). Eight years after disease onset, 15% of sufferers were in complete remission, 50% were improved, and 21% had worsened.

Prevention

Athletes with cholinergic urticaria should routinely take antihistamines. A program by which the athlete gradually increases the level of exertion and activity may help inhibit the development of hives (Adams, 2001a; Briner, 1993).

Cold Urticaria

Epidemiology

At least one study identifies cold urticaria as the most common of all urticaria types found in athletes (50% of overall numbers) (Mikhailov et al., 1977). Swimmers (and other athletes exposed to cold water) and winter sport athletes most commonly develop cold urticaria (Adams; Sarnaik et al., 1986). Most athletes first notice they have the condition while swimming during childhood.

The most common cause of cold urticaria is idiopathic (essential acquired cold urticaria), but other types of the condition must be considered. These include secondary cold urticaria from cold hemolysins, cryoglobulins, and connective tissue disorders (Sarnaik et al., 1986). The amount of cooling necessary to induce cold urticaria varies among individual athletes. The key to generation of cold urticaria directly relates to the change in skin temperature and not the absolute temperature.

Clinical Presentation

Like cholinergic urticaria, cold urticaria exhibits very well-defined, intensely pruritic, small, 1- to 5-mm, erythematous, edematous papules. The lesions typically are distributed on body surfaces exposed to the cold environment.

Systemic findings are of concern in this type of physical urticaria. Probably one of the most alarming aspects of the condition is the reported associated loss of consciousness (Sarnaik et al., 1987). Diving into cold water may be sufficient

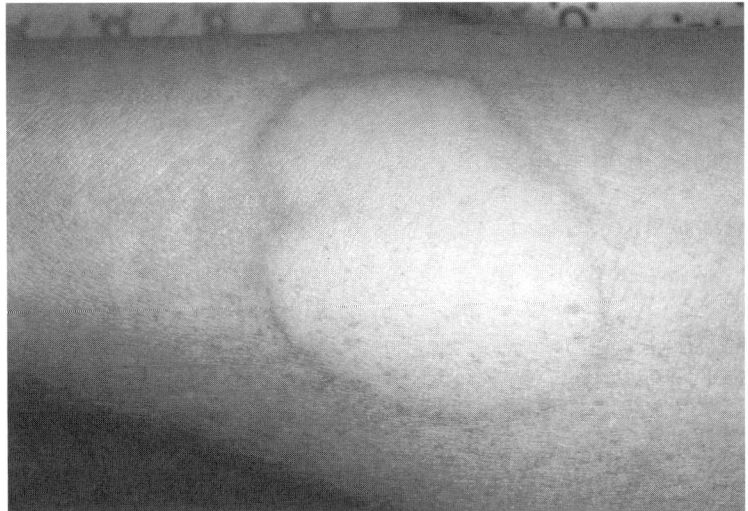

Figure 10-2. After an ice cube is placed on the forearm of an affected athlete, a square urticarial plaque is observed.

to trigger cold urticaria and its systemic findings; therefore, drowning is a serious concern.

Diagnosis

To confirm the diagnosis, a clinician can place an ice cube on the athlete's skin for 5 minutes. Upon rewarming, a hive developing in the area where the ice cube was placed signals a positive test result (Figure 10-2) (Table 10-1) (Adams, 2001a). Use of varying temperatures of water still may be necessary to confirm the diagnosis if the result of the ice cube test is negative (Pharis et al., 1997).

Treatment

Antihistamines should be given to athletes with cold urticaria (Adams, 2001b). The clinician must be wary about the secondary causes for cold urticaria and the need to treat the underlying condition.

Prevention

Protective clothing should be worn by susceptible athletes who will be exposed to outdoor winter environments. Several authors have noted that oral cyproheptadine hydrochloride is the antihistamine of choice to prevent cold urticaria. Elite swimmers who have used this particular antihistamine have been able to continue competition in cool pools (Briner, 1993).

Dermatographism

Epidemiology

One study showed that 17% of athletes with physical urticaria had dermatographism, which is the third most common urticaria in athletes (Mikhailov et al., 1977). This condition has formally been reported in football players, but any athlete can develop dermatographism. In one report, football players seemingly had dermatographism under rubbing equipment pads (Briner, 1993). Athletes with dermatographism acquire hives when the skin is scratched or vigorously rubbed. People with this condition are believed to have sensitive mast cells that degranulate upon trauma to the skin.

Clinical Presentation

Distinctive edematous, erythematous, well-defined plaques occur in the areas of trauma within seconds and dissipate soon thereafter (Figure 10-3).

Diagnosis

Scratching the athlete's back and observing the typical wheal confirm the diagnosis.

Treatment

The treatment of dermatographism rests mainly in its prevention.

Prevention

Several oral antihistamines have been suggested for prevention, including hydroxyzine, diphenhydramine, and cyproheptadine (Adams, 2001b; Briner, 1993).

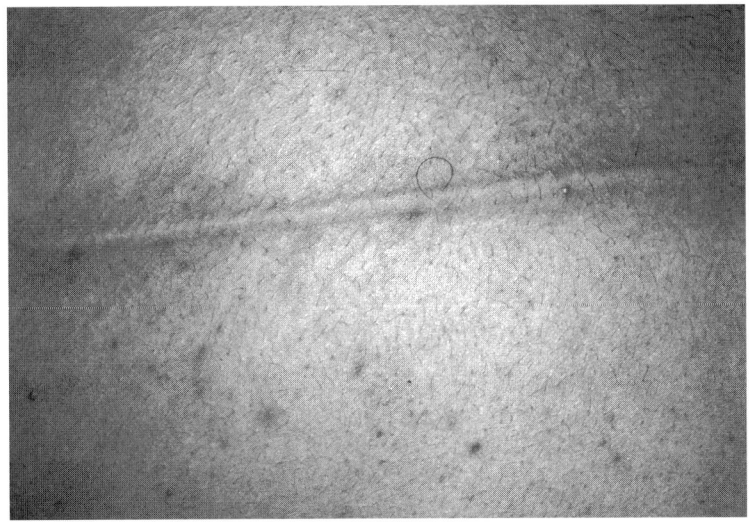

Figure 10-3. Linear and erythematous wheals illustrate dermatographism.

Solar Urticaria

Epidemiology

Solar urticaria is an uncommon cause of physical urticaria in athletes. Seven percent of athletes with urticaria had solar urticaria. No specific sport type has been identified as placing athletes more at risk. Clearly any outdoor sport with exposure to ultraviolet rays places athletes at risk for developing solar urticaria if they were genetically predisposed. Females are more likely to have solar urticaria. The median age of onset is 25 years, but many cases occur very early or much later in life.

Clinical Presentation

Solar urticaria is induced by ultraviolet A, ultraviolet B, or visible light. The history of lesion development is highly characteristic. Exposed skin develops hives within minutes of exposure to the light source, and the hives resolve spontaneously in 1 hour. The lesions typically are distributed on sun-exposed areas of the skin that are not constantly exposed to the sun. Individual lesions are well-

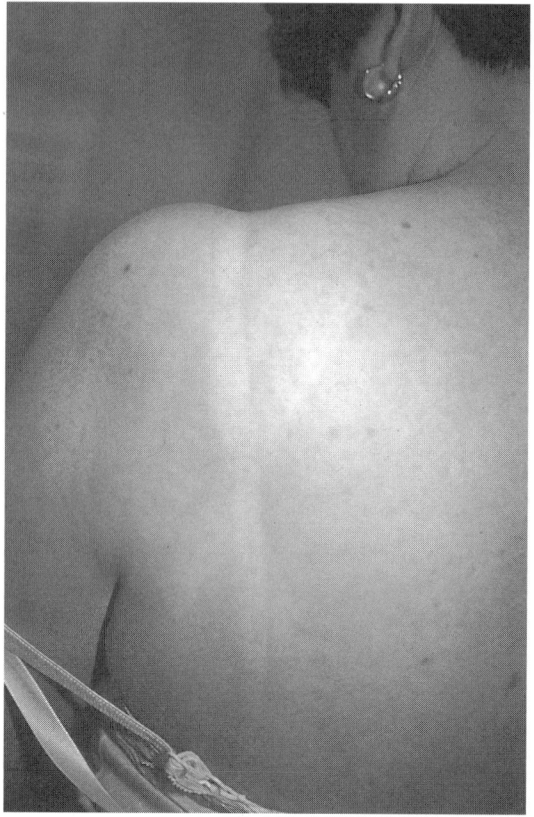

Figure 10-4. Erythematous and edematous plaques develop on sun-exposed skin minutes after exposure to ultraviolet light.

defined, erythematous, edematous papules and plaques (Figures 10-4 and 10-5). Systemic findings are uncommon but may include headache, nausea, and, very rarely, respiratory distress.

Diagnosis

The history given by the athlete with solar urticaria should clinch the diagnosis, but phototesting can be used to confirm the diagnosis (Figure 10-6) (Table 10-1). Athletes with solar urticaria will not only develop hives in areas tested but display a reaction at much lower doses of ultraviolet radiation than expected for their skin type.

10. Pruritus and Urticaria 189

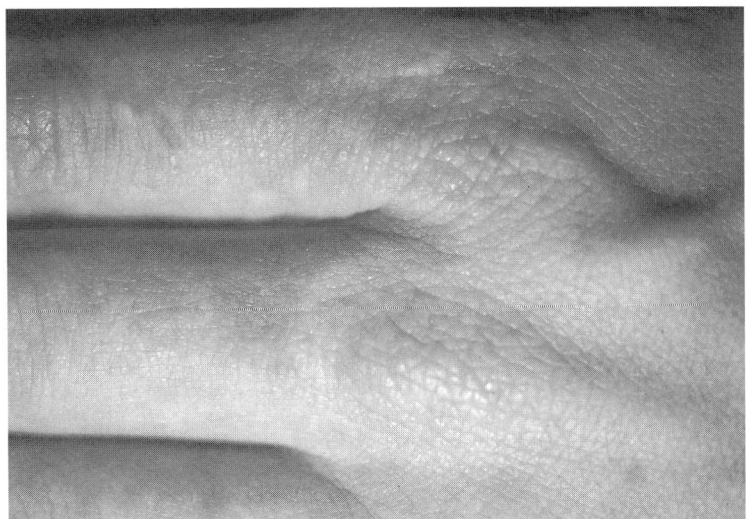

Figure 10-5. Erythematous, edematous plaques develop on sun-exposed skin minutes after exposure to ultraviolet light.

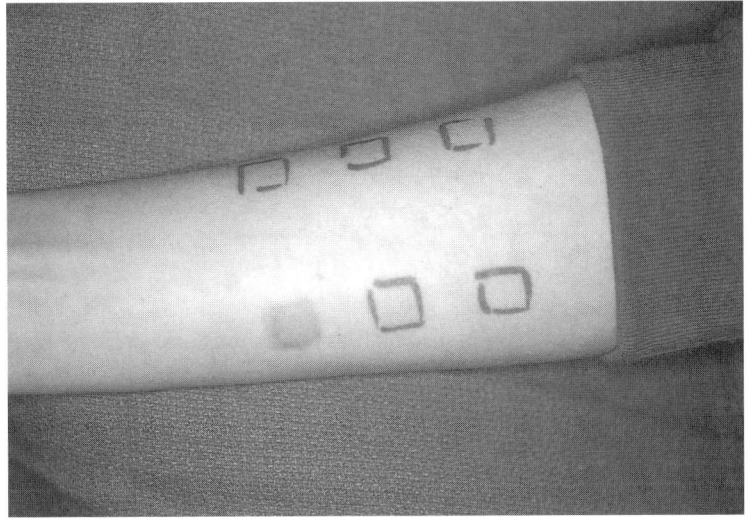

Figure 10-6. Phototesting confirms the diagnosis of solar urticaria.

Treatment

Antihistamines can be tried but are not universally effective. In the case of solar urticaria, the best therapy is a good defense with sunscreen. Spontaneous remission often occurs after several years.

Prevention

The key to therapy is broadband sunscreen that blocks both ultraviolet A and ultraviolet B. Athletes should attempt to use clothing as much as practical to block the ultraviolet radiation. Antimalarial agents have been successful in some cases (Adams, 2001a). Clinicians may consult with an expert dermatologist who may be able to prevent outbreaks by desensitizing the athlete. The dermatologist will expose the athlete to ever-increasing doses of ultraviolet radiation. It is important to remind the athlete whose solar urticaria is induced by ultraviolet A that ultraviolet A radiation passes through windows.

Aquagenic Urticaria

Epidemiology

True aquagenic urticaria is exceedingly rare. Most cases of suspected aquagenic urticaria are actually cold urticaria related to water temperature. Aquagenic urticaria was first reported in 1964, but only a handful of cases have been reported since (Panconesi and Lotti, 1987). At-risk sports include any sport that involves water exposure.

Clinical Presentation

Why water causes hives in some athletes is not clear. Some authors suggest that water mixes with sebum, creating a substance that induces histamine release from mast cells (Nichols. 1999).

Athletes with the condition note distinct, intensely pruritic, small (1-to 3-mm), well-defined, erythematous, edematous papules. The lesions may appear very similar to the hives seen in cholinergic urticaria. The lesions occur most commonly on the neck, trunk, and arms and appear relatively soon after contact with water (2–30 minutes). Pruritus precedes the hives. The water temperature is not involved in the production of the hives.

Diagnosis

The diagnosis of aquagenic urticaria is a serious one and must be differentiated from aquagenic pruritus, cold urticaria, and cholinergic urticaria. Athletes with aquagenic pruritus do not develop hives. Unlike cold urticaria, direct contact with ice will not create hives in an athlete with aquagenic urticaria. Intradermal injections of acetylcholine will not produce hives in athletes with aquagenic urticaria, so this test may be helpful to distinguish aquagenic from cholinergic urticaria (Panconesi and Lotti, 1987).

To confirm the diagnosis, the clinician can apply a warm-water compress at 35°C to the athlete's back. If an urticarial plaque forms in the area, the patient has aquagenic urticaria. This procedure takes less than 30 minutes (Table 10-1).

Treatment

Antihistamines are not universally effective for athletes with aquagenic urticaria.

Prevention

Inert oily substances can be applied to areas that will come in contact with water. This protective barrier decreases the penetration of water into the athlete's skin (Panconesi and Lotti, 1987).

Contact Urticaria

Epidemiology

One case report of contact urticaria exists (Neering, 1977). At-risk sports include diving, synchronized swimming, swimming, water polo, watersliding, scuba diving, and jet skiing.

Clinical Presentation

Swimmers allergic to chlorine may develop urticarial plaques on submerged surfaces 1 to 5 hours after exposure.

Diagnosis

The diagnosis of contact urticaria can be very challenging because the condition can be mistaken for aquagenic pruritus, cold urticaria, or aquagenic urticaria. Patch tests with NaOCL and $CaOCL_2$ are positive after several hours. None of the other types of sports-related urticaria demonstrate a positive patch test.

Treatment

Antihistamines can be tried.

Prevention

Inert oily substances can be applied to areas that will come in contact with water. This protective barrier decreases the penetration of water into the athlete's skin (Panconesi and Lotti, 1987).

Traumatic Plantar Urticaria

Epidemiology

Five cases of this unusual skin condition were originally reported in 1988 (Metzker and Brodsky, 1988). Basketball players and runners seem particularly susceptible.

Clinical Presentation

Five children aged 8 to 11 years developed sudden pain on the soles after playing basketball or running while wearing sneakers. The pain was limited to the soles and continued to increase over 3 to 4 days. Examination reveals very tender, well-defined, small (<0.5 cm), erythematous to violaceous macules and papules on the soles of both feet.

Diagnosis

The diagnosis of traumatic plantar urticaria is challenging and the uniqueness of the condition may be questioned; however, a sufficient number of characteristic findings probably differentiate it from other similar conditions in athletes. Biopsy is required to help differentiate it from other conditions. Biopsy reveals perivascular neutrophilic infiltration in the superficial and deep dermis in the acute stage. Results of all systemic tests are normal. The differential diagnosis includes painful piezogenic pedal papules that appear as skin-colored to white protrusions on the heel. Neutrophilic eccrine hidradenitis may appear morphologically similar on the feet with similar pain after physical activity. Biopsy also reveals neutrophils, but in this case the infiltrate is concentrated around the eccrine glands. Delayed pressure urticaria may have a similar appearance (Figure 10-7), but the limited anatomic involvement, resolution with rest, and low recurrence rate of traumatic plantar urticaria seem to help differentiate it and support its unique diagnosis.

Treatment

The lesions and symptoms spontaneously regress after the physical activity is discontinued.

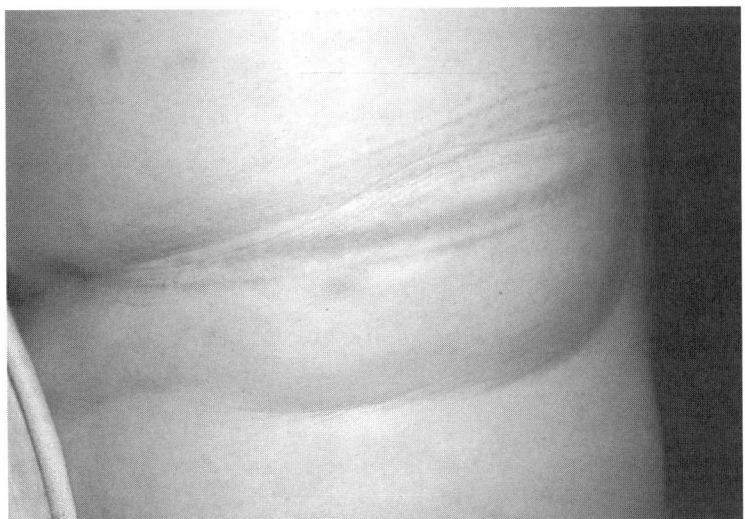

Figure 10-7. Pressure urticaria may occur in creases of skin, as in catchers.

Prevention

No adequate prevention exists. It does not always recur.

Bibliography

Adams BB. Sports dermatology. Adolesc Med 2001a;12:305–322.
Adams BB. Sports dermatology. Dermatol Nurs 2001b;13:347–363.
Briner WW. Physical allergies and exercise. Sport Med 1993;15:365–373.
Hirschmann JV, Lawlor F, English JSC, et al. Cholinergic urticaria. Arch Dermatol 1987;123:462–467.
Metzker A, Brodsky F. Traumatic plantar urticaria—an unrecognized entity? J Am Acad Dermatol 1988;18:144–146.
Mikhailov P, Berova N, Andreev VC. Physical urticaria and sport. Cutis 1977;20:381–390.
Momas I, Brette F, Spinasse A, et al. Health effects of attending a public swimming pool. J Epidemiol Commun Health 1993;47:464–468.
Neering H. Contact urticaria from chlorinated swimming pool water. Contact Dermatitis 1977;3:279.
Nichols AW. Nonorthopaedic problems in the aquatic athlete. Clin Sports Med 1999;18:395–411.
Panconesi E, Lotti T. Aquagenic urticaria. Clin Dermatol 1987;5:49–51.
Pharis DB, Teller C, Wolf JE. Cutaneous manifestations of sports participation. J Am Acad Dermatol 1997;36:448–459.
Sarnaik AP, Vohra MP, Sturman SW, et al. Medical problems of the swimmer. Clin Sports Med 1986;5:47–64.
Steinman HK. Water-induced pruritus. Clin Dermatol 1987;5:41.

11. Exercise-Induced Angioedema/Anaphylaxis

This last chapter on sports-related inflammatory reactions discusses probably one of the only potential sports dermatology-related emergencies. Athletes with a predisposition for exercise-induced angioedema/anaphylaxis (EIA) must be extremely cautious because their participation in exercise may lead to respiratory or vascular collapse. It is important to remember that the term exercise-induced "anaphylaxis" is found throughout the literature, but its nomenclature is a bit misleading. This condition represents a spectrum of disease, and many authors draw parallels with cholinergic urticaria discussed in Chapter 10. Not all athletes with this disease present with vascular or respiratory collapse.

Exercise-Induced Angioedema/Anaphylaxis

Epidemiology

Runners seem particularly prone to develop EIA. One study of 278 athletes with the disease noted that 78% experienced outbreaks while running (Shadick et al., 1999). A wide variety of athletes with the condition are reported, including cyclists, downhill skiers, and basketball, handball, racquetball, and tennis players (Adams, 2004; Nichols, 1992; Shadick et al., 1999; Sheffer and Austen, 1980). It is possible that runners have disproportionately developed EIA because there are a greater numbers of runners. Although most runners exhibit symptoms after at least moderate activity, some runners develop signs and symptoms with even mild exertion. The mean age of onset of the disease was between 4 and 74 years (mean age 25 years). Females are more likely than males to develop EIA (ratio 2:1).

The cause of EIA is unclear. The symptoms of EIA are believed to result from histaminemia after mast cell degranulation (Nichols, 1992; Sheffer and Austen, 1984). The cause of this degranulation is debatable. The list of possible degranulating promoters includes creatinine phosphokinase, immunoglobulin E, and lactate (Nichols, 1992; Sheffer and Austen, 1980). Activation of the alternative complement pathway also may be a factor (Stephansson et al., 1991).

Clinical Presentation

Several authors noted a range of signs and symptoms in EIA (Adams, 2002, 2004; Shadick et al., 1999). More than 90% of patients complain of pruritus.

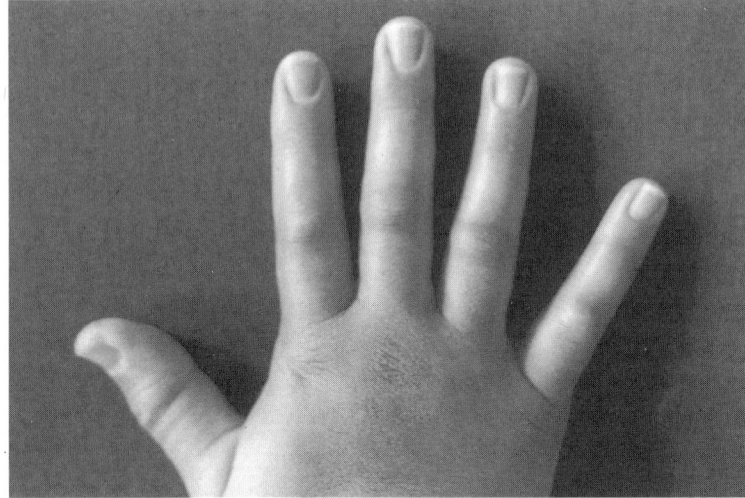

Figure 11-1. Athletes with exercise-induced angioedema/anaphylaxis may demonstrate diffuse angioedema on the hands.

Urticaria is present in 86% of athletes. Angioedema occurs in 70% to 80% of cases and typically is located on the face, palms, and hands (Figure 11-1). Respiratory symptoms are found in nearly half of the athletes with evanescent wheezing. One third of athletes develop chest tightness and syncope. Less commonly (25%), athletes experience nausea, diarrhea, and hoarseness. Headache and flushing are seen.

Symptoms can begin within the first 5 minutes of exercise but also can start after exercise is completed. Typical angioedema usually persists, but the angioedema related to EIA resolves in 30 minutes to 4 hours. EIA-related headaches might persist for days.

Diagnosis

The diagnosis of EIA is based on a constellation of clinical findings, including angioedema and pruritus, with or without respiratory or vascular collapse. No serologic test can confirm EIA. Patients with angioedema and at least mental status changes, laryngeal edema or hypotension should rapidly be recognized as having EIA and emergently referred for appropriate care.

The differential diagnosis primarily includes cholinergic urticaria (Table 11-1). Athletes with cholinergic urticaria may, like those with EIA, present with respiratory distress. The two conditions differ in two major ways.

Table 11-1. Differentiating Exercise-Induced Angioedema/Anaphylaxis from Cholinergic Urticaria

Disease	Complaint	Findings on Physical Examination
Cholinergic urticaria	Shortness of breath Skin rash	1. Expiratory lung wheezes 2. Small discrete red papules 3. Appropriate blood pressure 4. Appropriate heart rate
Exercise-induced angioedema/ anaphylaxis	Shortness of breath Skin rash Lightheaded Heart racing	1. Inspiratory stridor at larynx 2. Large areas of angioedema 3. Hypotension 4. Tachycardia

EIA exhibits angioedema, whereas cholinergic urticaria produces smaller (few mm to 1 cm), discrete, erythematous papules that may or may not coalesce into larger plaques. Second, although both conditions may present with respiratory distress, the reason for dyspnea in cholinergic urticaria stems from bronchospasm (Adams, 2004), whereas laryngeal edema causes shortness of breath in EIA. Hypotension occurs only in EIA. It is important to distinguish vascular and respiratory difficulties related to EIA from those related to participation in the sport itself, such as overexertion in hot and humid conditions during a marathon. Another slightly more subtle way to distinguish the two conditions is the fact that sweating seems to exacerbate cholinergic urticaria but has little effect on EIA (Sayama et al., 2002). Furthermore, simple passive warming will not induce EIA but may induce cholinergic urticaria. Provocative tests may be necessary to confirm the diagnosis. Some authors have used a test of cold stimulation before and after exercise to confirm the diagnosis of cold-dependent exercise-induced anaphylaxis in athletes (Sayama et al., 2002).

A condition called *vibratory angioedema* should be included in the differential diagnosis of EIA. Vibratory angioedema, reported in runners, presents with angioedema alone on the thighs and no associated systemic manifestations (Adams, 2002; Lawlor et al., 1989; Patterson et al., 1972). Like EIA, the angioedema in this sports-related variant does not persist and is caused by the constant vibration experienced during running.

Treatment

The primary treatment for EIA must resolve any respiratory or cardiovascular collapse. Athletes may require oxygen, intravenous fluids, and transfer to an emergency facility if an airway cannot be maintained. The subacute treatment of EIA includes antihistamines and epinephrine (Adams, 2002; Sheffer, 1980). No solid evidence indicates β-agonist inhalers or corticosteroids are helpful.

Table 11-2. Critical History Questions to Ask the Athlete with Suspected Exercise-Induced Angioedema/Anaphylaxis

---

Do you experience exercise-induced angioedema/anaphylaxis flares more frequently when you . . .

1. Exercise in very cold or very hot conditions?
2. Eat certain foods before exercising?
3. Take aspirin, ibuprofen (or other nonsteroidal antiinflammatory drugs), or antibiotics before exercising?

Interestingly, more than 25% of athletes with EIA do not use medicine to manage their disease (Shadick et al., 1999).

Prevention

Prevention of EIA is crucial given its potential serious consequences. Obviously avoiding exercise will prevent EIA; however, special techniques make continued participation possible. Several factors increase the risk that an athlete with a predisposition for EIA will develop signs and symptoms (Adams, 2002; Nichols, 1992; Shadick et al., 1999). Approximately 50% of athletes can prevent EIA attacks by not exercising in extreme hot or cold temperatures. Thirty percent of athletes can exercise without difficulty by not eating before their activity. Several foods are particularly implicated, such as barley, beans, broccoli, cheese, chicken, egg, garlic, grapes, lettuce, peaches, peanuts, rye, shellfish, tomatoes, and wheat (Adams, 2004). Ingestion of various medicines is associated with EIA flares. These medicines include aspirin, β-lactam antibiotics, and nonsteroidal antiinflammatory drugs. It is important for athletes to avoid these products before competing (Table 11-2).

Regular use of antihistamines seems prudent during exercise and is recommended by many authors, although no evidence-based data support this practice (Adams, 2002; Briner and Sheffer, 1992; Kato et al., 1997; Fisher et al., 1999). Ketotifen has been used to prevent the angioedema of EIA (Nichols, 1992), and cromolyn has been used to help prevent respiratory symptoms of EIA (Adams, 2002; Briner, 1993; Katz et al., 1989).

Athletes with EIA do not experience its signs and symptoms each time they exercise and may have a false sense of security. Afflicted athletes should not practice alone and should be cautioned to carry an epinephrine injectable.

Bibliography

Adams BB. Exercise-induced anaphylaxis in a marathon runner. Int J Dermatol 2002;41:394–396.

Adams ES. Identifying and controlling metabolic skin disorders. Phys Sportsmed 2004;32:29–40.

Briner WW, Sheffer AL. Exercise-induced anaphylaxis. Med Sci Sports Exerc 1992;24:849–850.

Briner WW. Physical allergies and exercise: clinical implications for those engaged in sports activities. Sports Med 1993;15:365–373.

Fisher AA. Sports-related cutaneous reactions: part I. Dermatoses due to physical agents. Cutis 1999;63:134–136.

Kato T, Komatsu H, Tagami H. Exercise-induced urticaria and angioedema. J Dermatol 1997;24:189–192.

Katz RM. Exercise-induced asthma/other allergic reactions in the athlete. Allergy Proc 1989;10:203–208.

Lawlor F, Black AK, Breathnach AS, et al. Vibratory angioedema: lesion induction, clinical features, laboratory and ultrastructural findings and response to therapy. Br J Dermatol 1989;120:93–99.

Nichols AW. Exercise-induced anaphylaxis and urticaria. Clin Sports Med 1992;11:303–312.

Patterson R, Mellies CJ, Blankenship ML, et al. Vibratory angioedema: a hereditary type of physical hypersensitivity. J Allergy Clin Immunol 1972;50:174–182.

Sayama M, Tohyama M, Hashimoto K. A case of cold-dependent exercise-induced anaphylaxis. Br J Dermatol 2002;147:368–370.

Shadick NA, Liang MH, Partridge AJ, et al. The natural history of exercise induced anaphylaxis: survey results from a 10-year follow-up study. J Allergy Clin Immunol 1999;104:123–127.

Sheffer AL, Austen KF. Exercise-induced anaphylaxis. J Allergy Clin Immunol 1980;66:106–111.

Sheffer AL, Austen KF. Exercise-induced anaphylaxis J Allergy Clin Immunol 1984;73:699–703.

Stephansson E, Koskimies S, Lokki M. Exercise-induced urticaria and anaphylaxis. Ann Dermatol Venereol 1991;71:138–142.

Section IV Sports-Related Traumatic Conditions

12. Friction Injuries to the Skin

This chapter begins Section IV on sports-related traumatic conditions. This section discusses the most common cause of all skin conditions in athletes, namely, trauma. This trauma most frequently affects the skin but does not spare the nails and hair. Although these cutaneous problems are the most common, they often are viewed as "just part of playing the game." Occasionally, however, athletes' performances are influenced by skin trauma. Although trauma will always be a part of the game, the athlete need not endure the results of trauma given the available methods of treatment and prevention.

Trauma comes from a variety of forces, which most often combine to create skin disease. However, for the sake of discussion, the predominating force causing skin disease categorizes each skin problem. *Pressure,* sufficient to cause skin and nail problems, generally occurs between athletes and their equipment. Chapter 14 of this section reviews the skin and nail changes in the athlete resulting from acute and chronic pressure forces. *Pounding trauma* tends to produce nail disease. Chapter 15 discusses pounding injuries to the nails. Some skin ailments in athletes result from a *combination of factors* (e.g., as seen in acne mechanica), as analyzed in Chapter 16.

Friction probably is the most common offending force to the athlete's skin and hair. Chronic frictional forces that create hair problems are discussed in Chapter 13. This first chapter in the section reviews the vast variety of skin problems related to acute and chronic friction. Some of the conditions are common to nearly all athletes, such as abrasions, blisters, callosities, and lacerations. On the other hand, many cutaneous conditions are specifically related to a specific sporting activity, such as powerlifter's patches.

Abrasions and Chafing
Epidemiology

Chafing and abrasions occur in 0.4% to 16% of marathon runners who present to the medical tent (Mailler and Adams, 2004). Authors have identified several sports with specific abrasions (Table 12-1). Scuba divers who are underwater for long periods develop significant chafing in the axillae, collar, groin, popliteal fossa, wrists, and along the seams of the suit. Skiers develop abrasions on the skin over the mid-tibia resulting from friction when skiers lean into their rigid ski boots. Water tubers develop abrasions on their hands, arms, and chest. In track and field, hurdlers and steeplechase runners may not make it cleanly over hurdles. Athletes abrade their skin not only on the track as they fall but also on the spikes of nearby competitors. Platform divers experience many abrasions

Table 12-1. Epidemiology of Abrasions and Lacerations in Several Sports

Sport or Event	Laceration Rate of Total Injuries	Abrasion Rate of Total Injuries	Total Affected Athletes (Lacerations)	Total Affected Athletes (Abrasions)
Cycling				
Mountain	65%, 75% (combined)	65%, 75% (combined)	41.5%	65.3%
Non-BMX	16.6%, 18%, 42%	9%, 28%	—	—
Road racing	16%	49%	11.5%	72.1%
BMX	6.9%	42.6%	—	—
Gymnastics	2%		0.7%	—
Hockey (ice)	13%		—	—
Ice skating	16%, 20%		0.5%	—
In-line skating (rollerblading)	—	—	—	18.4%, 31%, 67%
Junior Olympics (1985)	3%			
Nordic ski jumping	4.2%, 4.3%	1.4%, 13.9%	6.4%, 6.8%	2.2%, 22.1%
Nordic skiing	7.8%, 9%, 10%, 11%, 12%	—	—	—
Soccer	3.3%			
Tennis	—	—	0.2%	1%
Track and field	—	—	2.4%	—

on their hands as a result of contact with the rough-surfaced platform as they push off to dive into the pool. Wrestlers commonly acquire mat burns as they rotate and push on the mats. Friction between the skin and any other surface (e.g., other skin, including their own) results in abrasions. Skin-to-skin related abrasions occur most commonly when the skin is moist and macerated.

Clinical Presentation

Most often abrasions are superficial and involve only the topmost layers of the epidermis (Figure 12-1, see color plate). Skin-to-skin abrasions (chafing) appear in the intertriginous areas such as the groin and axillae. Skin abrasions from the playing surface commonly occur on the upper and lower extremities (especially the knees and elbows). When a large abrasion occurs with scattered pinpoints of bleeding (representing exposure of the superficial dermal papillae), the lesion is affectionately called a *raspberry* or *strawberry.*

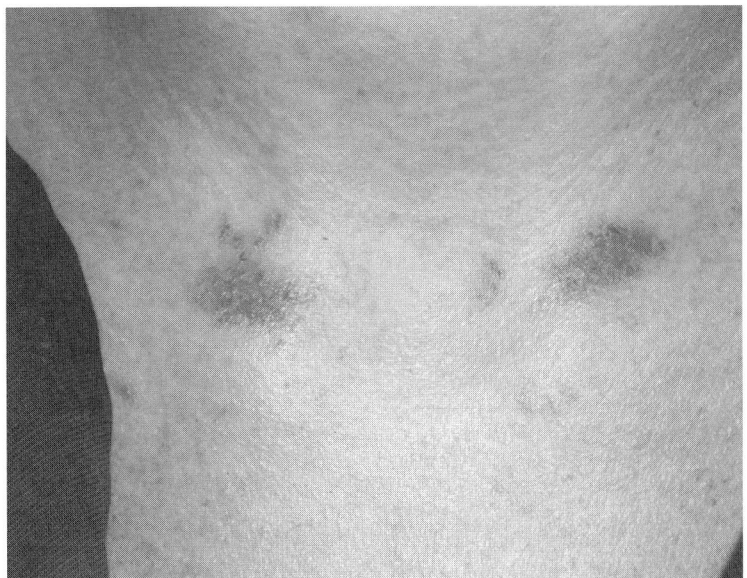

Figure 12-1. Symmetrical abrasions developed over a marathoner's upper chest as a result of friction from her running top. (See color plate.)

Diagnosis

The diagnosis is straightforward.

Treatment

Initial wounds should be cleaned as soon as possible. It is best to clean these abrasions with lukewarm tap water and a mild soap such as Lever 2000. Soap is not necessary for clean wounds (i.e., as occur with chafing). Flushing debris from the wound with a water-filled syringe is preferable to scrubbing with a cloth, brush, or other instrument. These objects can cause increased mechanical trauma to the viable tissue. For this same reason, hydrogen peroxide should not be used.

It is important to assess the pain level before debridement. Moderate or greater pain may necessitate injection of lidocaine 2% with epinephrine before thorough debridement. For decades dermatologists and dermatologic surgeons have safely used epinephrine on the nose, ears, feet, and hands. Epinephrine should *not* be used (or it should be used with great caution) on the penis or the distal tips of the fingers.

Once a wound is clean and tolerant of manipulation, the clinician should achieve hemostasis using aluminum chloride 20%. This solution stings but remarkably curtails bleeding by causing vasoconstriction. In rare cases where this substance does not work, the clinician should sparingly apply Monsel solution to the wound. The downside to this solution, which causes local clotting, is that the solution can permanently stain the skin.

Subsequent to cleaning, controlling pain, and stopping bleeding, the clinician must cover the wound. Moist wounds heal better and faster than dry and scabbed wounds. Every effort should be made to ensure that a wound does not desiccate. Chafing areas require topical antibiotic ointments or petroleum jelly. Moderate-potency topical steroids can significantly decrease any associated irritation.

Multiple surgical dressings for wounds are available and have various advantages and disadvantages. For very simple small abrasions, clinicians can apply cyanoacrylate to the area. A thin layer of this glue will keep the underlying abrasion moist and protected from the environment. The traditional method has been to cover the wound with Polysporin ointment or petroleum jelly, followed by a nonadherent barrier such as a Telfa pad. To keep the Telfa pad in place, Kerlix (gauze roll) can be wrapped around the area and taped to itself. Clinicians may need to lightly apply Coban (self-adherent wrap) if the injured area experiences a great deal of movement. This dressing must be changed at least daily.

More modern coverings include semipermeable and hydrocolloid dressings. These dressings speed healing and decrease scarring. Both can be left on the skin for prolonged periods (even up to 5–7 days). For this reason, the dressings must be applied to clean wounds; however, not uncommonly the dressings come off in 3 days. Clinicians should remove the dressing and replace it with another if excess exudate is present. Tegaderm is a type of semipermeable dressing that keeps the wound moist; bacteria and water cannot penetrate it and wound exudate evaporates. It is important to warn athletes that accumulation of colored fluid under the dressing is normal. On the other hand, hydrocolloid dressings absorb excess exudate and offer more protection because they are thicker than semipermeable dressings.

Tetanus shots should be given to individuals who cannot remember their last immunization for tetanus or those who last received a tetanus shot more than 10 years ago. If the wound is major or is not clean, tetanus shots should be given to athletes who last received their tetanus shot 5 or more years ago. In most athletic leagues, bleeding must be stopped and the lesion covered before the athlete may return to play.

Prevention

Athletes with chafing should use drying powders to decrease sweating in problem areas. These athletes also can apply petroleum jelly (or combination products, such as lanolin and benzocaine ("runner's lube") or aloe vera and natural wax ("Bodyglide")) to friction-prone areas. Synthetic moisture-wicking underclothes help to prevent chafing. Basketball players, cyclists, rowers (of all types), and runners can wear Lycra biking tights to prevent chafing. To prevent abrasions related to contact with the playing field, athletes can wear elbow pads, kneepads, and helmets. Education is still needed, as several studies note that at least 50% of in-line skaters (rollerbladers) do not wear any protective equipment. Skiers can place padding between their anterior shin and the rigid boot to decrease abrasions.

Archery Arms

Epidemiology

One small case series in archers is reported (Rayan, 1992).

Clinical Presentation

During an arrow launch, the bowstring recoils to the bow with great velocity. Repeated trauma between the recoiling bowstring and the volar aspect of the forearm holding the bow produces a well-defined, edematous, erythematous, variably eroded patch. Eventually, ecchymotic patches develop in the same area.

Diagnosis

The diagnosis is made clinically while obtaining the history of archery activity.

Treatment

The affected area requires topical petroleum jelly or topical antibiotic ointments (e.g., Polysporin or silver sulfadiazine). Warm-water soaks for 5 to 10 minutes several times per day assuage symptoms. Moderate-potency topical steroids can be used for a brief period if pruritus or irritation is present. Nonsteroidal antiinflammatory drugs also may be required, depending on the pain.

Prevention

Arm guards attached to the volar aspect of the arm protect it from repeated bowstring insults.

Bicyclist's Nipples

Epidemiology

Unlike its counterpart, jogger's nipples, no epidemiologic studies on bicyclist's nipples are available. In contrast to jogger's nipples, which are caused by friction, bicyclist's nipples result from thermal injury (Powell, 1983).

Clinical Presentation

Sweat, rain, and the intense wind chill (inherent with high bike speeds) combine to cause very tender, erythematous nipples. This eruption reflects cold damage to the nipples.

Diagnosis

The diagnosis is straightforward. The nipple is very sensitive to temperature changes.

Treatment

Treatment may include petroleum jelly or topical antibiotics and warm compresses.

Prevention

Prevention is paramount. The first layer of clothing should be composed of moisture-wicking synthetic material. The outermost clothing must be wind and rain resistant.

Bullae

Epidemiology

Although nearly every athlete, from the neophyte to the professional, suffers from blisters (bullae), their epidemiology, specifically on the feet, is well investigated in military personnel and marathon runners. The prevalence of blisters in military personnel, especially new recruits, is greater than 40% (Ressman, 1975). More than 20 studies on the prevalence of bullae have investigated marathon runners in the past three decades. The range of prevalence is between 0.2% and 25% of marathoners, with a median of 16%, which probably is the best estimation. The large range results from different study methodologies (Mailler and Adams, 2004).

Several clinicians have noticed the development of small painful blisters on the fingers of the throwing hand of baseball and softball pitchers. This condition is related to the fact that these pitchers experience great frictional forces especially when they apply torque to the ball to alter its rotation (e.g., the curve ball). Kayakers and canoers develop "soft skin" related to their repeated water immersions. This "soft skin" predisposes the athlete to blisters. Blisters are the most common injury noted in tennis players at the US Open.

Blisters are caused by constant friction between the skin and the shoe and sock or, in the case of hands, between the skin and equipment. The probability of blister formation is related to both the magnitude of the frictional force and the number of times an object cycles across the epidermis. This friction creates a split in the epidermis always in the granular layer (the layer just beneath the stratum corneum, which is the topmost layer of skin) or just beneath it. This space then fills with transudate and sweat from the body, forming a blister (Akers and Sulzberger, 1972). If the stratum corneum is not particularly thick or is held tightly to underlying structures, as it is on the palms and soles, then friction may lead to an erosion rather than a fluid-filled blister.

Several factors can influence the production of these blisters. Moist epidermis is more likely to become a blister after it is exposed to shearing forces. Very dry skin and very wet skin decrease the frictional forces. Increased temperatures also are related to increasing probability of blister production. Athletic footwear worn during sporting activities creates these environmental conditions. Ill-fitting footwear worsens the situation by increasing shearing forces (Levine, 1982). Duration and intensity of activity are other important factors.

Clinical Presentation

Athletes generally can sense early blisters as areas experiencing sufficient shearing forces. Athletes who sense warm areas occasionally refer to the lesions as *hot spots* (Figure 12-2). Mature blisters are well-defined bulla with peripheral tender erythema. Occasionally the blister cavity also fills with blood, appearing dark brown to black. Even the mature blister may not be self-evident or may appear "deep," especially on very thick skin. In this scenario, the blister cleft is still located at the granular layer.

After 6 hours, the cells in the blister base begin to actively repair the damaged skin. By 48 hours, a new granular layer is formed, and by 5 days the repair mechanism slows down and a new stratum corneum is formed.

Diagnosis

The diagnosis usually is not in question. Very early blisters may appear as tender, erythematous macules or patches. It is important to identify underlying disorders that place athletes at risk for blisters on their feet. For example, not uncommonly the genetic blistering disorder epidermolysis bullosa simplex (Weber-Cockayne) presents initially when young basketball players get many severe blisters on the soles. In addition, it is important to exclude bony abnormalities such as hammertoe deformity, which can predispose the athlete to friction blisters over the dorsal aspects of the foot.

Color Plate   I

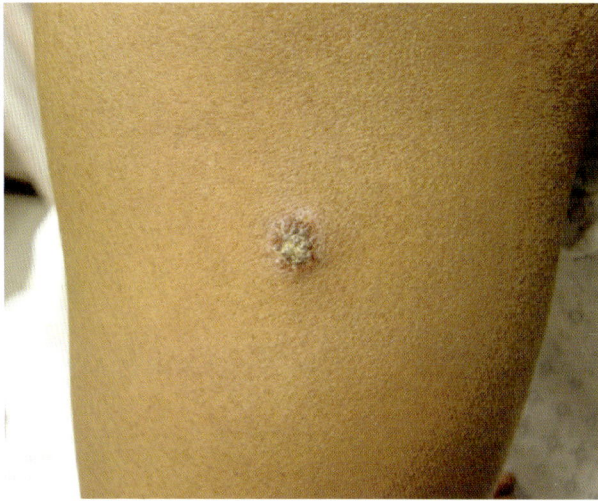

Figure 1-1. Well-defined, erythematous, centrally crusted papule characteristic of impetigo located on an arm.

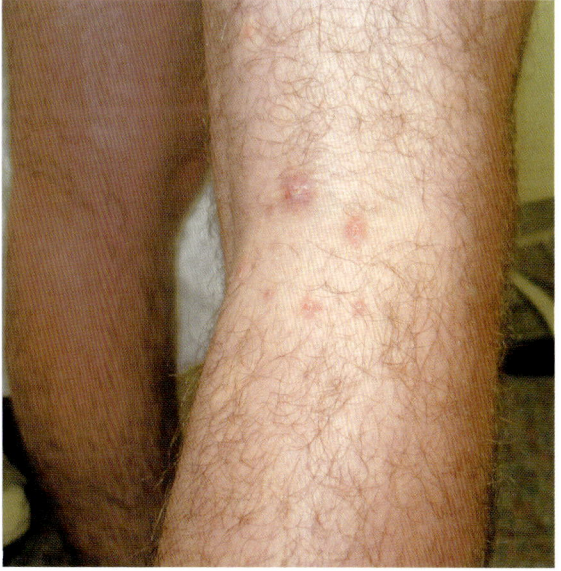

Figure 1-4. Well-defined, scattered, red, follicular papules and pustules that are classic for folliculitis occurring under occlusive knee pads.

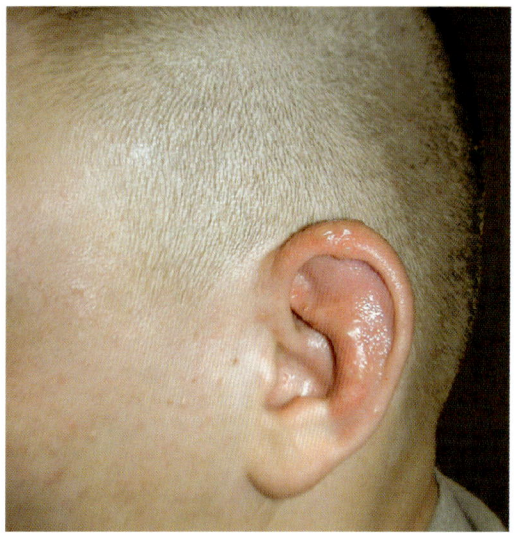

Figure 2-2. Grouped vesicles on an erythematous base are characteristic of herpes gladiatorum or herpes rugbeiorum. The ears are commonly affected in wrestlers.

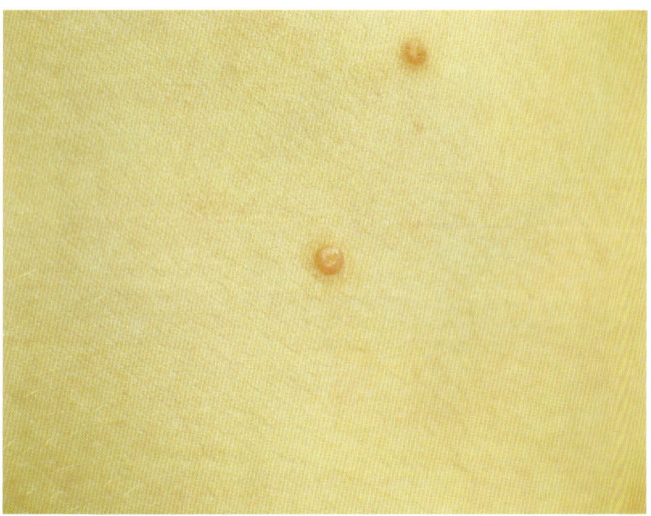

Figure 2-5. Molluscum contagiosum is characterized by a white well-circumscribed papule with a central dell.

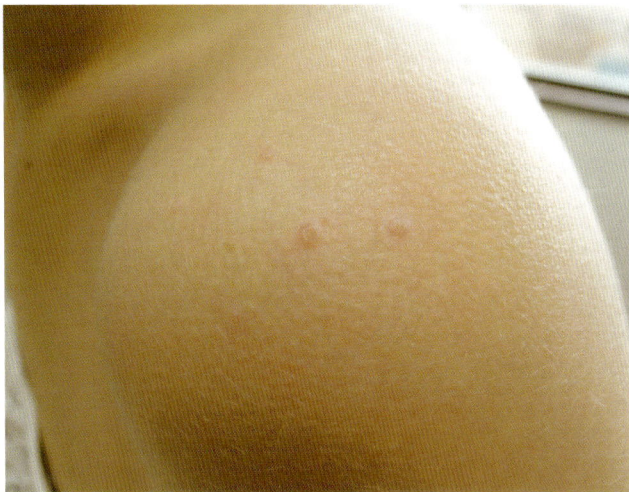

Figure 2-6. Very small lesions of molluscum contagiosum not uncommonly mimic folliculitis in athletes.

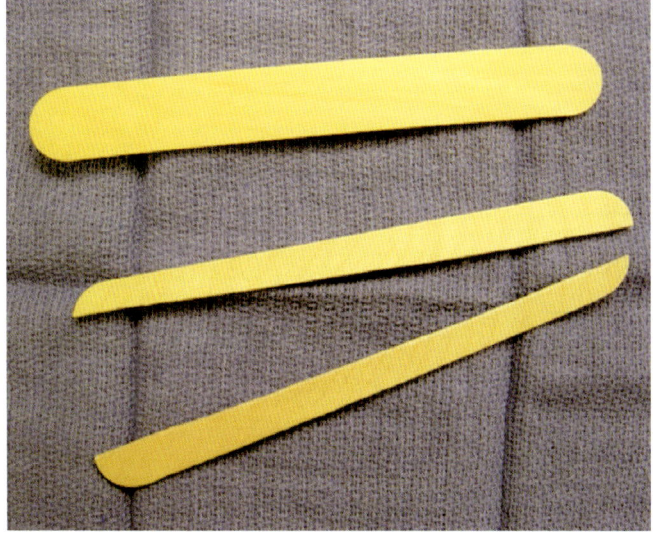

Figure 2-7. A tongue depressor can double as a makeshift curette when a formal surgical instrument is unavailable. The tongue depressor should be broken longitudinally and the rounded end used as the "scooper."

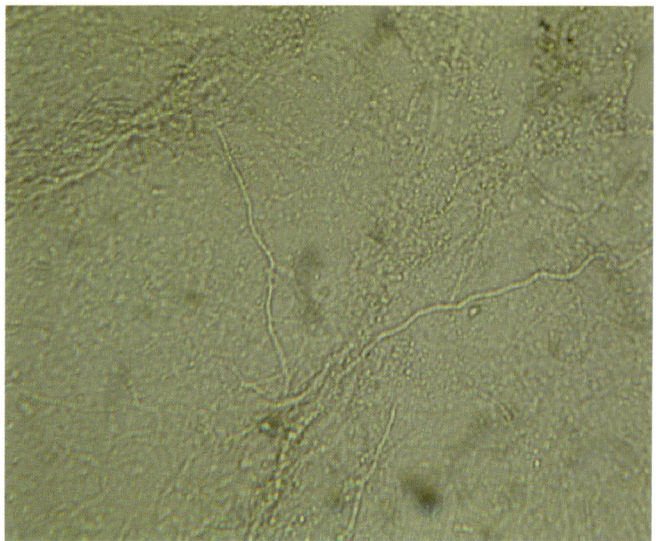

Figure 3-4. Microscopic examination of scale shows multiple hyphal structures traversing the normal cells of the skin (corneocytes).

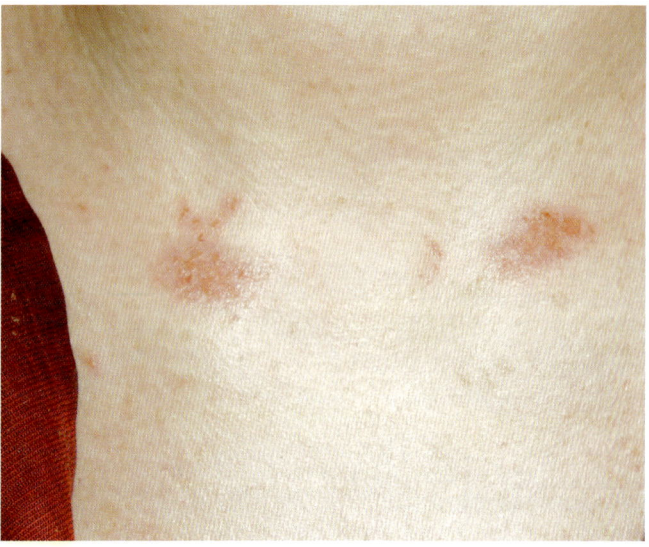

Figure 12-1. Symmetrical abrasions developed over a marathoner's upper chest as a result of friction from her running top.

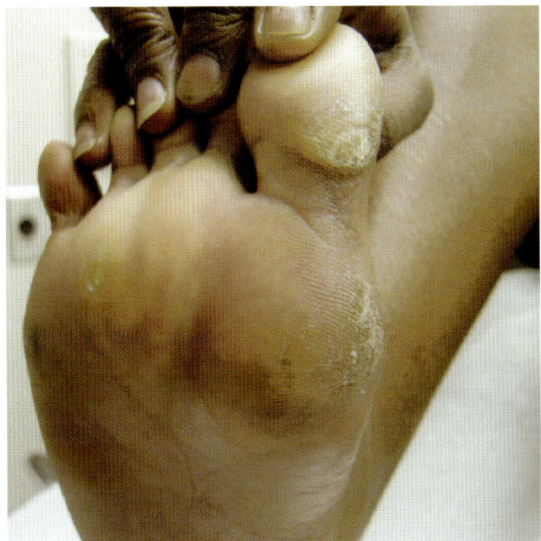

Figure 12-7. Callosities frequently develop on the lateral aspects of the first toe and the ball of the foot.

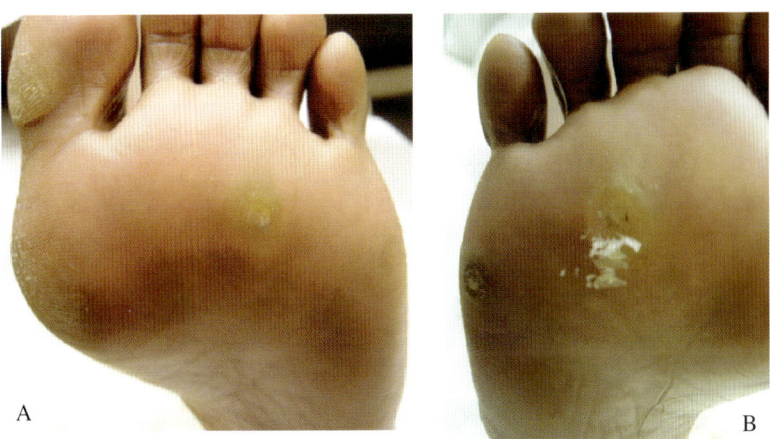

Figure 12-8. **A**: Corns are painful, thick plaques on pressure points of the sole. They may appear to be warts or callosities. **B**: Paring thick scaling plaques on the feet reveals a core characteristic of a corn. There are no normal skin markings or "black dots".

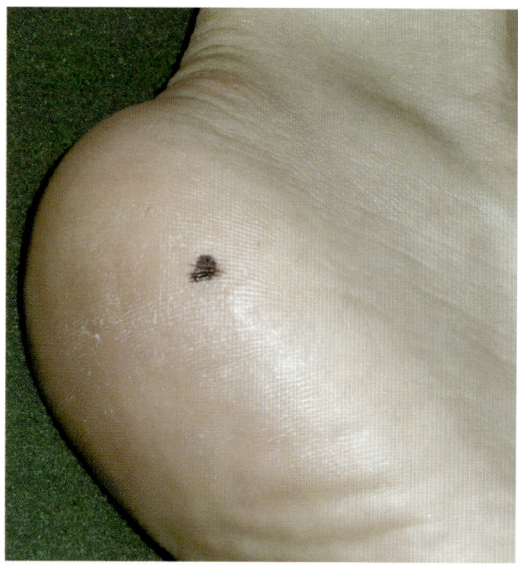

Figure 14-1. Irregularly shaped black macules and patches on the sole may be black heel or melanoma. Linear streaks and punctate lesions favor the former diagnosis. This lesion displays a black lesion typical of melanoma on the sole.

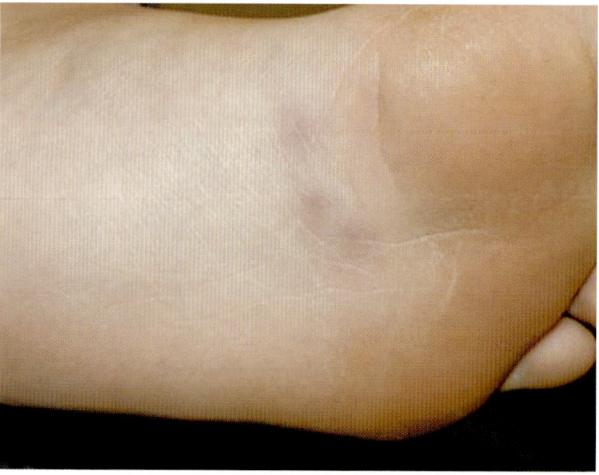

Figure 14-2. Eruption on the sole illustrates palmoplantar eccrine hidradenitis.

Color Plate   VII

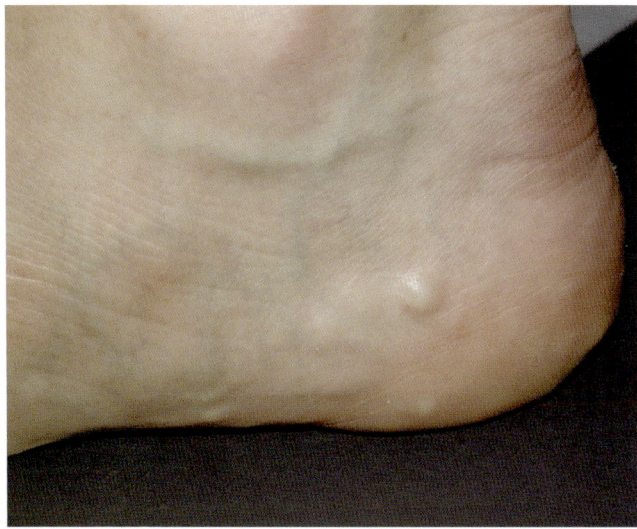

Figure 14-3. Medial and yellow to skin-colored papulonodules portray piezogenic pedal papules.

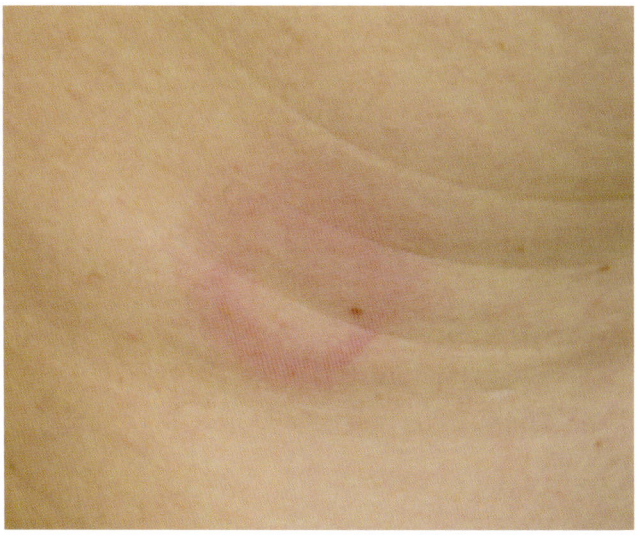

Figure 14-4. Erythematous plaque depicts one of the racquet sport patches. Note the central clearing.

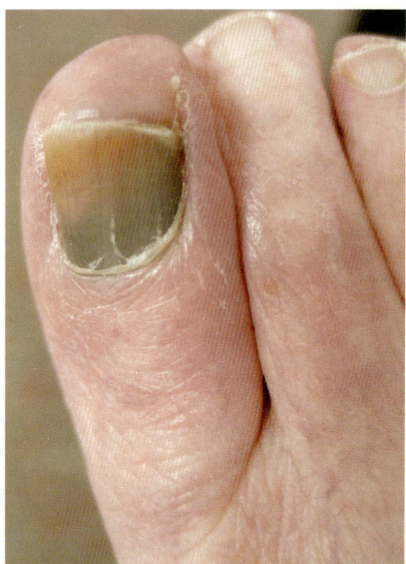

Figure 15-6. Skier's toenail.

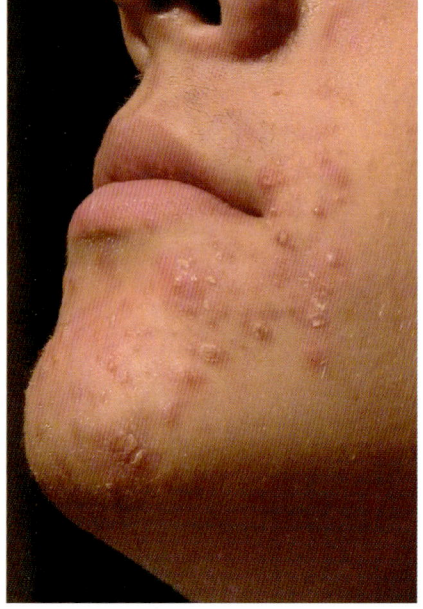

Figure 16-1. Football players frequently develop acne mechanica beneath the chin strap. This type of acne is much more difficult to treat than typical acne vulgaris.

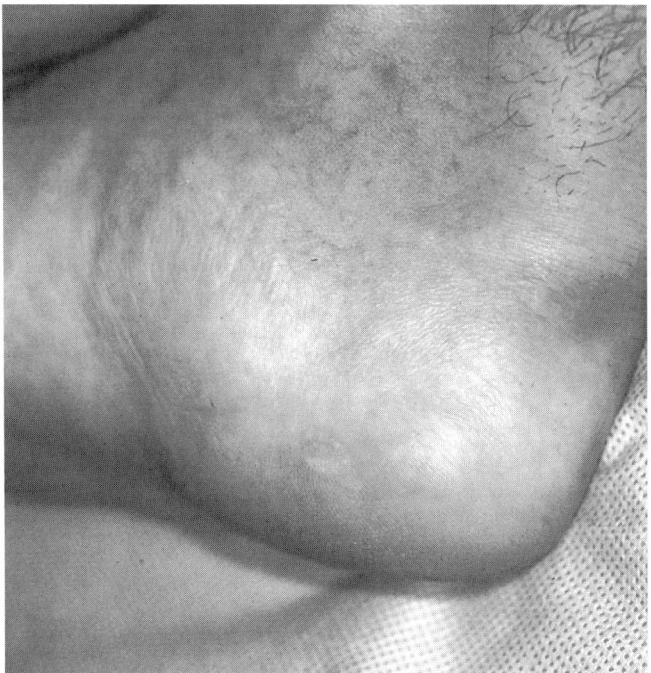

Figure 12-2. This athlete's foot demonstrates erythematous patches representing "hot spots." These "hot spots" likely will develop frank blisters with continued activity.

Treatment

Investigators wrote the seminal article on the proper therapy of blisters in 1968 (Cortese et al., 1968). These investigators showed that a blister should be drained without disturbing the roof (Figure 12-3). If this procedure is performed up to three times in the first 24 hours, the athlete experiences the greatest chance that the blister roof will adhere to the base of the blister. A drained blister with an intact blister roof decreases pain and infection. Furthermore, studies reveal that a drained blister with an intact blister roof heals faster than if the roof is removed.

Once the blister is drained, topical dressings should be applied if continued athletic activity is planned. Without added protection, the flaccid blister likely will expand with minor shearing forces. Petroleum jelly should be applied to the blister and then covered with a padded occlusive dressing, such as moleskin or Duoderm. The clinician should ensure that the dressing not only covers the wound but also attaches to a considerable portion of the margin of unaffected skin.

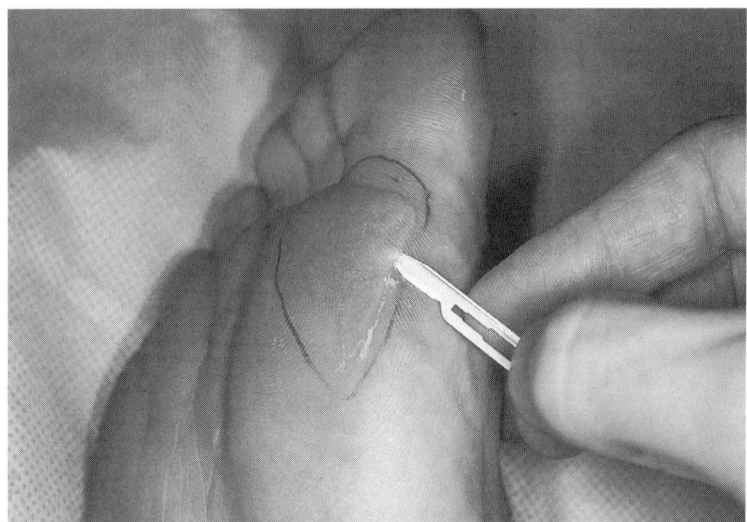

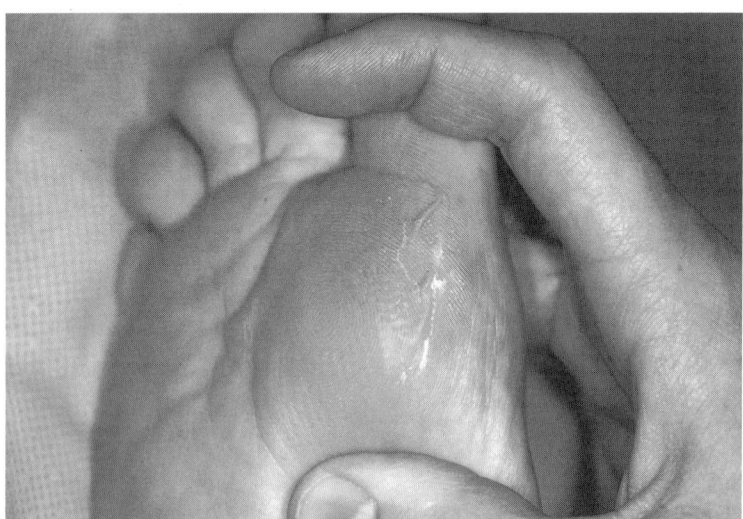

Figure 12-3. **A**: Blisters should be lanced at the periphery using a sterile needle, paying special attention to keeping the blister roof intact and on the skin. **B**: Pressure should be applied to the blister to drain all fluid. This procedure can be taught to athletes so that they can do it themselves.

Some athletes may not be able to stop their play so that they can tend to early or mature blisters. Thus, the aftermath of the sporting activity may be an already ruptured blister. These blisters can be quite painful and may hinder continued activity. With the blister roof removed, it is important to apply petroleum jelly and subsequently cover with Duoderm or moleskin. Some studies note decreased pain with these procedures.

Topical tissue adhesives also can be used. Liquid cyanoacrylates, applied to the exposed skin, act as a "second skin" and add protection for continued activity. One study showed that cyanoacrylates were superior therapy than antibiotic creams with moleskin. The isoamyl and pentyl cyanoacrylates resist cracking on the skin for up to 6 days. Other forms of cyanoacrylates provide only 2 to 3 days of protection (Akers et al., 1973). For competitors who are three fourths of the way into the race, some marathons provide "blister stops" where many of these procedures can be performed. Topical antibiotics are not necessary for treatment of uncomplicated blisters.

Prevention

Because the pain and inconvenience of blisters can inhibit athletic activities, prevention is paramount. Several approaches can be used to decrease the prevalence of blisters. First, the athlete must have the proper equipment (Figure 12-4). Athletic shoes should be professionally fitted. For example, runners should

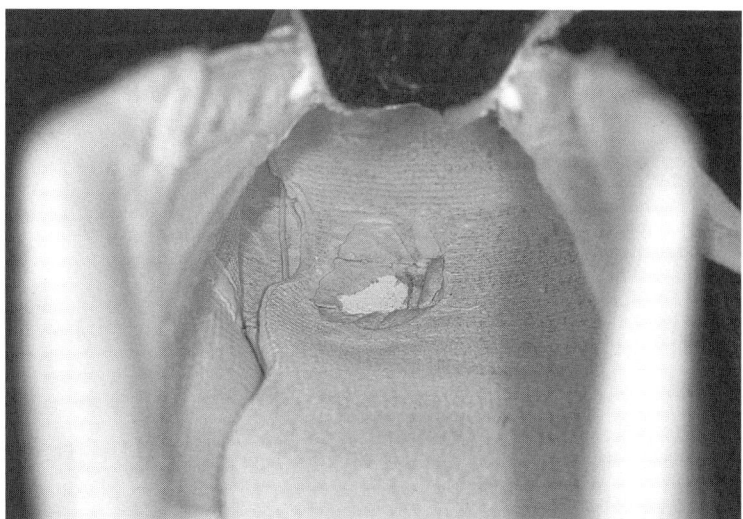

Figure 12-4. Athletic insoles sustain a great deal of trauma that necessitates frequent replacement. Malfunctioning insoles eventuate in blisters.

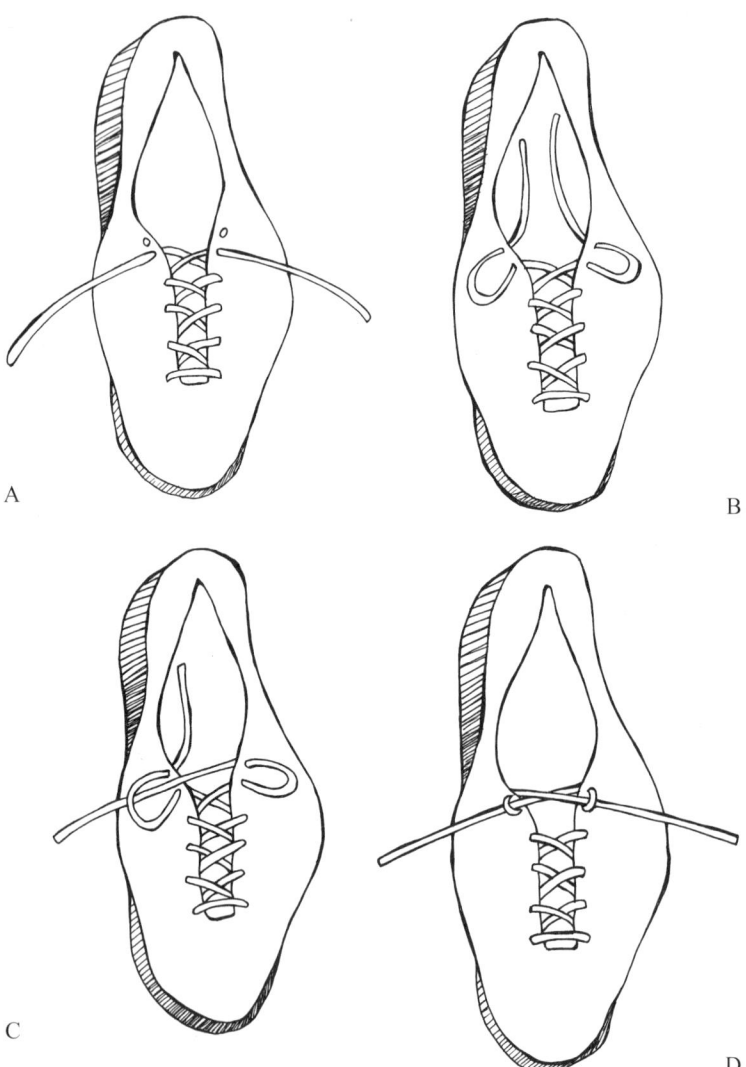

Figure 12-5. Proper lacing of athletic footwear to prevent heel slippage and resultant blisters. **A**: Lace as normal, but leave the last holes undone. **B**: Rather than lacing across to the opposite hole, lace the shoestring through the hole on the same side. **C**: Through each of the loops made by the lacing procedure in B, lace across to the opposite side. **D**: Finally pull up and out and tight. This snuggly stabilizes the heel and ankle for athletic participation.

not purchase shoes at department stores but rather should visit specialty running stores; most cities have at least one. Shoes should be snug but not tight; there should be 2 to 3 cm between the toes and the toe box. On the other hand, shoes that are too big may cause Achilles heel blisters. Special lacing can keep the heel firmly in place even if the toe box is too roomy. Instead of crossing the laces into the last hole on the opposite side, the athlete or trainer should make an outside loop by lacing the last hole on the same side (Figure 12-5). Once the loops are formed on both sides, then the free end of the lace is crossed through each loop. The athlete then pulls firmly and ties as usual.

Slip-resistant shoe insoles can decrease the movement of the athlete's foot within the shoe. New shoes should never be worn first in competition or in a practice when the athlete may not quickly switch shoes. It is best to slowly break in new shoes because invariably they initially are a bit firm in places.

Socks must be synthetic and moisture wicking. Cotton socks retain moisture and increase the likelihood of blistering, whereas synthetic socks keep the sole dry. Studies have shown that athletes who wear synthetic socks develop fewer and smaller blisters (Herring and Richie, 1990). New technologic designs have led to the production of socks with extra padding in "hot spots" and socks without seams (Figure 12-6). Some athletes whose sport includes rapid stops and starts find it helpful to wear two pairs of socks. The shearing forces from their

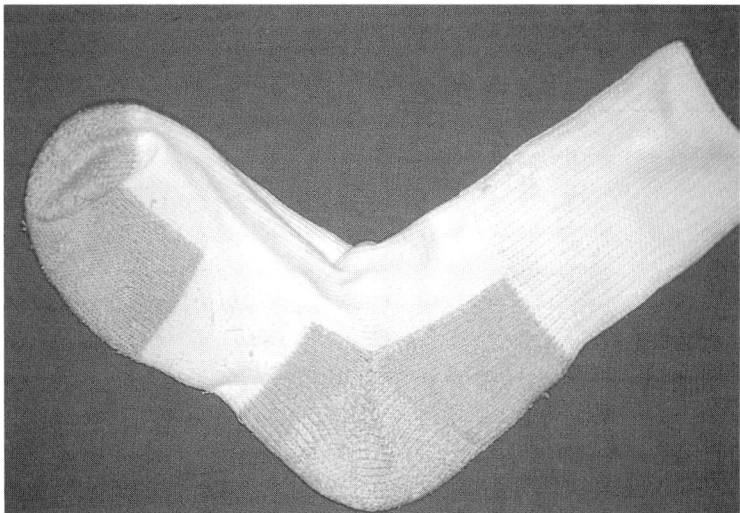

Figure 12-6. Some companies manufacture socks with extra padding at locations that experience increased friction.

activity are distributed across the pairs of socks rather than on the epidermis. Protective gloves work in the same manner to prevent blisters on the hands. Baseball, softball, and racquet sport players and weightlifters are examples of athletes who would benefit from gloves. Unfortunately, gloves decrease an athlete's fine touch and decrease their finesse play.

Clinicians can apply a variety of inert and chemical substances to athletes' "hot spots". Like the addition of an extra sock, application of petroleum jelly to problem areas distributes the shearing forces associated with friction. One aspect of petroleum jelly's role in preventing friction blisters needs some explanation. Some studies have shown that after 3 hours of application of petroleum jelly, the coefficient of friction actually increased. It is believed that, over time, the petroleum jelly decreases transepidermal water loss, thus hydrating the skin (Knapik et al., 2000). This unique property of petroleum jelly may explain in part why marathon runners who successfully use the jelly in practice still develop blisters after 3 or more hours of running.

The same tissue adhesives used for blister treatment can be used as an extra layer of skin protection. These adhesives may be particularly helpful for blisters on the hands; however, pitchers must be careful about what they apply to their fingers. Foreign substances are not allowed on the fingers because they may provide an unfair advantage in creating rotational forces on the pitched ball.

Athletes can decrease the production of blisters by applying aluminum chloride or drying powders to areas that develop blisters when moist. One study showed that the incidence of foot blisters after cross-country hiking was significantly decreased when individuals applied 20% aluminum chloride (Knapik et al., 1998). Unfortunately, this preparation can be quite irritating. Another commercially available agent is called *blister shield*. This product is a micronized wax and silicone powder formula. The athlete places one teaspoon of the powder in each sock and then shakes the sock. These agents decrease the amount of moisture and hence decrease the incidence of blisters (Table 12-2).

Athletes, of course, develop calluses in areas of chronic blistering. These athletes may use these calluses as protection against blisters. This technique is not universally effective, because athletes may still develop blisters beneath the callus.

Callosities (Calluses)

Epidemiology

No prevalence studies exist, although authors note specific callosities in various sports (Table 12-3). Improper footwear or anatomic abnormalities in the foot predispose certain athletes to development of callosities.

Table 12-2. Prevention of Friction Bullae

Category	Method
Equipment	Gloves
Shoes	Adequate-size toe box
	Nonslip insoles
	Supple shoes
	Unique lacing techniques
Socks	Double-layered
	Padded
	Synthetic moisture wicking
Topical agents	Aluminum chloride
	Drying powders
	Micronized wax and silicone powder
	Petroleum jelly
	Tissue adhesives

Clinical Presentation

Callosities are thick, well-defined, hyperkeratotic plaques created by the skin's reaction to repeated frictional trauma (usually causing blisters). Most callosities are found on the hands and feet and are related to the athlete's interaction with the playing field and equipment (Figure 12-7, see color plate). Callosities are generally not painful unless they become extremely thick or fissure (crack).

Diagnosis

The diagnosis can be confused with verruca vulgaris (warts), corns, and "dry skin." Lesions of verruca vulgaris contain the characteristic "black dots" after paring. In the case of callosities, upon paring the lesion, the clinician notes normal skin markings and no "black dots." A pared corn reveals a central core. Paring should be done carefully using a no. 15 surgical blade. A clinician with a touch that is too gentle may confuse the diagnosis, whereas a clinician who is too aggressive may cause bleeding.

Treatment

Often, athletes prefer to keep callosities because they are relatively protective against trauma and eventual blistering. Undesired or painful callosities can be removed using the following series of procedures in the morning and at

Table 12-3. Sport-Specific Callosities

Sport	Location	Etiology
Archery	Fourth fingertip	Releasing bowstring
Baseball	Palms First finger	Batting Pitching
Billiards	Nondominant, palmar aspect thumb and first finger; dorsal aspect of second finger	Holding the cue
Bowling (no holes)	Throwing hand, third and fourth fingers	Throwing ball
Bowling (with holes)	Throwing hand, second, third and fourth lateral fingers	Throwing ball
Canoeing/crew/kayaking/rowing	Palms (depending on oar type)	Rowing
Cycling	Ischial tuberosities	Peddling
Dance	Distal toes	Dancing ballet
Equestrian	Fingers and palms	Holding on to reins
Fishing	Thumb and opposite first finger	Reeling in fish
Golf	Dominant hand, first finger and opposite palm, and opposite third finger	Swinging club
Gymnastics	Palms	Using horse, parallel bar, rings
In-line skating	Legs	Pushing off while skating
Karate/judo	Lateral sides of hands and heels	Performing blows, chops, kicks
Tennis (badminton, racquetball, squash)	Dominant palm and thumb	Swinging racquet
Track and field (discus)	Throwing hand, all palmar aspects of fingers except thumb	Throwing discus
Track and field (shot put)	Hypothenar eminence	Throwing shot
Distance running	Heel ("runner's bump"), medial aspect of first toe	Running
Weightlifting	Palms, web spaces between thumb and first fingers	Lifting

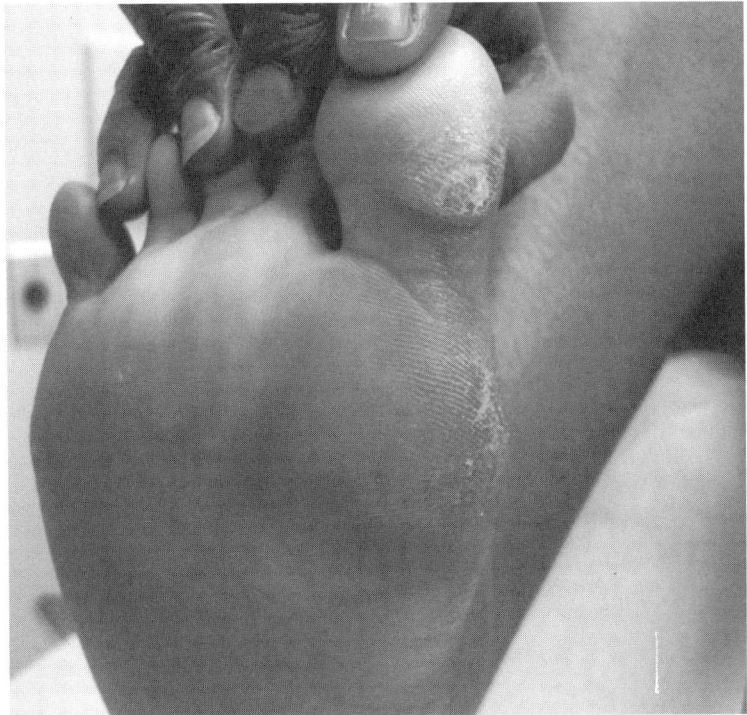

Figure 12-7. Callosities frequently develop on the medial aspects of the first toe and the ball of the foot. (See color plate.)

bedtime. Soak the callosities in warm water for 10 minutes. Rub a pumice stone on the lesion for several minutes. Apply urea cream 20% or 40% and cover with duct tape.

Prevention

Synthetic socks, petroleum jelly, and well-fitted athletic wear decrease friction and help to prevent calluses (Adams, 2002). When athletes develop callosities due to anatomic abnormalities, orthotic devices may be helpful. These pads equilibrate frictional forces, thereby preventing callosities. Athletes must use professional athletic shoe salespeople to avoid purchasing improperly fitted shoes.

Corns

Epidemiology

No prevalence data of corns exist. Corns result from unequal forces experienced by focal areas of the foot.

Clinical Presentation

Corns come in two varieties: hard corns (clavus durus) and soft corns (clavus mollis). Hard corns are located on the sole and tend to be quite painful, which hinder athletic activity. Hard corns resemble callosities but are smaller and more focal. Soft corns are produced by pressure of one toe upon another and typically are located in the interdigital area. Soft corns are characterized by white macerated plaques.

Diagnosis

To make an accurate diagnosis, the clinician must pare the lesion. Paring reveals black dots, a central core, and normal skin in warts, corns, and callosities, respectively (Figure 12-8, see color plate). Patients with corns often complain that they feel like they have a "pebble in their shoe."

Treatment

Paring corns produces the most effective immediate pain relief. Paring should be done carefully using a no. 15 surgical blade. A clinician with a touch that is too gentle may confuse the diagnosis. Multiple over-the-counter pads are available to decrease pressure from hard cores. Over-the-counter toe separators or moleskin products relieve soft corn pain and may prevent recurrence. Shoe inserts may alleviate some pressure points related to structural abnormalities. Surgical intervention for anatomic irregularities may be required if conservative measures fail.

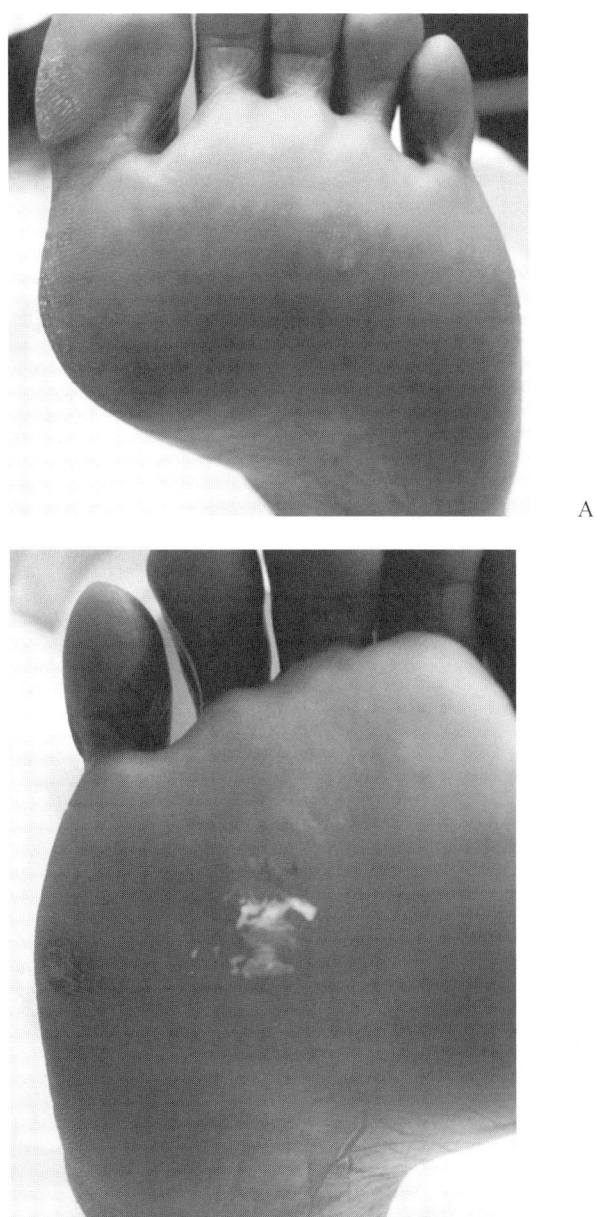

Figure 12-8. **A**: Corns are painful, thick plaques on pressure points of the sole. They may appear to be warts or callosities. **B**: Paring thick scaling plaques on the feet reveals a core characteristic of a corn. There are no normal skin markings or "black dots". (See color plate.)

Prevention

In addition to preexisting bony and soft tissue problems, ill-fitting shoes produce corns. Athletes must have their shoes professionally fitted; the toe box must be adequate. To prevent hard corns, shoe inserts or referral to a podiatrist specialist may be necessary. Toe separators or surgical intervention may be required to prevent soft corns (Katchis and Hershman, 1993).

Foosball Finger

Epidemiology

One case report of foosball finger exists (Mathias, 1982). Foosball is a table-top soccer game. Most people experience this game in the family room and recreation centers, but professional foosball exists. Players spin a hard plastic grip that controls plastic-mounted players on the field. The direction of the attack is always to the right.

Clinical Presentation

To increase the force kicking the ball, the player places their wrist on the plastic grip, rolls the hand upward (keeping constant contact between the skin and the grip), and abruptly stops the rotational movement of the rod with the fingers. This repeated procedure produces painful bullae on those fingers (Figure 12-9).

Diagnosis

The diagnosis is obvious to the player.

Treatment

Treatment includes lancing the bulla and keeping the roof as a biologic dressing (see Bullae: Treatment).

12. Friction Injuries to the Skin   223

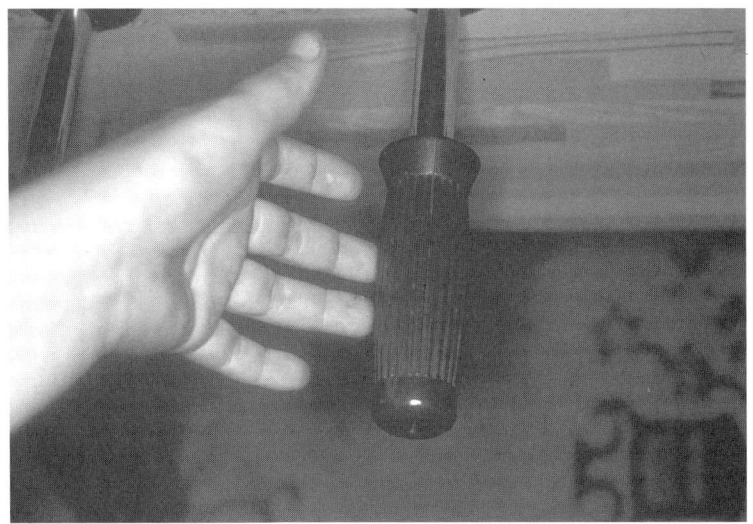

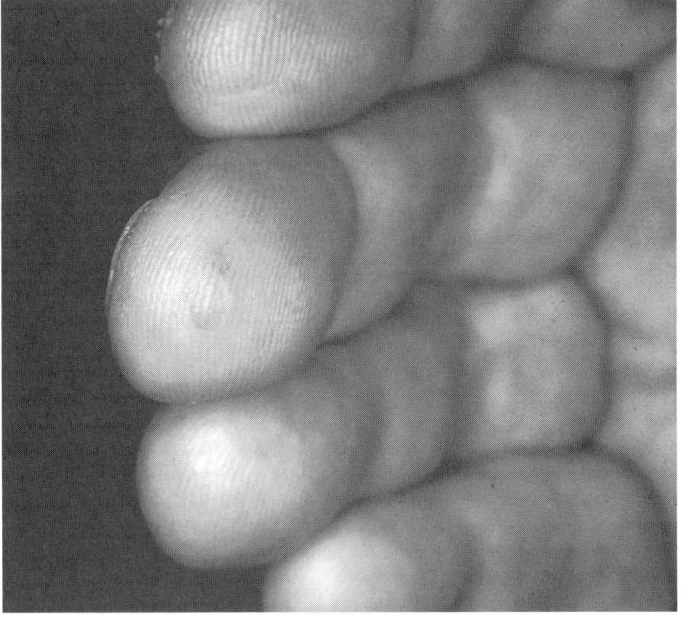

Figure 12-9. **A**: Foosball players grip firmly the handles and rotate them vigorously. **B**: Painful and erythematous blisters form on the fingertips.

Prevention

A leather athletic glove helps prevent foosball finger.

Jazz Ballet Bottom

Epidemiology

One small case series of dancers exists (Radford and Greatorex, 1987). Repeated friction and the force of the entire dancer's weight placed between the sacrococcygeal region and the floor can produce abscesses of *Staphylococcus aureus*.

Clinical Presentation

The dancer exhibits well-defined, erythematous, tender papules and nodules on the gluteal cleft.

Diagnosis

The diagnosis is based on clinical findings and the historical note of participation in jazz ballet. Cursory evaluation may lead to a mistaken diagnosis of pilonidal sinus and other infections. Jazz ballet bottom reveals no features of pilonidal origin. Cultures are necessary.

Treatment

Warm compresses soaks for 5 to 10 minutes several times per day assuage symptoms. After injection of local anesthetic, clinicians should lance the abscess, especially if it is tender. Oral dicloxacillin or cephalexin combined with topical mupirocin is indicated. Dancers should avoid the contributing activity until the lesions are completely clear.

Prevention

Predisposed dancers may need to apply extra padding to the sacrococcygeal region.

Jogger's Nipples

Epidemiology

Three studies have examined the prevalence of jogger's nipples in marathon runners (Mailler and Adams, 2004). The lowest prevalence was noted in a study that sent a questionnaire to runners 1 month after the marathon was complete. Two percent of the runners had jogger's nipples. An informal study of runners at a marathon noted the highest prevalence of 16.3%, and a survey of the actual injuries presenting to the medical tent at a marathon noted a prevalence of 5.4%. A weighted analysis of these three studies reveals an overall prevalence of 6.7%.

Men who wear shirts made of coarse fibers, such as cotton, and women who do not wear a bra while running develop this condition most commonly. Unfortunately, these coarse fiber cotton shirts are by far the most common type of shirt given as "gifts" by running race organizers. Neophytes often wear these cotton T-shirts at race time and ultimately find themselves in the medical tent before the day is over. The first individual to enter the medical tent at the inaugural running of the Cincinnati marathon (now in its seventh year) required medical attention for his bleeding and painful nipples.

Clinical Presentations

Repeated friction between nonsynthetic shirts and the nipple produces very painful, erythematous, bleeding erosions on the areola and nipple. In an extended run, such as a marathon, the lesions not uncommonly bleed and produce a vivid image of vertical lines of blood most visible on white T-shirts (the most common color of shirts given as "gifts" to the participants). The intense pain frequently is out of proportion to the clinical findings and should not be underestimated by the clinician (Figure 12-10).

Diagnosis

The diagnosis is straightforward.

Treatment

Treatment includes warm-water soaks (2–3 times per day for 5 minutes each), petroleum jelly, or topical antibiotic ointment.

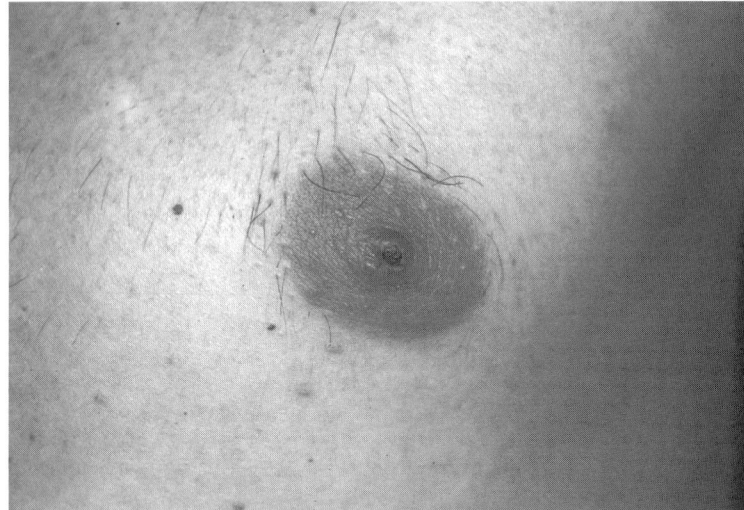

Figure 12-10. Jogger's nipples, although visually unimpressive, are intensely painful and can bleed profusely.

Prevention

Prevention is paramount. Participants should avoid wearing coarse fiber shirts until after the marathon is complete. Various synthetic shirts are available and should be worn during long runs. Athletic companies manufacture different synthetic shirts to be used in nearly every environmental condition (from frigid and cold to hot and humid). For women, silk, semisynthetic, and other soft fiber bras should be worn. Specialty running stores, which can be found in most major cities, sell this state-of-the-art clothing. In addition to the advanced equipment, runners should apply petroleum jelly, commercially available patches, or adhesive tape before very long runs (Adams, 2002).

Karate Cicatrices

Epidemiology

Twenty-five percent of karate contests result in some type of injury. Most injuries occur on the head and neck, abdomen, and extremities. Only one case report describes this condition (Adams, 2001). Practitioners of karate perform physical moves such as brick and block breaking and punching over a period of years. The dorsal aspects of the hands receive repeated acute pressure trauma from irregularly surfaced blocks, nails, and teeth.

Clinical Presentation

The actions of karate practitioners lead to lacerations that heal with scars. On physical examination, well-defined, scattered, linear, hypopigmented, atrophic patches over the dorsal aspects of the hands are observed. There is no hypertrichosis, milia, or blistering.

Diagnosis

The diagnosis is made clinically after obtaining an appropriate history. The differential diagnosis includes epidermolysis bullosa acquisita and porphyria cutanea tarda. The lack of blisters, milia, and hypertrichosis help differentiate karate cicatrices from these other disorders.

Treatment

Lacerations lead to these atrophic scars, so impeccable wound care is paramount.

Prevention

The nature of the sport results in these lacerations. Regular use of hand protection and mouth guards decreases the likelihood of karate cicatrices.

Lacerations
Epidemiology

Lacerations are among the most common injuries experienced by athletes. For instance, rugby players experience 2.75 lacerations per 1000 playing hours

(Garraway and Macleod, 1975). Lacerations acquired during cycling result in 3.2 days of missed work (Tucci and Barrone, 1988). Careless cycling (25%), cars (25%), and potholes (15%) cause these cycling accidents. Lacerations, the second most common injury experienced by wind surfers, relate to contact with not only fins and other equipment but also rocks, coral, and other water obstacles.

Some studies reveal that not only athletes experience lacerations. Children who ride in carriers on the back of bicycles develop bicycle spoke injuries at great rates. In one emergency room, spoke injuries accounted for 4% of all orthopedic problems in 1 year (Roffman et al., 1980). Of those who sustain spoke injuries, up to 95% experience abrasions or lacerations. The epidemiology of lacerations in many sports and events are detailed (Table 12-1).

Clinical Presentation

Lacerations occur in the normal routine of athletic participation, and tears in the skin range from superficial to deep (extending past the subcutaneous tissue). The clinician should first assess tendon and nerve function relative to the laceration. With either of these complications, immediate referral to a surgical specialist is necessary (Bouchard, 2005).

Diagnosis

The diagnosis is not in question.

Treatment

Large, deep, or facial lacerations require physician involvement. Superficial lacerations are common and can be treated by other nonphysician, athletically trained medical staff.

Initial lacerations should be cleaned as soon as possible. It is best to clean these lacerations with lukewarm tap water and a mild soap such as Lever 2000. Flushing debris from the wound with a water-filled syringe is preferable to scrubbing with a cloth, brush, or other instrument. These last objects can cause increased mechanical trauma to the viable tissue. For this same reason, hydrogen peroxide should not be used.

It is important to assess the pain level before debridement. Moderate or greater pain may necessitate the injection of lidocaine 2% with epinephrine before thorough debridement. For decades dermatologists and dermatologic surgeons have safely used epinephrine on the nose, ears, foot, and hand. Epinephrine should *not* be used (or should be used with great caution) on the penis or the distal tips of the fingers.

Once a laceration is clean and tolerant of manipulation, the clinician should achieve hemostasis using aluminum chloride 20%. This solution stings but remarkably curtails bleeding by causing vasoconstriction. In rare cases where this substance does not work, the clinician should sparingly apply Monsel solution to the wound. The downside to this solution, which causes local clotting, is that the solution can permanently stain the skin.

For the past 7 years, tissue adhesives (e.g., butyl cyanoacrylates and 2-octyl cyanoacrylates) have been used to hold together superficial wounds. The face and areas with low tension on the extremities and trunk are optimal sites for tissue adhesive use; the wound must not be infected.

Deeper wounds without subcutaneous involvement require suturing. If lidocaine 2% with epinephrine was not used for debridement, the anesthetic should be used before suturing. The type of suture depends on the anatomic site of the laceration. Lips and eyelids require 6-0 silk suture; other facial lacerations require 6-0 nylon. All other parts of the body, including the scalp, can be adequately sutured with 4-0 nylon. Facial sutures must be removed in 5 days; all other sutures can be removed in 10 to 14 days.

Tetanus shots should be given to individuals who cannot remember their last tetanus immunization or those who last had their tetanus shot more than 10 years ago. If the wound is major or is not clean, tetanus shots should be given to athletes who last received their tetanus shot 5 or more years ago. In most athletic leagues, bleeding must be stopped and the lesion covered before the athlete may return to play.

Prevention

Reasonable protective equipment should be worn in all sports. Many sports require gloves, suits, and helmets. Water sports enthusiasts should wear neoprene booties to prevent unanticipated lacerations.

Pool Palms

Epidemiology

One small case series of pool palms exists (Blauvelt et al., 1992). Repeated rubbing of the palms on rough pool wall and floor surfaces produces pool palms.

Swimmers rub against the pool surfaces to help navigate while they are underwater.

Clinical Presentation

Swimmers ultimately develop erythematous and linear plaques on both palms.

Diagnosis

The diagnosis is straightforward if the clinician obtains the history of swimming in a pool having rough wall surfaces. Otherwise the differential diagnosis includes perniosis, neutrophilic eccrine hidradenitis, and other sports-related traumatic conditions.

Treatment

No treatment is necessary.

Prevention

Use of pools with smoother-surfaced walls and floors prevents pool palms.

Powerlifter's Patches

Epidemiology

No studies of powerlifter's patches exist. During the "clean and jerk" maneuver used by some weightlifters, the rough-surfaced barbell rests upon the anterior aspect of the neck and sternoclavicular areas. As the lifter forcefully thrusts the barbell over the head, the barbell abrades the same areas. While dropping the barbell, the athlete's shins bear the brunt of the force (Scott et al., 1992).

Clinical Presentation

Well-defined, erythematous, occasionally purpuric patches and abrasions on the anterior aspects of the neck and sternoclavicular areas and the shins are observed. Lichenified plaques occur in the same locations over the long term.

Diagnosis

The diagnosis is based on clinical findings and the history of weightlifting.

Treatment

The affected area requires topical petroleum jelly or topical antibiotic ointments (e.g., Polysporin or silver sulfadiazine). Warm-water soaks for 5 to 10 minutes several times per day assuage symptoms. Treatment should be commensurate with the degree of severity. Moderate-potency topical steroids can be used for the lichenified plaques; concomitant use with significant erosions is discouraged.

Prevention

The application of petroleum jelly to frictional points on at-risk areas decreases the dermatologic manifestations. In competition, lifters may not apply foreign substances to their skin.

Rower's Rump

Epidemiology

One case report of rower's rump exists (Tomecki and Mikesell, 1987). Frictional contact between the buttocks and the metal seat of a rowing machine produces rower's rump (Figure 12-11).

Clinical Presentation

Affected individuals have a well-defined and lichenified plaque on both buttocks.

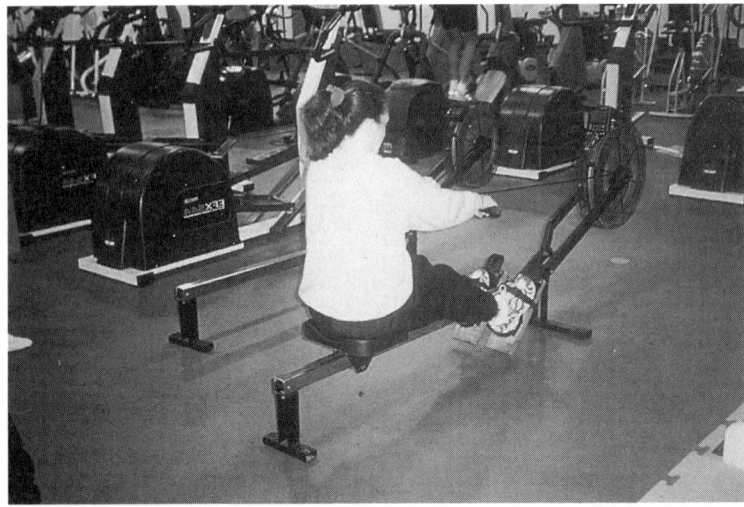

Figure 12-11. Rower's rump is created by repeated friction between the buttock and the seat.

Diagnosis

Assessing the involvement in rowing clinches the diagnosis. The differential diagnosis includes maceration intertrigo, tinea cruris, saddle sores, and extramammary Paget's disease. A biopsy may be required to differentiate among these conditions.

Treatment

Potent topical steroids or intralesional steroids (e.g., triamcinolone at a concentration of 10 mg/ml) improves rower's rump.

Prevention

Rowers may use a padded seat that conforms to the size of the buttocks. A seat that is too large results in increased movement and friction. Petroleum jelly can be applied to frictional areas.

Runner's Rump

Epidemiology

No studies of runner's rump exist.

Clinical Presentation

Distance runners develop small asymptomatic ecchymoses on the superior gluteal cleft as a result of repeated friction during long runs.

Diagnosis

The diagnosis is based on clinical findings and the history of long-distance running.

Treatment

No treatment is necessary.

Prevention

Application of petroleum jelly to frictional points on the buttock may decrease signs of runner's rump.

Saddle Sores

Epidemiology

No epidemiologic studies of saddle sores exist, but this condition, to varying degrees, is not uncommon among cyclists (Mellion, 1991).

Clinical Presentation

Frictional contact between the rocking buttocks and the bicycle seat produces saddle sores. The affected individual has tender, well-defined, erythematous patches and plaques in the perineum (Figure 12-12); when the eruption is severe, maceration and erosions are also present. Over a long period, lichen simplex chronicus (chronic lichenified dermatitis) can occur.

Diagnosis

Assessing cycling activity without a protective cushion clinches the diagnosis. The differential diagnosis includes maceration intertrigo, tinea cruris, extramammary Paget's disease, and rower's rump. A biopsy may be required to differentiate among these conditions.

Treatment

The affected area requires topical petroleum jelly or topical antibiotic ointments (e.g., Polysporin or silver sulfadiazine). Warm-water soaks for 5 to 10

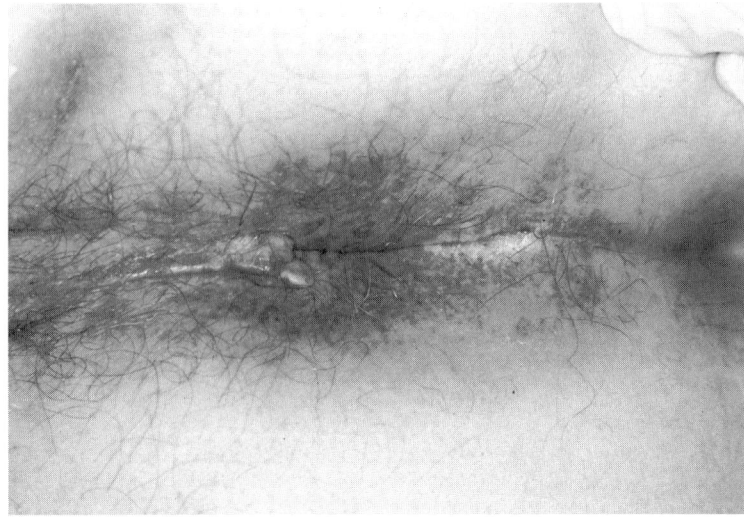

Figure 12-12. Perianal erythema, petechiae, and erosions occur in the perineum of a cyclist.

minutes several times per day assuage symptoms. Treatment should be commensurate with the degree of severity. Moderate-potency topical steroids can be used for a brief period if pruritus or irritation is present. Concomitant use with significant erosions is discouraged.

Prevention

Preventive measures include adjusting the height and angle of the bicycle seat, wearing padded shorts (synthetic moisture-wicking material), using a saddle pad, obtaining a different shaped saddle, and shaving surrounding hair. To further decrease friction, cyclists can apply petroleum jelly or Bodyglide to susceptible areas.

Stringer's Fingers

Epidemiology

No epidemiologic studies of stringer's fingers exist. Racquet sport athletes frequently adjust misaligned strings on their racquet between points.

Clinical Presentation

Friction between the middle three fingers and the strings create well-defined, thick scaling plaques on the distal tips of those fingers (Basler and Garcia, 1998).

Diagnosis

The diagnosis is based on clinical findings and the history of fastidious string adjustment.

Treatment

Topical urea cream (20% or 40%) applied daily, along with routine paring with sharp instruments, clears stringer's fingers.

Prevention

Newer racquets whose strings move much less after hard or spin shots can be used.

Tennis Thighs

Epidemiology

One case note of tennis thighs exists (Basler and Garcia, 1998). Continuous rubbing between the medial thighs of tennis players produces tennis thighs.

Clinical Presentation

The eruption is characterized by tender, well-defined, brightly erythematous patches and plaques on the medial thighs.

Diagnosis

The diagnosis is based on clinical findings and the historical note of athletic activity resulting in muscular medial thighs rubbing against each other. Cursory evaluation may lead to a mistaken diagnosis of tinea cruris or allergic contact dermatitis.

Treatment

Sore areas can be treated with moderate-potency topical steroids in an ointment base. Warm compresses for 5 to 10 minutes several times per day assuage symptoms.

Prevention

Athletes with hypertrophic vastus medialis muscles should consider applying petroleum jelly to the medial thighs before activity.

Track Bites

Epidemiology

No studies of rowers exists (Karlson, 2000).

Clinical Presentation

Repeated friction between the posterior leg and the track in which the seat rolls back and forth causes tender, well-defined, erythematous, abraded patches. These abrasions scar and can become secondarily infected.

Diagnosis

The diagnosis is based on clinical findings and the history of rowing.

Treatment

The affected area requires topical petroleum jelly or topical antibiotic ointments (e.g., Polysporin or silver sulfadiazine). Warm-water soaks for 5 to 10 minutes several times per day assuage symptoms. Treatment should be commensurate with the degree of severity. Moderate-potency topical steroids can be used for a brief period if pruritus or irritation is present. Concomitant use with significant erosions is discouraged.

Prevention

Application of long socks or circumferential gauze or tape to the at-risk area will protect the lower legs.

Treadmill Tracks

Epidemiology

One case series exists in runners (Attalla et al., 1991).

Clinical Presentation

The fast, warm, moving conveyor belt can create abrasions and full-thickness ulcers on the hands. These lesions occur when children fall off the treadmill or erroneously put their hands in the gap between the belt and the supporting structure.

Diagnosis

The diagnosis is immediately evident.

Treatment

The affected area requires topical petroleum jelly or topical antibiotic ointments (e.g., Polysporin or silver sulfadiazine). Warm-water soaks for 5 to 10 minutes several times per day assuage symptoms. Treatment should be commensurate with the degree of severity. Moderate-potency topical steroids can be used for a brief period if pruritus or irritation is present. Concomitant use with significant erosions is discouraged.

Prevention

Children should not use treadmills without close adult supervision. Athletes should use the installed safety equipment that cuts power to the machine if they lose their balance.

Waterskiing Welts

Epidemiology

One case series of waterskiers exists, although the presence of lesions is not uncommon (Scott and Scott, 1995).

Clinical Presentation

The rope attached to the speedboat that tugs the waterskier splits into two and inserts into the skier's handle (the yoke). The initial forceful tug to pull the skier to an upright position or the failure to release the yoke upon falling into the water allows the rope to rapidly abrade the medial aspects of the thighs. This area of the thighs demonstrates linear, erythematous, (initially) edematous, variably eroded plaques. The lesions become increasingly more tender after the injury.

Diagnosis

The diagnosis is immediately evident.

Treatment

The affected area requires topical petroleum jelly or topical antibiotic ointments (e.g., Polysporin or silver sulfadiazine). Warm-water soaks for 5 to 10 minutes several times per day assuage symptoms. Treatment should be commensurate with the degree of severity. Moderate-potency topical steroids can be used for a brief period if pruritus or irritation is present. Concomitant use with significant erosions is discouraged.

Prevention

Waterskiers can wear longer swimsuits to cover the legs where the yoke ropes rub. Alternatively, the skiers can apply padding to the at-risk area of the legs.

Bibliography

Adams BB. Dermatologic disorders of the athlete. Sport Med 2002;32:309–321.
Adams BB, Mutasim DF. Karate cicatrices. Cutis 2001;67:499–500.
Akers WA, Sulzberger MB. The friction blister. Mil Med 1972;137:1–7.
Akers WA, Leonard F, Ousterhout DK, et al. Treating friction blisters with alkyl-cyanoacrylates. Arch Dermatol 1973;107:544–547.
Attalla MF, Al-Baker AA, Al-Ekiabi SA. Friction burns of the hand caused by jogging machines: a potential hazard to children. Burns 1991;17:170–171.
Basler RSW, Garcia MA. Acing common skin problems in tennis players. Phys Sportsmed 1998;26:37–44.
Blauvelt A, Duarte AM, Schachner LA. Pool palms. J Am Acad Dermatol 1992;27:111.
Bouchard M. Sideline care of abrasions and lacerations. Phys Sportsmed 2005;33:21–29.
Cortese TA, Fukuyama K, Epstein W, et al. Treatment of friction blisters. Arch Dermatol 1968;97:717–721.

Garraway M, Macleod D. Epidemiology of rugby football injuries. Lancet 1995;345: 1485–1487.

Herring KM, Richie DH. Friction blisters and sock fiber composition. J Am Pod Med Assoc 1990;80:63–71.

Karlson KA. Rowing injuries. Phys Sportsmed 2000;28:40–50.

Katchis SD, Hershman EB. Broken nails to blistered heels. Phys Sportmed 1993;21: 95–104.

Knapik JJ, Reynolds K, Barson J. Influence of an antiperspirant on foot blister incidence during cross-country hiking. J Am Acad Dermatol 1998;39:202–206.

Knapik, JJ, Reynolds KL, Duplantis KL, et al. Friction blisters. Sports Med 2000; 20:136–147.

Levine N. Friction blisters. Phys Sportsmed 1982;10:84–92.

Mailler EA, Adams BB. The wear and tear of 26.2: dermatological injuries reported on marathon day. Br J Sports Med 2004;38:498–501.

Mathias CGT. Foos ball finger. Can Med J 1982;127:953.

Mellion MB. Common cycling injuries. Sport Med 1991;11:52–70.

Powell B. Bicyclist's nipples. JAMA 1983;249:2457.

Radford PJ, Greatorex RA. Jazz ballet bottom. Br Med J 1987;295:1173–1174.

Rayan GM. Archery-related injuries of the hand, forearm, and elbow. S Med J 1992;85:961–962.

Ressman RJ. Epidemiology of friction blisters. J Assoc Mil Dermatol 1975;2:13–17.

Roffman M, Moshel M, Mendes DG. Bicycle spoke injuries. J Trauma 1980;20:325–326.

Scott MJ, Scott MJ. Dermatologic stigmata in sports: water skiing. Cutis 1995;55:353–354.

Scott MJ, Scott NI, Scott LM. Dermatologic stigmata in sports: weightlifting. Cutis 1992;50:141–145.

Tomecki KJ, Mikesell JF. Rower's rump. J Am Acad Dermatol 1987;16:890–891.

Tucci JJ, Barone JE. A study of urban bicycling accidents. Am J Sport Med 1988; 16:181–184.

13. Friction Injuries to the Hair

This chapter on sports-related traumatic conditions focuses on frictional effects on the hair. Skin almost always is the only interface between athletes and their equipment, competitor, or environment. The hair plays the primary interface role in only a few scenarios. In these situations, the hair may bear the brunt of intense friction. Skin can accommodate these frictional forces over time (i.e., by adapting with calluses). Hair is much more fragile and has no ability to adjust; it simply falls out. Thus, frictional forces from all varieties of athletic activity result in the common endpoint of alopecia.

Aquaslide Alopecia

Epidemiology

Whereas epidemiologic studies of skin infections at water parks exist, none has examined the incidence of alopecia caused by waterslide friction. Only one report of alopecia from a day at the water park is reported in the literature (Adams, 2001). This condition is the direct result of repeated friction between the waterslide and the hair. To increase the speed down the slide, enthusiasts arch their backs, hold their hands on their stomach, and tense their legs so that only a small portion of the back of the head and the outside edges of the legs touch the slide. In this position, very small areas receive all the friction.

Clinical Presentation

On examination, well-defined, symmetrical, round, nonscarring, alopecic patches are observed over the posterolateral aspects of both legs (Figure 13-1). Theoretically, alopecic areas also can occur on the posterior scalp, although this has not been observed.

Diagnosis

Without taking a proper history, the clinician may confuse these round patches for alopecia areata. No exclamation point hairs are seen, which sets this condition apart from alopecia areata.

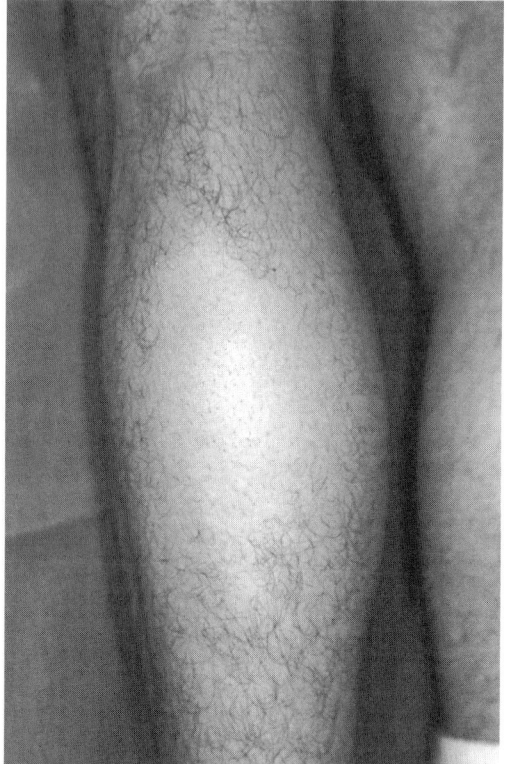

Figure 13-1. Round alopecic patches that could be mistaken for alopecia areata actually are the result of friction from a waterslide.

Treatment

The water enthusiast should be reassured that the hair will regrow and will be back to normal length within 1 to 2 months (depending on the original length of the leg hair).

Prevention

If speed is the goal for the water park visitor, then the practice of limiting the amount of direct connection to the slide will always produce, over several downhill trips, enough friction to cause alopecia. If the hair loss is disturbing, then they should be encouraged to allow as much as their posterior body to touch the slide to distribute the frictional forces and to slow their descent speed. In this way, no alopecia will occur.

Balance Beam Alopecia

Epidemiology

No studies have systematically reviewed patterned hair loss in gymnastics; however, this condition has been observed on multiple occasions (Adams, 2001; Ely, 1978).

Clinical Presentation

A patterned thinning alopecia develops from the centrofrontal scalp to the occiput due to tremendous frictional forces between the balance beam and the gymnast's hair during head stands and rollovers.

Diagnosis

The first time this condition was reported, the clinician believed the patterned alopecia was the result of tension from the athlete's hairstyle. This condition underscores the importance of relating skin and hair abnormalities to an athlete's activity.

Treatment

No treatment is necessary. The hair loss will decrease as the gymnast decreases use of the beam. Acutely, this is not a scarring process, so all the hair should return. Scalp hair grows quite slowly and may take many months to attain the pre-alopecia length.

Prevention

There is no satisfactory preventative action.

Jogger's Alopecia

Epidemiology

There has been one case report of jogger's alopecia (Copperman, 1978).

Clinical Presentation

A female jogger developed linear, transverse, nonscarring alopecia due to the daily friction of a very heavy, tight-banded, wide headphone worn upon her scalp.

Diagnosis

Any pattern (especially unusual) should prompt the clinician to search for a connection to the athlete's environment and activities.

Treatment

Discontinuation of the heavy Walkman is curative (see Prevention).

Prevention

In the age of iPods and very small, compact, athletic radios, this condition likely will not be a problem.

Bibliography

Adams BB. Water-slide alopecia. Cutis 2001;67:399–400.
Copperman SM. Two new cause of alopecia. JAMA 1984;252:3367.
Ely PH. Balance beam alopecia. Arch Dermatol 1978;114:968.

14. Pressure Injuries

This third chapter in the section on sports-related traumatic conditions reviews the effects of pressure. Generally, pressure, in this context, produces maximal damage to the skin when it is powerful and acute. Each sport creates different forces on the integument, so many of the disorders in this chapter are sport specific.

Black Heel

Epidemiology

Otherwise known as "talon noire," black heel has been reported more than 125 times in young individuals ranging in age from 12 to 24 years. The condition more rarely has been referred to as calcaneal petechiae, chromidrose plantaire, pseudochromidrose plantaire, and posttraumatic punctate hemorrhage of the skin. Basketball, football, lacrosse, soccer, and tennis players and weightlifters have developed black heel. In total, the male-to-female ratio is 1 : 1 (Wilkinson, 1977). Sheering forces, related to quick stops, starts, and jumps produce rupture of tiny blood vessels within the papillary dermis (superficial dermis).

Clinical Presentation

An asymptomatic, well-defined, linear, irregularly shaped, somewhat speckled black macule, varying in size but mostly less than 1 cm, is observed on the posterior heel of the athlete (Figure 14-1, see color plate). The plantar aspects of the toes can rarely be affected.

Diagnosis

The diagnosis can be challenging, especially when the clinician fails to incorporate the individual's sport. Athletes have undergone wide local excision of these lesions when the clinician mistook the black heel for melanoma. The differential diagnosis includes junctional melanocytic nevus (mole), melanoma, tinea nigra, and resolving verruca vulgaris (Levit, 1968; Nabai and Mehregan, 1970). Paring the edge of the lesion reveals the hemorrhage's very superficial nature. If melanoma is strongly suspected, a punch biopsy must be performed.

246   Sports Dermatology

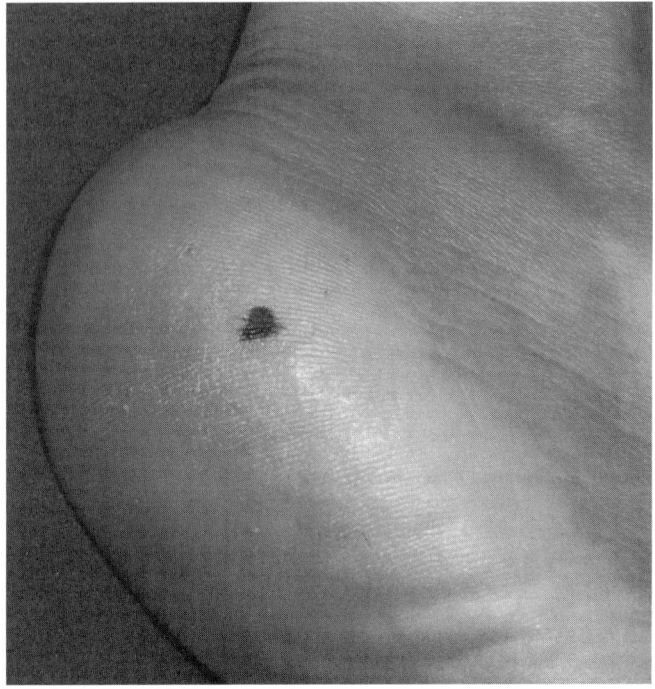

Figure 14-1. Irregularly shaped black macules and patches on the sole may be black heel or melanoma. Linear streaks and punctate lesions favor the former diagnosis. This lesion displays a black lesion typical of melanoma on the sole. (See color plate.)

Histopathologically, melanoma and black heel are easily differentiated. Black heel demonstrates "lakes of pigment" that stain for blood. A great deal of the hemorrhage escapes to the epidermis through sweat ducts (Casas and Woscoff, 1974).

Treatment

No treatment is needed. Paring the stratum corneum removes the hemorrhage.

Prevention

Some authors prevent black heel by placing a felt pad under the heel.

Black Palm

Epidemiology

Otherwise known as "mogul skier's palm," only one case report exists. Mogul skiers repeatedly and vigorously plant their poles in the snow as they make their tight turns. The hypothenar eminence experiences all the pressure from the plant as the skier speeds down the hill (Swinehart, 1992). Tennis and racquetball players and weightlifters can also develop black palm.

Clinical Presentation

In mogul skiers, the intense pressure exerted on the palm, especially the hypothenar eminence, produces a tender, ill-defined, large (several centimeters), golden brown, violaceous-red patch surrounded by ill-defined erythema. Over a period of days the lesion can become darker and more painful.

In tennis and racquetball players, the powerful ground strokes and serves result in sheering forces in the palm that produce well-defined, linear, speckled brown to black macules. Weightlifters develop the same clinical lesions as a result of abrupt and forceful trauma related to lifting huge weights (Izumi, 1974). These lesions on tennis and racquetball player's palms are most similar to that of black heel (talon noire).

Diagnosis

The diagnosis is made after discovering the correlation with mogul skiing, racquet sport, or weightlifting trauma. The differential diagnosis for mogal skiiers includes cold panniculitis, erythema multiforme, fixed drug eruption, insect bite reaction, lichen aureus, and neutrophilic eccrine hidradenitis. The differential diagnosis for black palm in racquet sport players is similar to that for black heel (talon noire).

Treatment

Localized heat, provided by over-the-counter warm packs, helps to clear the eruption. With discontinuation of mogul skiing, the skier will observe lesion clearance in 2 weeks. Treatment for black palm in racquet sport players is not necessary.

Prevention

Skiers can prevent these lesions by wearing padded gloves, changing their grip on the pole, and using less aggressive skiing moves.

Palmoplantar Eccrine Hidradenitis

Epidemiology

Also known as "idiopathic plantar hidradenitis," "neutrophilic eccrine hidradenitis" and "recurrent palmoplantar hidradenitis," fewer than 50 cases have been noted in the literature (Robinson et al., 2004). Athletes with intense physical activity have developed the condition. Reported athletes with this condition include baseball players, dancers, and mountaineers. I have seen these lesions in in-line skaters (rollerbladers) and runners. Young and otherwise very healthy children aged 4 to 12 years seem particularly vulnerable. Intense trauma on the soles or palms from sports combined with sweating may cause the rupture of eccrine glands. The rupture may activate the complement pathway and trigger a neutrophilic inflammatory response to the eccrine gland.

Clinical Presentation

Clinically, most lesions occur suddenly on either or both soles (rarely on the palms in baseball players) and appear as very tender, well-defined, erythematous, edematous plaques and nodules (Figure 14-2, see color plate). Young athletes may experience so much pain that they cannot walk. Relapses occur in 50%, and spontaneous remission is the rule.

Diagnosis

The diagnosis is dependent on the acumen of the clinician in inquiring about the sporting activity. Without this information, the diagnosis can be quite challenging. The differential diagnosis includes bacterial infection, chilblains, erythema elevatum diutinum, erythema nodosum, insect bite reaction, traumatic plantar urticaria, and vasculitis.

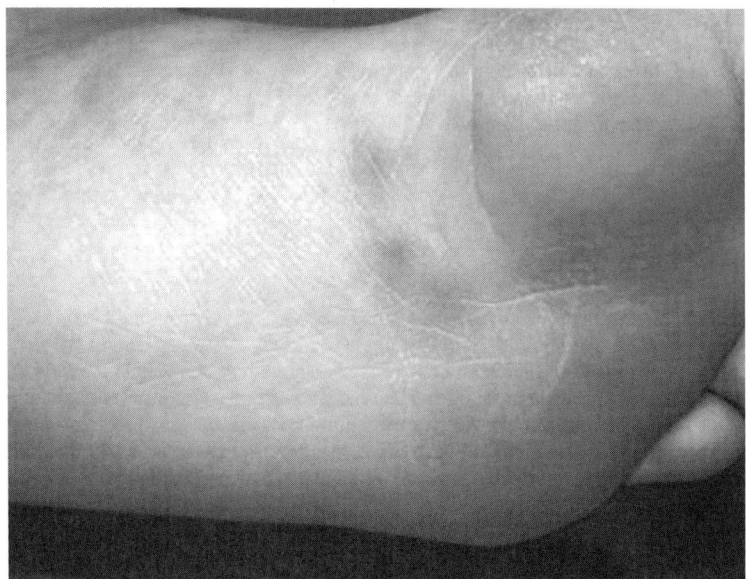

Figure 14-2. Eruption on the sole illustrates palmoplantar eccrine hidradenitis. (See color plate.)

Treatment

Palmoplantar eccrine hidradenitis clears spontaneously in 1 to 4 weeks. Warm compresses may assuage symptoms. However, the athlete may need to rest and take nonsteroidal antiinflammatory drugs (e.g., ibuprofen) because of severe pain.

Prevention

There are no effective preventative strategies.

Paintball Purpura

Epidemiology

No studies exist. Paintballs rocket at fast speeds (300 feet per second). The kinetic energy of a paintball is nearly five times as much as a speeding table tennis ball.

Clinical Presentation

A paintball's impact creates a 3-cm urticarial, hemorrhagic, well-defined plaque with central clearing. The pain associated with these lesions relates to the proximity of the shot. In general, close range shots result in greater pain. The lesions eventuate in ecchymoses that may not resolve for 10 to 14 days (Schnirring, 2004). Postinflammatory hypopigmentation or hyperpigmentation may result.

Diagnosis

The diagnosis is dependent on the acumen of the clinician in inquiring about the sporting activity. Without the history, the differential diagnosis includes erythema chronica migrans, erythema multiforme, fixed drug eruption, gyrate erythema, racquet sport patches, tinea corporis, and urticaria.

Treatment

Warm compresses water soaks for 5 to 10 minutes two or three times per day may assuage the pain. Nonsteroidal antiinflammatory drugs also may be required, depending on the pain.

Prevention

Individuals should wear loose-fitting clothes while playing paintball. Goggles, helmets, gloves, athletic cups, padded bras, elbow pads, and kneepads are a must.

Piezogenic Pedal Papules

Epidemiology

First reported in 1968 (Shelley and Rawnsley, 1968), piezogenic pedal papules have been reported nearly 400 times in the literature, with 4.4% of these cases sports-related (Redbord and Adams, 2006). In one study, the authors examined 412 consecutive patients and found that 2.5% had piezogenic pedal papules;

100% of these individuals had a history of vigorous physical activity (Kohn and Blasi, 1972). *Piezo* means "pressure" and *genic* means "giving rise to," which relates to the etiology of these papules. Long-distance runners demonstrate this condition.

Clinical Presentation

Piezogenic pedal papules are only recognizable upon application of pressure to the foot. Most piezogenic papules are not painful (90%), but they may be more apparent after prolonged exercise (e.g., during marathon training). The painful minority results from ischemia to blood vessels and nerves as the fat lobules herniate into the papillary dermis. It is believed that structural weaknesses in the connective tissue allow the fat to push into the upper layers of the skin. With this pressure, athletes notice multiple, less than 5-mm, well-defined, skin-colored, firm papules on the medial and lateral aspects of the heel (Figure 14-3, see color plate).

Diagnosis

The diagnosis of the painful variety of piezogenic pedal papules can be very challenging. In the case of painful piezogenic pedal papules, often clinicians perform an exhaustive search for a musculoskeletal cause. The diagnostic maneuver for piezogenic pedal papules may not be included in the typical evaluation of an athlete's foot pain. During this maneuver, the clinician observes the protrusion of the fat lobules through the skin on the heel as the athlete stands on one foot, applying as much force as possible. This maneuver not only may reveal the fat pad protrusion but also may reproduce the athlete's pain.

A biopsy is rarely performed but demonstrates thickened dermis, loss of the typical compartmentalization of the fat lobules, and thinning trabeculae in the subcutaneous fat.

Treatment

Successful treatment for symptomatic piezogenic pedal papules often is unsatisfactory. Strategies used include heel cups, compression stockings, acupuncture, intralesional steroids and anesthetics, avoidance of repeated foot trauma, and surgical excision (Woodrow et al., 1997).

Prevention

No satisfactory prevention exists, but some recommend heel cups.

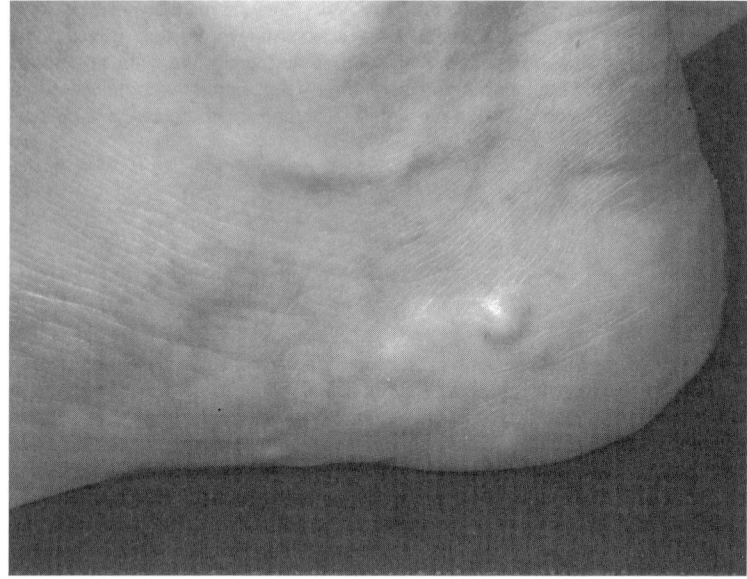

Figure 14-3. Medial and yellow to skin-colored papulonodules portray piezogenic pedal papules. (See color plate.)

Ping-Pong Patches

Epidemiology

Only one case of ping-pong patches exists (Scott and Scott, 1989). Table tennis balls move at speeds up to 100 miles/hour in elite play. Upon impact of the projectile on the skin, the ball indents centrally and the edges of the ball create intense pressure on the skin.

Clinical Presentation

The resulting skin lesion is an approximately 12- to 15-mm, annular (ring-shaped), erythematous plaque. The erythematous rim is less than 5 mm. Because the ball indents upon skin impact, a central clearing or zone of no erythema exists. With enough velocity and force, the rim may also be purpuric. Most lesions resolve in 2 to 5 days.

Diagnosis

The diagnosis is dependent on the acumen of the clinician in inquiring about the sporting activity. Ping-pong patches and racquet sport patches may appear similar but vary in size. The size of a ping-pong ball is 38 mm, which creates a 12- to 15-mm diameter lesion. Squash ball patches are a bit larger, reflecting the ball's larger diameter (44 mm). Racquetball patches are the largest because the ball is the largest (55 mm). Without the history, the differential diagnosis includes erythema chronica migrans, erythema multiforme, fixed drug eruption, gyrate erythema, paintball purpura, tinea corporis, and urticaria.

Treatment

Warm compresses for 5–10 minutes two or three times per day may assuage the pain. Nonsteroidal antiinflammatory drugs may also be required, depending on the pain.

Prevention

No prevention exists.

Platform Purpura

Epidemiology

No epidemiologic studies of platform purpura exist. The force with which the diver enters the pool may transmit to the skin on the thighs in a missed dive.

Clinical Presentation

The resulting skin lesions are relatively symmetrical, variably painful, erythematous plaques. Depending on the force experienced by the thighs, purpura may develop. Most lesions resolve in several days.

Diagnosis

The diagnosis is dependent on the acumen of the clinician in inquiring about the sporting activity. Without the history, the differential diagnosis includes erythema multiforme, fixed drug eruption, a rare type of pigmented purpuric dermatosis, and urticaria.

Treatment

Warm compresses for 5 to 10 minutes two or three times per day may assuage the pain. Nonsteroidal antiinflammatory drugs may also be required, depending on the pain.

Prevention

Only dives with a perpendicular entry into the water will prevent the slapping force onto the thighs.

Port-Wine Stains

Epidemiology

Port-wine stains typically appear at birth; however, 59 cases of acquired portwine stains are reported. Twenty-nine percent of the cases were related to antecedent trauma, of which 30% could be attributed to sports-related trauma (Adams and Lucky, 2000). It is believed that trauma results in either abnormal vascular repair or altered vascular innervation.

Clinical Presentation

Susceptible athletes may develop well-defined, violaceous, pink, or erythematous patches in areas of trauma. The patches are most commonly located on the face and less commonly on the extremities.

Diagnosis

The diagnosis often is made clinically, and the history of trauma supports the diagnosis. Biopsy may be necessary. The differential diagnosis includes arteriovenous malformations and cutis marmorata telangiectatica congenita, though neither of these is associated with sports trauma.

Treatment

Patients treated with pulsed-dye lasers have experienced an excellence response or complete clearance in 54% of the cases.

Prevention

Only avoidance of trauma can prevent acquired port-wine stains in predisposed individuals.

Powerlifter's Purpura

Epidemiology

One case report of powerlifter's purpura exists (Pierson and Suh, 2002).

Clinical Presentation

Purpura and petechiae result from ruptured blood vessels that can occur when powerlifting athletes increase their arterial pressure to levels as high as 450/380 mmHg. Weightlifters subsequently develop asymptomatic, numerous purpura and petechiae on the eyelids and anterior and lateral neck.

Diagnosis

The diagnosis often is made clinically, and the history of weightlifting exacerbating the condition supports the diagnosis. If the athlete has a history of fever, chills, or night sweats, a complete blood count should be performed to help evaluate for a blood disorder, such as lymphoma.

Treatment

No treatment but reassurance is required.

Prevention

No prevention exists.

Purpura of Prolonged Running

Epidemiology

Two case reports of purpura of prolonged running exist (Cohen, 1968; Latenser and Hempstead, 1985). Purpura and petechiae result from ruptured blood vessels. The factor that produce petechiae or purpura in runners includes increased transmural capillary pressure from the repetitive and intense pressure with every step of running. Preexisting solar damage results in decreased collagen and places small skin capillaries at increased risk for rupture.

Clinical Presentation

Well-defined, purpuric patches or petechial macules have been reported on the faces and ankles of runners. One runner developed subsequent facial purpura after his cheeks became bright red during a 20-mile run.

Diagnosis

The diagnosis often is made clinically, and the history of running exacerbating the condition supports the diagnosis. When this eruption occurs on the face, the condition may be confused for acne rosacea, lupus erythematosus, and seborrheic dermatitis. When this eruption occurs on the legs, the condition could be confused with pigmented purpuric dermatosis (a rare, often idiopathic skin disease). If the athlete has a history of fever, chills, or night sweats, a complete blood count should be performed to help evaluate for a blood disorder, such as lymphoma.

Treatment

No treatment exists.

Prevention

For the long term, patients should wear sunscreen to prevent thinning of the connective tissue that protects the tiny blood vessels in the superficial dermis.

Purpura Gogglorum

Epidemiology

Only one case report of purpura gogglorum in swimmers exists. Overtightening of elastic straps on leaky goggles leads to this skin problem.

Clinical Presentation

One swimmer developed an extensive, well-defined, purpuric patch over one eyelid after wearing new swimming goggles. The opposite eye piece started to leak during a swimming practice. Each time water entered the leaky eyepiece, the swimmer incrementally tightened the elastic band and pulled both eyepieces from her head to empty the water on the leaky side. After repeating this process several times, the swimmer effectively created significant negative pressure in the functioning eyepiece. This enormous suction broke the superficial blood vessels and produced purpura.

Diagnosis

The diagnosis could be quite challenging unless the history of swimming with goggles is obtained. Although the morphology of the lesions will be different, some clinicians might confuse purpura gogglorum with contact dermatitis related to the cushion seals.

Treatment

Treatment consists of a cool compress applied to the area for several minutes, several times per day. Swelling and purpura resolve within 1 day.

Prevention

Swimmers must discard goggles with inadequate seals. If the seal leaks during a swim, the swimmer should not incrementally pull tightly the elastic strap while also pulling on the goggles to empty them of water. Low-elasticity straps are helpful.

Racquet Sport Patches

Epidemiology

No studies of racquet sport patches exist.

Clinical Presentation

Hollow, firm rubber balls used in racquet sports travel at great speeds. Upon contact with the skin, the ball indents and creates a strong force along the edge of the ball that is in contact with the skin. All the energy of the ball is transferred to the skin in a ring (annular) pattern. The central area (the location of the ball's indentation) remains relatively unscathed (Figure 14-4, see color plate). The urticarial plaque usually resolves in a few hours. Hemorrhage, induced by an exceptional force, may take days or 1 week to resolve.

Diagnosis

The diagnosis is dependent on the acumen of the clinician in inquiring about the sporting activity. Ping-pong patches and racquet sport patches may appear similar but vary in size. The size of a ping-pong ball is 38 mm, which creates a 12- to 15-mm diameter lesion. Squash ball patches are a bit larger, reflecting the ball's larger diameter (44 mm). Racquetball patches are the largest because the ball is the largest (55 mm). Without the history, the differential diagnosis includes erythema chronica migrans, erythema multiforme, fixed drug eruption, gyrate erythema, paintball purpura, tinea corporis, and urticaria.

Treatment

Warm compresses for 5 to 10 minutes two or three times per day may assuage the pain. Nonsteroidal antiinflammatory drugs may also be required, depending on the pain.

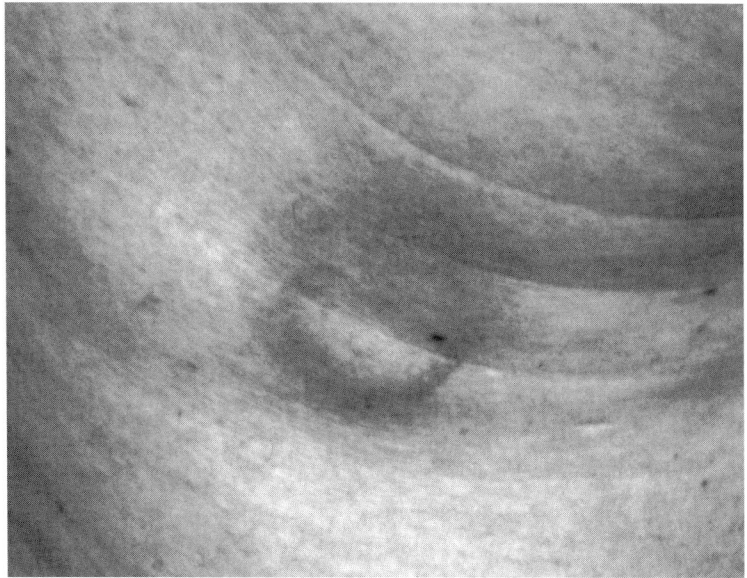

Figure 14-4. An erythematous plaque depicts one of the racquet sport patches. Note the central clearing. (See color plate.)

Prevention

Loose-fitting clothing may dampen the force of the ball, but welts may still develop beneath these clothes.

Stria Migrans
Epidemiology

One report of stria migrans in a weightlifter exists (Shelley and Cohen, 1964). This disorder contrasts with striae distensae, which is a relatively more common disorder representing wider and more numerous stretch scars in areas of high skin tension.

Clinical Presentation

From repeated trauma of lifting heavy weights, a linear, narrow, atrophic band extended symmetrically from a central portion on the lower back. The eventual length was 35 cm.

Diagnosis

The diagnosis is made clinically, in conjunction with a history of weightlifting.

Treatment

No successful treatments for striae exist. Topical retinoids, topical and intralesional steroids, and laser therapy have been used, with variable results.

Prevention

No evidence-based recommendation for prevention can be made. Athletes should not abruptly increase the amount of weightlifted.

Bibliography

Adams BB, Lucky AW. Acquired port-wine stains and antecedent trauma: case report and review of the literature. Arch Dermatol 2000;65:367–370.

Casas JG, Woscoff A. Calcaneal petechiae. Arch Dermatol 1974;109:571.

Cohen HJ. Jogger's petechiae. N Engl J Med 1968;279:109.

Izumi AK. Pigmented palmar petechiae. Arch Dermatol 1974;109:261.

Kohn SR, Blasi JM. Piezogenic pedal papules. Arch Dermatol 1972;106:597–598.

Latenser BA, Hempstead RW. Exercise-associated solar purpura in an atypical location. Cutis 1985;35:365–366.

Levit F. Plantar pseudochromidrosis. JAMA 1968;203:807–808.

Nabai H, Mehregan AH. Black heel. Cutis 1970;July:751–753.

Pierson JC, Suh PS. Powerlifter's purpura: a valsalva-associated phenomenon. Cutis 2002;70:93–94.

Redbord KP, Adams BB. Piezo genic pedal papules in a marathon runner. Clin J Sport Med 2006;14:81-83.

Robinson R, Larralde M, Santos-Munoz A, et al. Palmoplantar eccrine hidradenitis: seven new cases. Pediatr Dermatol 2004;21:466–468.
Schnirring L. Paintball popularity explodes. Phys Sportsmed 2004;32:11–12.
Scott MJ, Scott MJ. Ping pong patches. Cutis 1989;43:363–364.
Shelley WB, Rawnsley HM. Painful feet due to herniation of fat. JAMA 1968;205:110–111.
Shelley WB, Cohen W. Stria migrans. Arch Dermatol 1964;90:193–194.
Swinehart JM. Mogul skier's palm. Cutis 1992;50:117–118.
Wilkinson DS. Black heel. Cutis 1977;20:393–396.
Woodrow SL, Brereton-Smith G, Handfield-Jones S. Painful piezogenic pedal papules: response to local electro-acupuncture. Br J Dermatol 1997;136:628–630.

15. Traumatic Injuries to the Nails and Toes

The fourth chapter in the section on sports-related traumatic conditions in the athlete discusses nail disorders. These nail changes in athletes are related to the great forces applied to the toes as they are forced into the athletic shoe's toe box. Some athletes are susceptible to nail problems resulting from repeated steady trauma, as expected with long-distance running. Other nail conditions relate to very abrupt and massive forces, as experienced from kicking a soccer ball or stopping suddenly after running at top speed on a basketball or tennis court. The three most commonly reported disorders—tennis toe, jogger's toenail, and ingrown nails (onychocryptosis)—are discussed separately, then miscellaneous fingernail and toenail conditions are reviewed.

Tennis Toe

Epidemiology

Investigators examined the epidemiology of tennis toe in 1000 tennis players occurring over a 6-year period at the United States Tennis Association National Boys' Tennis Championships. Tennis toe was rare and occurred only 0.4 per 100 athletes (Hutchinson et al., 1995). The authors believed that players at the elite level of tennis used high-quality and properly fitted shoes. Tennis toe results from the strong force applied to the longest toes (usually the first two toes) when the player's foot rapidly thrusts into the toe box during abrupt stops and starts.

Clinical Presentation

Tennis toe is characterized by nail darkening secondary to subungual hemorrhage.

Diagnosis

The diagnosis can be challenging. Tennis toe can be mistaken for melanoma, psoriasis, and onychomycosis, especially because athletes appear to develop fungus more frequently than do nonathletes. The lack of subungual hyperker-

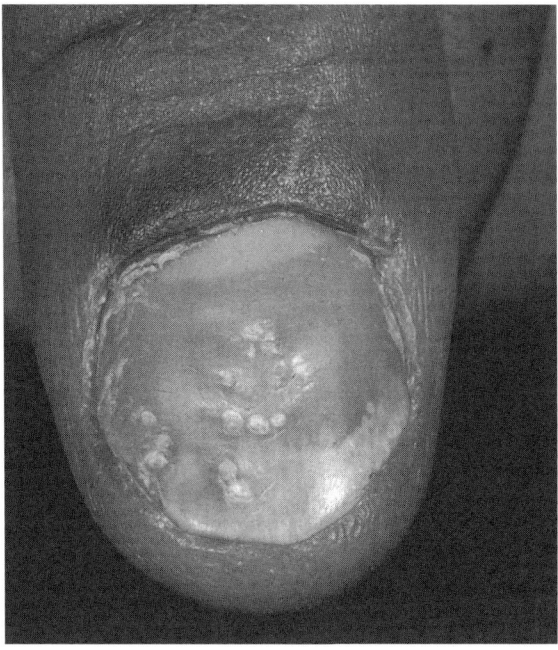

Figure 15-1. Yellow discoloration and pits in the nail exemplify psoriasis. There is no nail darkening suggestive of tennis toe.

atosis and the yellow discoloration differentiate tennis toe from psoriasis and onychomycosis (Figure 15-1). If the diagnosis is unclear, culture or periodic acid–Schiff (PAS) staining of subungual debris by the dermatopathology laboratory is recommended. Potassium hydroxide examination may be useful but can be technically challenging. A biopsy should be performed if melanoma is suspected.

The differential diagnosis also includes other sports-related nail abnormalities, such as center's callosities, jogger's toe, and the nail conditions associated with football, dancing, skating, skiing, and soccer.

Treatment

Tennis toe resolves without therapy when tennis playing is stopped. Some tennis players simply paint their toes to cover the discoloration. Acute and painful subungual hematomas may require treatment. A heated paper clip or needle bores through the nail plate and promptly relieves the pressure and pain. Sterile dressings and topical wound care are mandatory thereafter until the nail heals (Katchis and Hershman, 1993).

Prevention

Wearing properly fitted shoes decreases the likelihood of tennis toe. Tennis shoes must be professionally fit. Orthotic devices help ameliorate the sliding effect of the foot in the tennis shoe. Lacing techniques can prevent the foot from freely slamming into the toe box. Athletes should cut their toenails straight across, without rounded edges. Straight nails allow equal distribution of forces when the nail hits the toe box. Athletes can use foam toe caps, which fit around the at-risk toe inside the shoe (Katchis and Hershman, 1993).

Jogger's Toenail

Epidemiology

Only one epidemiologic study has examined jogger's toenail. In the 1979 New York City marathon, the incidence of jogger's toenail was 2.5%. The incidence of jogger's toenail very likely is much higher (Mailler and Adams, 2004). Although this condition is reported only three times in the literature, jogger's toenail is a frequent observation at the high school, collegiate, and professional levels.

The incidence of the skin condition relates to the intensity and duration of workouts. Long-distance runners or race walkers are more likely to develop lesions. Novices often purchase ill-fitting shoes that predispose them for jogger's nail. However, distance runners still develop nail problems even with proper-fitting shoes. Downhill courses result in a great deal of force transmission to the most distal toe and toenail (Adams, 2003; Mailler and Adams, 2004). Repeated pounding of the distal most nail (many people's second toe is the longest) into the toe box produces jogger's toenail.

Clinical Presentation

The first reported case of jogger's toe involved the third, fourth, and fifth toenails and demonstrated subungual hemorrhage (and subsequent nail discoloration), onycholysis (separation of the nail plate from the nail bed), and erythema (Figure 15-2). The second reported case noted second toenail changes only with transverse ridging in addition to the first description's changes (Figure 15-3). Subungual hyperkeratosis is generally not seen, and the Hutchinson sign (pigmentation not only of the nail but also of the proximal nail fold, suggesting melanoma) is not present.

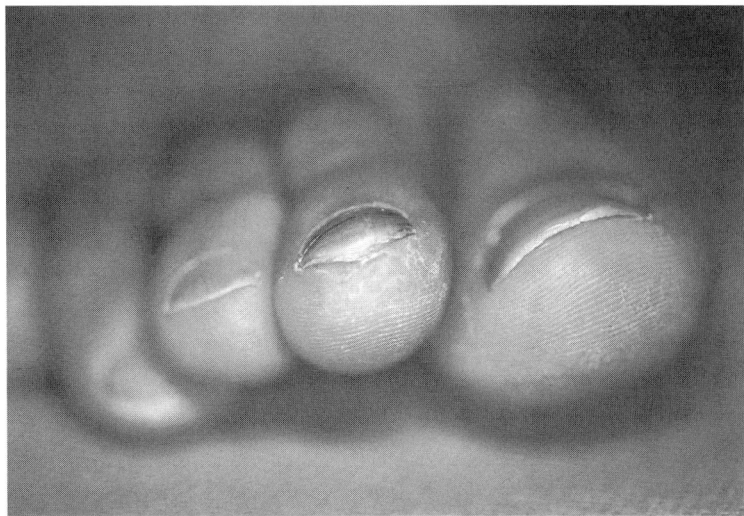

Figure 15-2. Runner's toe demonstrates black discoloration, distal callosity, and onycholysis (nail separation). These findings are classic for jogger's toenail.

Diagnosis

The diagnosis can be challenging. Jogger's toenail frequently is misdiagnosed as onychomycosis, especially because athletes appear to develop fungus more frequently than do nonathletes. The lack of subungual hyperkeratosis and the yellow discoloration differentiate jogger's toenail from onychomycosis. If the

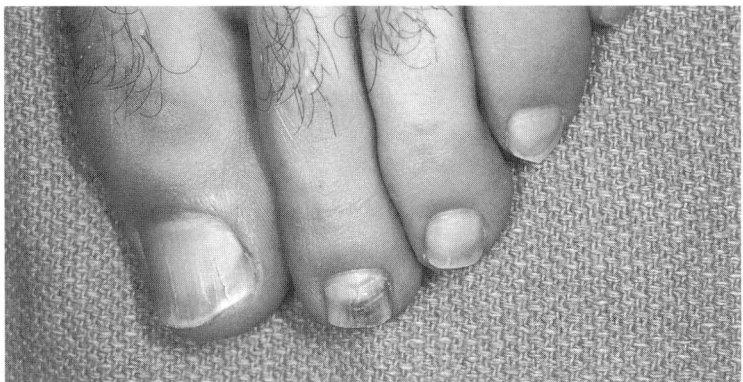

Figure 15-3. Jogger's toenail can reveal transverse ridging.

diagnosis is unclear, culture or PAS staining of subungual debris by the dermatopathology laboratory is recommended. Potassium hydroxide examination may be useful but can be technically challenging. A biopsy should be performed if melanoma is suspected.

The differential diagnosis also includes nail psoriasis and other sports-related nail abnormalities, such as center's callosities, tennis toe, and the nail conditions associated with dancing, football, skating, skiing, and soccer.

Treatment

Jogger's toenail resolves without therapy when running is stopped. Some runners simply paint their toes to cover the discoloration. A heated paper clip or needle bores through the nail plate and promptly relieves the pressure and the pain of a subungual hematoma. Sterile dressings and topical wound care are mandatory until the nail heals.

Prevention

Wearing properly fitted shoes decreases the likelihood of jogger's toenail. Most major cities have specialty running stores staffed by experts in fitting shoes for myriad foot and body shapes and running abilities. Orthotic devices help ameliorate the sliding effect of the foot in the running shoe. Lacing techniques can prevent the foot from freely slamming into the toe box, especially on downhill courses when there is a great deal of force pushing the toenail into the end of the shoe. Athletes should cut their toenails straight across, without rounded edges. Straight nails allow equal distribution of forces when the nail hits the toe box. Athletes can use foam toe caps, which fit around the at-risk toe inside the shoe (Adams, 2003).

Onychocryptosis

Epidemiology

This condition is also known as "ingrown toenail." No epidemiologic studies of onychocryptosis exist. It is specifically reported in basketball, football, and tennis players and dancers.

15. Traumatic Injuries to the Nails and Toes 267

Clinical Presentation

A particularly curved (not flat) nail produces force between the first toe nail and the surrounding soft tissue. Individuals who cut their nails too short and curve the edges develop onychocryptosis. The surrounding tissue (most commonly around the first toenail) can become extremely painful, edematous, and erythematous (Ronzca and Lupo, 1989).

Diagnosis

Upon careful inspection of the nail and surrounding tissue, the clinician observes penetration of the sharp edge of the nail into the surrounding skin (Figure 15-4). The differential diagnosis includes bacterial infection, gout, and subungual exostosis. Radiographic examination is necessary if subungual exostosis, which is a benign growth on the surface on bone related to trauma, is suspected (Howse, 1983).

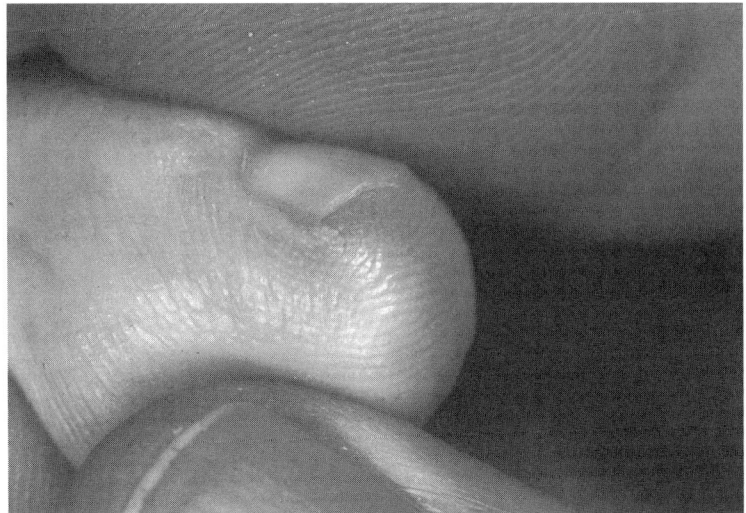

Figure 15-4. Growth of the nail into surrounding soft tissue characterizes onychocryptosis. There is associated erythema and edema.

Treatment

Athletes should soak their toes for 5 to 10 minutes, three times per day. A longitudinal incision should be made from the distal end to the mid-nail plate near the soft tissue penetration. The clinician then lifts this linear nail flap and places a piece of wool beneath the flap. The wool prevents the nail from continuing to penetrate the surrounding skin. Some surgeons also encircle the linear nail flap with the plastic protective covering on the small surgical scissors tips. Surgical excision of the embedded nail occasionally is required.

Prevention

Athletes should cut their toenails straight across, without rounded edges. Straight nails allow equal distribution of forces when the nail hits the toe box. Shoes that do not fit properly and are too tight will exacerbate onychocryptosis. Athletes can use foam toe caps, which fit around the at-risk toe inside the shoe.

Miscellaneous Sports and Activities Associated with Nail Changes

Fingernails

Bowler's Fingernail

Epidemiology

No studies of bowler's fingernail exist.

Clinical Presentation

Bowlers who use balls with holes develop thin fingernails (except the thumb) on the throwing hand. Callosities arise on the lateral aspects of the second, third, and fifth fingers. Bowlers who use balls without holes do not experience nail abnormalities but acquire callosities on the third and fourth fingers of the throwing hand (Spoor, 1977).

Diagnosis

The diagnosis is straightforward after a history is obtained.

Treatment

For undesired callosities, topical urea cream 20% or 40% should be applied after the area is soaked with water for 5 to 10 minutes twice per day.

Prevention

Some bowlers prefer to have the callosities. Lacquers can be applied to the nail, but this may alter a bowler's throwing motion.

Frisbee Nail

Epidemiology

No studies of frisbee nail exist.

Clinical Presentation

Acute or repeated trauma to the fingernail generates splinter hemorrhages in the affected nail (Tanzi and Scher, 1999).

Diagnosis

The diagnosis is straightforward but should be distinguished from golfer's nail. Splinter hemorrhages also are seen in patients with cardiac abnormalities.

Treatment

No treatment is necessary.

Prevention

Cutting the nails short, squarely, and even with the hyponychium prevents Frisbee nails.

Golfer's Nail

Epidemiology

One case report of this condition exists (Ryan and Goldsmith, 1995). The collision between the head of the club and the ball produces 3000 lb of pressure for 1/1000 second. This force is generally not transmitted to the hands because of the flexibility of the club. However, an excessively tight grip on the club results in transfer of the powerful force to the hands, specifically the nails.

Clinical Presentation

The enormous force transferred to the nails when a golfer grasps the golf club too firmly damages the vascular bed, resulting in splinter hemorrhages. Chronically, the nail may become thickened (onychauxis).

Diagnosis

The diagnosis is straightforward but should be distinguished from Frisbee nail. Splinter hemorrhages also are seen in patients with cardiac abnormalities.

Treatment

No treatment is necessary.

Prevention

Loosening the grip on the club prevents golfer's nail (and likely improves the player's shots).

Karate Nail

Epidemiology

No studies of Karate nail exist.

Clinical Presentation

Acute blows to the hands and nails create multiple transverse white bands (Ronzca and Lupo, 1989).

Diagnosis

The diagnosis is straightforward.

Treatment

No treatment is necessary.

Prevention

None is necessary.

Weightlifter's Nail

Epidemiology

One case report of this condition exists (Scott et al., 1992). Hooking is a barbell gripping method during which the weightlifter covers the distal portion of the thumbs with the second and third fingers. This gripping method ensures a secure grasp.

Clinical Presentation

The gripping method used exerts enormous force on the thumbnail. Subungual hematomas and onychoptosis defluvium (complete loss of nail) can occur.

Diagnosis

The diagnosis is straightforward after an appropriate history is obtained.

Treatment

A heated paper clip or needle bores through the nail plate and promptly relieves the pressure and pain of a subungual hematoma. Sterile dressings and topical wound care are mandatory until the nail heals. In cases of onychoptosis defluvium where the nail is loose but still attached, the clinician should encircle the toe and nail with adhesive tape. The nail acts as an excellent biologic dressing as the new nail plate is manufactured.

In the unfortunate scenario where the nail is completely shed, a sterile petroleum jelly or antibiotic impregnated gauze should be inserted into the proximal nail fold. The dressing should also cover the bare nail matrix. The nail plate typically provides protection for the nail matrix; without this protection, damage to the matrix may lead to permanent nail plate deformity. The dressing should be changed daily until the nail begins to return.

Prevention

If weightlifters do not use the hooking method, they will not develop the nail changes but will have a less firm grip on the bar.

Toenails

Center's Callosities

Epidemiology

No epidemiologic studies of center's callosities exist, but one case report noted the presence of these specific callosities in a basketball player (Adams and

Lucky, 2001). Basketball players' toes, especially the most distal ones, experience a great deal of chronic friction between the skin and the toe box. Basketball floors (regardless of indoor or outdoor venue) do not allow the soles of basketball shoes to freely move. Thus, the basketball player's distal toe rams into the shoe with every abrupt stop and start.

Clinical Presentation

The most distal toe (the second toe in the only reported case) reveals well-defined and hyperkeratotic plaques extending from the hyponychium to the distal tip of the toe. The distal nail also may demonstrate changes that include splinter hemorrhages. No subungual debris, yellow discoloration of the nail plate, or scaling of the soles is observed.

Diagnosis

It is important for the clinician to obtain the sports participation history because this condition is commonly mistaken for onychomycosis or psoriasis. When the nail changes in center's callosities predominate, the differential diagnosis includes other sports-related nail abnormalities, such as jogger's toe, tennis toe, and the nail conditions associated with football, dancing, skating, skiing, and soccer.

Treatment

The only effective treatment is obtaining larger shoes so that the toe does not constantly jam into the toe box. Topical urea at concentrations of 20% or 40% applied twice per day after soaking the area in water for 5 to 10 minutes will clear the hyperkeratosis. The hyperkeratosis clears during the off season.

Prevention

Wearing properly fitted shoes decreases the likelihood of center's callosities. Orthotic devices help ameliorate the sliding effect of the foot in the basketball shoe. Lacing techniques can prevent the foot from freely slamming into the toe box. Athletes can use foam toe caps, which fit around the at-risk toe inside the shoe.

Football Toenail

Epidemiology

No epidemiologic studies of football toenail exist. Acute blunt forces create enough energy to shed the nail (onychoptosis defluvium). These blunt forces may result from kicking the ball or from trauma upon contact with grass or artificial turf.

Clinical Presentation

Subungual hematomas, typically on the second and third toenails, lead to discoloration of the nail (Figure 15-5) (Ronzca and Lupo, 1989). Occassionally, strong forces will remove the nail entirely.

Diagnosis

The differential diagnosis includes other sports-related nail abnormalities, such as center's callosities, jogger's toenail, tennis toe, and the nail conditions associated with dancing, skating, skiing and soccer. Subungual hematomas may also be confused for melanoma.

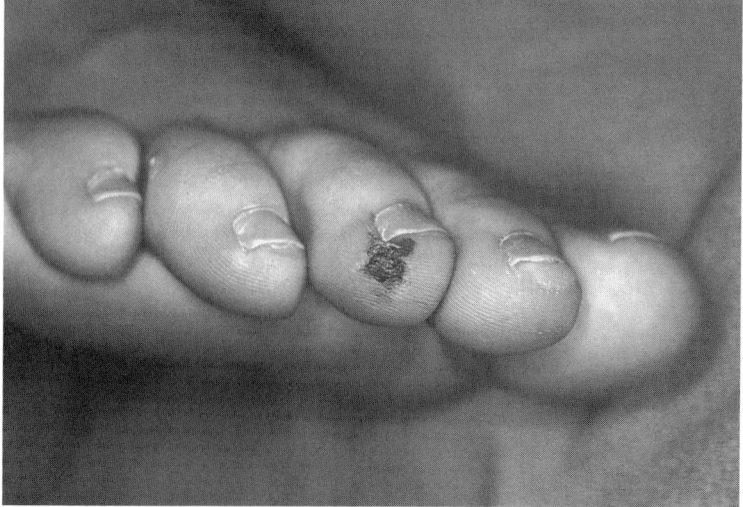

Figure 15-5. Hemorrhage on the third toe, as would occur from kicking a ball. This lesion may mimic melanoma.

Treatment

Football nail resolves without therapy when football is stopped. A heated paper clip or needle bores through the nail plate and promptly relieves the pressure and pain of a subungual hematoma. Sterile dressings and topical wound care are mandatory until the nail heals. In cases of onychoptosis defluvium where the nail is loose but still attached, the clinician should encircle the toe and nail with adhesive tape. The nail acts as an excellent biologic dressing as the new nail plate is manufactured.

In the unfortunate scenario where the nail is completely shed, a sterile petroleum jelly or antibiotic impregnated gauze should be inserted into the proximal nail fold. The dressing should also cover the bare nail matrix. The nail plate typically provides protection for the nail matrix; without this protection, damage to the matrix may lead to permanent nail plate deformity. The dressing should be changed daily until the nail begins to return.

Prevention

Wearing properly fitted shoes decreases the likelihood of football toenail. Football cleats should be professionally fitted. Orthotic devices help ameliorate the sliding effect of the foot in the shoe. Lacing techniques can prevent the foot from freely slamming into the toe box. Athletes should cut their toenails straight across, without rounded edges. Straight nails allow equal distribution of forces when the nail hits the toe box. Athletes can use foam toe caps, which fit around the at-risk toe inside the shoe.

Skier's Toenail

Epidemiology

No studies of skier's toenail exist. By leaning forward in ski boots, the skier places increased force upon the most distal toenails as they hit the end of the very firm boot (Basler, 1990). Ill-fitting boots are problematic, but the nail changes can occur in adequately sized boots as well.

Clinical Presentation

The first toes develop subungual hematomas that eventuate in discoloration of the nail plate (Figure 15-6, see color plate).

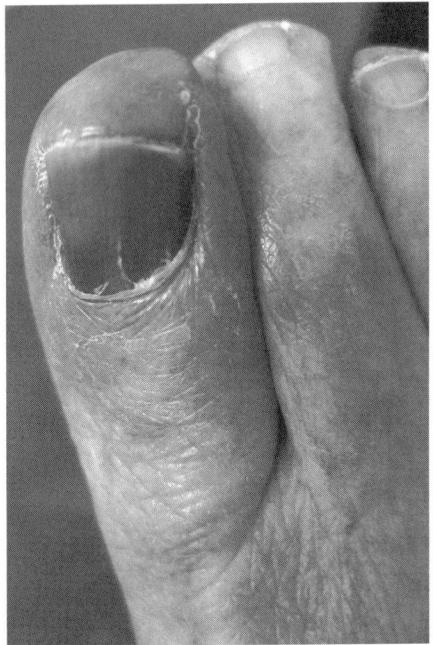

Figure 15-6. Skier's toenail. (See color plate.)

Diagnosis

The differential diagnosis includes other sports-related nail abnormalities, such as center's callosities, jogger's toenail, tennis toe, and the nail conditions associated with dancing, football, skating, and soccer. Subungual hematomas may also be confused for melanoma.

Treatment

A heated paper clip or needle bores through the nail plate and promptly relieves the pressure and the pain of a subungual hematoma. Sterile dressings and topical wound care are mandatory until the nail heals.

Prevention

Wearing properly fitted boots decreases the likelihood of skier's toenail. Athletes should cut their toenails straight across, without rounded edges. Straight nails allow equal distribution of forces when the nail hits the toe box. Athletes can use foam toe caps, which fit around the at-risk toe inside the boot.

Soccer Toenail

Epidemiology

No epidemiologic studies of soccer toenail exist.

Clinical Presentation

Acute blunt forces from a swift kick of the ball may result in onycholysis or onychoptosis defluvium (complete loss of nail) (Ronzca and Lupo, 1989). Chronic repetitive kicks produce transverse ridging and subungual hemorrhage through damage to the nail matrix (Mortimer and Dawber, 1985).

Diagnosis

The diagnosis is straightforward after a history is obtained. The differential diagnosis includes other sports-related nail abnormalities, such as center's callosities, jogger's toenail, tennis toe, and the nail conditions associated with dancing, football, skating, and skiing. Subungual hematomas may also be confused for melanoma.

Treatment

A heated paper clip or needle bores through the nail plate and promptly relieves the pressure and pain of a subungual hematoma. Sterile dressings and topical wound care are mandatory until the nail heals. In cases of onychoptosis defluvium where the nail is loose but still attached, the clinician should encircle the toe and nail with adhesive tape. The nail acts as an excellent biologic dressing as the new nail plate is manufactured.

In the unfortunate scenario where the nail is completely shed, a sterile petroleum jelly or antibiotic impregnated gauze should be inserted into the proximal nail fold. The dressing should also cover the bare nail matrix. The nail plate typically provides protection for the nail matrix; without this protection, damage to the matrix may lead to permanent nail plate deformity. The dressing should be changed daily until the nail begins to return.

Prevention

These nail changes can be prevented by taping the toes together or by using soccer shoes with a very firm toe box (Ronzca and Lupo, 1989). Athletes can use foam toe caps, which fit around the at-risk toe inside the shoe.

Skater's Toenail

Epidemiology

No studies of skater's toenail exist. Improperly fitted skates allow the feet to thrust into the toe box during the myriad movements involved with skating in hockey or figure skating.

Clinical Presentation

Onychauxis (thickened nail), splinter hemorrhages, subungual hematoma, subungual hyperkeratosis, and onycholysis (separation of the nail plate from the nail bed, which appears as a white part of the nail) occur. A pincer nail deformity, in which both lateral edges of the nail curve down into the underlying soft tissue, can occur and is quite painful (Scher, 1988).

Diagnosis

The diagnosis is straightforward after a history is obtained. The differential diagnosis includes psoriasis, onycholysis, other sports-related nail abnormalities, such as center's callosities, jogger's toenail, tennis toe, and the nail conditions associated with dancing, football, and soccer. Subungual hematomas may also be confused for melanoma.

Treatment

Nail abnormalities resolve once the skater discontinues skating or wears properly fitted skates. Surgery may be necessary to alleviate the pincer nail deformity. A heated paper clip or needle bores through the nail plate and promptly relieves the pressure and the pain of a subungual hematoma. Sterile dressings and topical wound care are mandatory until the nail heals.

In cases of onycholysis, the clinician should encircle the toe and nail with adhesive tape. The nail acts as an excellent biologic dressing as the new nail plate is manufactured.

Prevention

Wearing properly fitted skates decreases the occurrence of hockey or skater's toenail. Orthotic devices help ameliorate the sliding effect of the foot in the skate. Furthermore, athletes should cut their toenails straight across, without rounded edges. Straight nails allow equal distribution of forces when the nail hits the end of the skate. Athletes can use foam toe caps, which fit around the at-risk toe inside the skate.

Subungual Exostosis

Epidemiology

No epidemiologic studies in athletes have been performed, but cyclists who use toe clips and ballet dancers who use toe shoes seem to be at particular risk (Young et al., 2001). Trauma precedes the onset of subungual exostosis in one fourth of cases. Irritation to the distal digit causes cartilage to proliferate and become ossified.

Clinical Presentation

Clinically a solitary, tender, skin-colored, less than 1-cm nodule occurs in the nail bed and eventually deforms the nail plate. Most cases (80%) occur on the big toe. Most lesions develop over a period of 2 to 5 months, and individuals complain of pain or throbbing.

Diagnosis

The diagnosis is challenging. The differential diagnosis includes epidermoid cyst, glomus tumor, melanoma, pyogenic granuloma, squamous cell carcinoma, subungual fibroma, and verruca vulgaris. Radiographic studies reveal ossified subungual exostosis arising from the phalanx. Biopsy confirms the diagnosis.

Treatment

Surgical excision, after digital block, clears the tumor. Recurrence occurs in 5% to 11% of cases.

Prevention

No prevention exists other than avoidance of trauma.

Windsurfer's Nail

Epidemiology

This condition is otherwise known as "toe jam." Only one brief case report exists.

Clinical Presentation

By planting their toes tightly on the surfboard, windsurfers develop subungual purpura on the first toe (Chiarello, 1985).

Diagnosis

The diagnosis is straightforward after a history is obtained. The differential diagnosis includes other sports-related nail abnormalities, such as center's callosities, jogger's toenail, tennis toe, and the nail conditions associated with dancing, football, skating, skiing, and soccer.

Treatment

No treatment is needed. Some athletes paint the toes to cover the discoloration.

Prevention

No prevention exists.

Bibliography

Adams BB, Lucky AW. A center's callosities. Cutis 2001;67:141–142.
Adams BB. Jogger's toenail. J Am Acad Dermatol 2003;48:S58–S59.
Basler RSW. Skin problems encountered in winter sports. In: Casey MJ, Foster C, Hixson EG, editors. Winter sports medicine. Philadelphia: FA Davis; 1990, p. 142–147.
Chiarello SE. Toe jam [letter]. Arch Dermatol 1985;121:591.
Howse J. Disorders of the great toe in dancers. Clin Sports Med 1983;2:499–505.
Hutchinson MR, Laprade RF, Burnett QM II, et al. Injury surveillance at the USTA Boys' Tennis Championships: a 6-yr study. Med Sci Sports Exerc 1995;27:826–830.
Katchis SD, Hershman EB. Broken nails to blistered heels. Phys Sportsmed 1993;21:95–104.
Mailler EA, Adams BB. The wear and tear of 26.2: dermatological injuries reported on marathon day. Br J Sports Med 2004;38:498–501.
Mortimer PS, Dawber RPR. Trauma to the nail unit including occupational sports injuries. Dermatol Clin 1985;3:415–420.
Ronzca EC, Lupo PJ. Pedal nail pathology. Clin Podiatr Med Surg 1989;6:327–337.
Ryan AM, Goldsmith LA. Golfer's nails. Arch Dermatol 1995;131:857–858.
Scher RK. Occupational nail disorders. Dermatol Clin 1988;6:27–33.
Scott MJ Jr, Scott NI, Scott LM. Dermatologic stigmata in sports: weightlifting. Cutis 1992;50:141–145.
Spoor HJ. Sports identification marks. Cutis 1977;19:453–456.
Tanzi EL, Scher RK. Managing common nail disorders in active patients and athletes. Phys Sportsmed 1999;27:35–47.
Young RJ, Wide JL, Sartori CR, et al. Solitary nodule of the great toe. Cutis 2001;68:57–58.

16. Combined Factors (Pressure, Friction, Occlusion, and Heat)

The first four chapters in the section on sports-related traumatic skin conditions examine the singular effect of friction, pressure, and pounding trauma on the skin, hair, and nails of athletes. This final chapter in the section examines two cutaneous conditions that result from a combination of the forces described in Chapters 12 through 15. Acne mechanica results from a multitude of elements on the skin, including pressure, friction, occlusion, and heat. Pulling boat hands result from the combination of pressure, friction, and a wet and cold environment. Acne keloidalis nuchae likewise develops after exposure to a combination of factors.

Acne Mechanica

Epidemiology

There have been no epidemiologic studies of acne mechanica in athletes. A variety of athletes with acne mechanica are reported, including football, tennis, and hockey players, dancers, golfers, shot putters, wrestlers, and weightlifters (Adams, 2001, 2002; Basler, 1992). The joint forces of pressure, occlusion, heat, and friction cause acne mechanica. Some believe that acne mechanica occurs in individuals who already had acne (Mills and Kligman, 1975), whereas others note that a prior history of acne is not necessary for development of acne mechanica (Basler, 1992).

Clinical Presentation

The lesions are well-defined, erythematous papules and pustules distributed in a pattern that relates to the athlete's causative clothing or equipment (often protective). The most common locations for lesions are the upper back, chin, and posterior scalp (Adams, 2001) (Figure 16-1, see color plate). These locations correlate to the areas of protective equipment used by football and hockey players (Basler, 1992). Helmets help to create the occipital scalp, cheek, and forehead lesions, shoulder pads contribute to the back lesions, and chin straps help to induce the chin and lower cheek lesions.

Tennis players can develop acne mechanica on the upper back, lower neck, and chest if they wear heavy clothes while practicing in the cold (Basler and

16. Combined Factors (Pressure, Friction, Occlusion, and Heat)   283

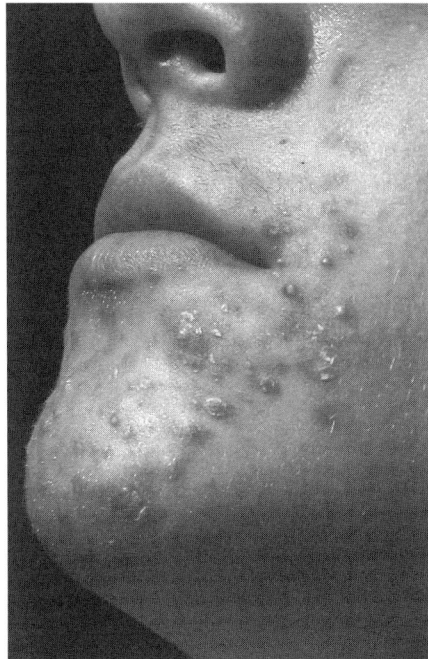

Figure 16-1. Football players frequently develop acne mechanica beneath the chin strap. This type of acne is much more difficult to treat than typical acne vulgaris. (See color plate.)

Garcia, 1998). Wrestlers develop acne mechanica beneath their headgear and knee and elbow pads (Adams, 2001, 2002). While walking, golfers acquire lesions on their lower lateral back corresponding to the area where the golf bag rests. Dancers get acne mechanica under their tight-fitting leotards.

Field event athletes, particularly those who throw the shot put, can develop acne mechanica. A shot putter's technique repetitively places the metal shot on a sweaty neck for hours on end. This method is the perfect recipe for development of acne mechanica. Weightlifters are also at risk to develop acne mechanica. While bench pressing and arching the back for extra support and power, athletes may experience a great deal of pressure and friction on their sweaty upper back. Weightlifters constantly bring the bar-bearing weights to their upper central chest. Not surprising then, acne mechanica occurs on the upper central back and chest in weightlifters (Adams, 2001, 2002) (Figure 16-2 and Table 16-1).

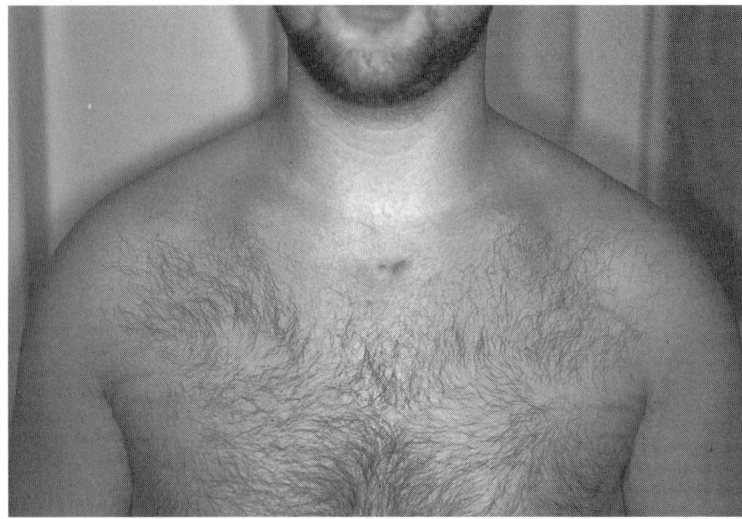

Figure 16-2. Weightlifters may develop acne mechanica on the central chest.

Table 16-1. Location and Cause of Acne Mechanica According to Sport

Sport	Acne Location	Etiology
Dancing	Trunk	Tight leotard
Football	Chin	Chin straps
	Shoulders	Shoulder pads
	Upper inner arm	Shoulder pad straps
	Forehead, cheeks	Helmet
Golf	Lower lateral back	Golf bag being carried
Hockey	Chin	Chin straps
	Shoulders	Shoulder pads
	Upper inner arm	Shoulder pad straps
	Forehead, cheeks	Helmet
Shot put	Neck	Shot put before launch
Tennis	Back	Heavy warm clothes
Weightlifting	Upper back	Plastic/vinyl bench cover
	Upper central chest	Weight bar
Wrestling	Chin, neck (periauricular)	Headgear
	Elbows, knees	Elbow and knee pads

Diagnosis

The clinician needs to astutely consider an athlete's equipment and clothing when confronted with acneiform papules. Upon questioning the athlete about sport activities, the sports clinician will be able to make the diagnosis. Very early lesions of tinea corporis gladiatorum, herpes gladiatorum, and impetigo may closely resemble early lesions of acne mechanica. On these very rare occasions, bacterial, fungal, and viral cultures and a punch biopsy may be necessary.

Treatment

Lesions improve after the season ends and the instigating clothing or equipment is no longer being used. Acne mechanica tends to be more resistant to therapy than typical acne vulgaris. Unless the clinician and athlete address the physical factors causing the acne, this condition will persist.

Topical therapy includes topical retinoids (e.g., tretinoin and tazarotene) and topical antibiotics (e.g., clindamycin solution, gel, or lotion). In my experience, tazarotene is the most effective, although no studies confirm this observation. Benzoyl peroxide products also are helpful. Topical compounds of keratolytics (3% salicylate and 8% resorcinol in 70% ethanol) also have been useful. Some clinicians add clindamycin to that compound (Basler, 1992). Systemic antibiotics may be effective, but not as effective as for typical acne vulgaris.

Prevention

Prevention of acne mechanica is critical because the treatment regimens are suboptimal. First, athletes should immediately shower after their sports activity. High school and collegiate athletes with their busy schedules frequently forego showering after practice. Use of mildly abrasive soaps in the areas of acne mechanica while bathing has been suggested (Adams, 2001; Basler, 1992). Athletes also can use keratolytic lotions (e.g., salicylic acid or urea cream) after showering to decrease the incidence of acne mechanica.

Athletes can wear synthetic moisture-wicking material beneath shoulder pads and other protective equipment. This relatively new technologic clothing decreases the influence of warmth, moisture, and occlusion, factors that are critical in the pathogenesis of acne mechanica.

Pulling Boat Hands

Epidemiology

A case series of 13 rowers/sailors noted a total of 30 episodes of this condition from May to October in 1982 in coastal New England (Toback et al., 1985). Each individual developed the condition while on a 30-foot rowing and sailing vessel called the "pulling boat" for 1 to 3 weeks at a time. The median age was 29 years, and 69% of the affected individuals were female. Individuals on similar boats in Florida have not developed this condition. Other at-risk sports include sailing, rafting, canoeing, crew, and kayaking. The combination of rowing's mechanical trauma and exposure to nonfreezing wet environments produces vasospasm and vascular injury.

Clinical Presentation

Individuals develop pulling boat hands after 3 days to 2 weeks aboard the pulling boat. Initially, well-defined, 1-mm to 1-cm, erythematous macules, papules, and plaques form on the distal dorsal aspect of the hand and proximal fingers, sparing the metacarpophalangeal joints. Subsequently, vesicles and bullae evolve within the lesions and ultimately become violaceous. More than 90% of subjects complain of pruritus, and 70% have associated burning and pain. Sixty-two percent demonstrate associated Raynaud's phenomenon. All lesions resolve with scarring after 7 days off the boat.

Diagnosis

The diagnosis can be challenging. Clinicians must remember this condition when watercraft athletes from cold climates present with erythematous papules or vesicles on the hands. Failure to appreciate the role of the sport leads to diagnostic failure. The differential diagnosis includes chilblains, epidermolysis bullosa acquisita, porphyria cutanea tarda, palmoplantar eccrine hidradenitis, irritant or allergic contact dermatitis, lupus erythematosus, photoallergic drug eruptions, and polymorphous light eruption.

Histopathologic examination reveals a superficial and deep perivascular lymphocytic infiltrate, subepidermal bullae, extravasated red blood cells, and capillary thromboses. Chilblains most resembles pulling boat hands but does not show histopathologic evidence of subepidermal blisters.

Treatment

A multitude of treatments, including oral antihistamines, topical steroids, and warm-water soaks, have failed to clear pulling boat hands. The only effective cure has been getting off the boat.

Prevention

Sunscreen does not prevent the condition. Rowers develop more episodes during May than August, which suggests that acclimatization and warmer temperatures can prevent pulling boat hands. Waterproof, windproof, and climate control gloves may help to prevent pulling boat hands.

Acne Keloidalis Nuchae

Epidemiology

One study investigated the incidence of acne keloidalis nuchae in football players ranging in age from 14 to 27 years. Fourteen percent of African-American football players exhibited the condition. Football players (college age and older) demonstrated more disease (9.4%) than younger players (5.2%) (Knable et al., 1997). Occlusion and friction with the football helmet initiate or exacerbate acne keloidalis.

Clinical Presentation

The athlete occasionally develops multiple, pruritic, grouped, discrete and confluent, erythematous to violaceous papules and plaques on the posterior neck and occipital scalp (Figure 16-3).

Diagnosis

The diagnosis is made based on the morphologic features and distribution.

Treatment

Treatment during the football season can be difficult. During the season, one National Football League (NFL) football player continued to develop lesions

288 Sports Dermatology

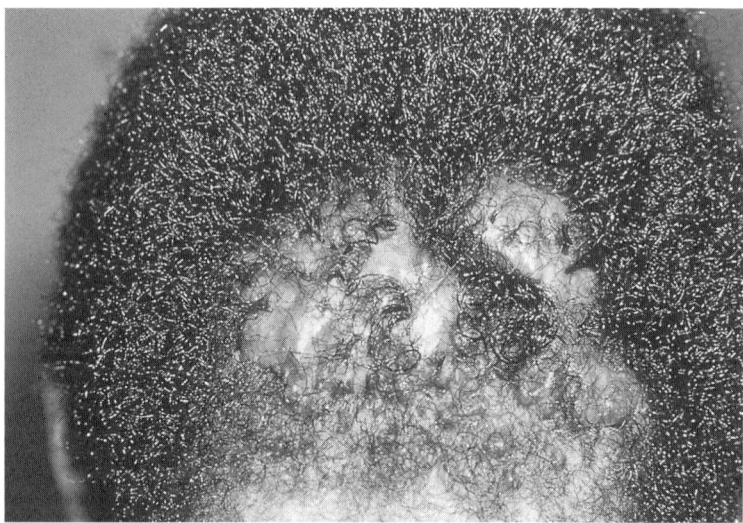

Figure 16-3. Athletes may develop many discrete or confluent, erythematous, violaceous papules and plaques on the back of the scalp, particularly aggravated by helmets.

despite therapy (Harris, 1992). The eruption cleared during the off season. The typical therapeutic modalities include topical and oral antibiotics (e.g., clindamycin and minocycline, respectively), topical retinoids, intralesional steroids, CO_2 laser, radiation therapy, and excision. Warm compresses for 10 minutes twice per day may be necessary for draining areas on the posterior neck or occipital scalp.

Prevention

Predisposed athletes must avoid very short haircuts on the occipital scalp. Players can place a thin pad between the scalp and the posterior portion of the helmet.

Bibliography

Adams BB. Sports dermatology. Adoles Clin 2001;12:305–322.
Adams BB. Dermatologic disorders of the athlete. Sports Med 2002;32:309–321.
Basler RSW. Acne mechanica in athletes. Cutis 1992;50:125–128.

Basler RSW, Garcia MA. Acing common skin problems in tennis players. Phys Sportsmed 1998;26:37–44.

Harris H. Acne keloidalis aggravated by football helmets. Cutis 1992;50:154.

Knable AL, Hanke WC, Gonin R. Prevalence of acne keloidalis nuchae in football players. J Am Acad Dermatol 1997;37:570–574.

Mills OH, Kligman A. Acne mechanica. Arch Dermatol 1975;111:4813.

Toback AC, Korson R, Krusinski PA. Pulling boat hands: a unique dermatosis from coastal New England. J Am Acad Dermatol 1985;12:649–655.

Section V Sports-Related Conditions Induced by the Environment

17. Chemical Deposition

This book reviews many diseases of athletes acquired through interaction with other competitors and their equipment. This section focuses on the interaction between athletes and the environment in which they compete. Even perfectly trained and prepared athletes are at the mercy of the venue's environment. Athletes are exposed to chemicals, anabolic steroids, thermal changes, and animals in the various venues. Some exposures are unique to specific sports, such as a swimmer's exposure to copper in the swimming pool. Other exposures, such as to cold temperatures, relate to sports that share only cold venues.

Chapter 18 reviews the cutaneous manifestations of anabolic steroid use. Chapter 19 focuses on the thermal effects of the environment on athletes' skin. Both acute and chronic extreme temperatures (cold or hot) pose difficulties for all athletes. Chapter 20, the last of this section and the last of the book, reviews the myriad encounters that athletes have with animals. Most of these encounters discussed occur in the sea or lakes. Land encounters with nonhuman competitors also are discussed.

Chapter 17, the first in this section, focuses on chemical deposition, the first of the four general categories of environmental exposure for athletes, specifically the effect of chlorine and copper on the hair of swimmers and nitrogen in the subcutaneous tissue of scuba divers.

Green Hair

Epidemiology

There have been no epidemiologic studies of green hair in swimmers. Clinicians have stated that the condition is more common than the rare cases reported in the literature (Sarnaik et al., 1986). Epidemics have occurred in pools with high levels of copper. One such epidemic occurred in Framingham, Massachusetts, when fluoridation treatment made the water much more acidic and the copper content in the water increased. Children and women are more likely to develop green hair after swimming (Basler et al., 2000). At-risk sports include diving, synchronized swimming, swimming, watersliding, and water polo.

The cause of green hair is copper and not chlorine, as is often mentioned. (In fact, one large cosmeceutical company even ran television advertisements incorrectly stating that their marketed shampoo protects swimmer's hair from becoming green by blocking the effects of chlorine.) Pools have varying levels of copper in the water. The copper originates as a naturally occurring ion in the water, from the copper pipes related to the pool, or from copper-containing algaecides. The acidity of water increases leaching from old pipes; hence, the level of copper in the water increases as the pH of the water decreases (Person, 1985).

Clinical Presentation

The greenish hue of hair is most easily appreciated in individuals with white, blonde, or very light hair.

Diagnosis

The diagnosis is unmistakable. Wet hair in bright light best demonstrates the greenish hue imparted on affected hair (Goette, 1978).

Treatment

Although there is no medical reason to treat the green hair, its appearance may disturb the athlete, who may wish to alter the hair color. Some have recommended heated vegetable [salad] oil (Goldschmidt, 1989). Over-the-counter copper chelating shampoos are readily available at any pharmacy. Applying 3% to 5% hydrogen peroxide to the green hair for 30 minutes also removes the color. This method essentially bleaches the hair. For treatment-resistant green hair, one author created a penicillamine shampoo by dissolving a 250-mg capsule of the medicine in 5 ml water and 5 ml shampoo. This shampoo cleared the green hair in several days (Person, 1985).

Prevention

Regular and immediate shampooing after swimming should be effective in preventing green hair. Athletes should fully rinse their hair after shampooing to ensure that the residual shampoo does not create an ideal microenvironment for precipitation of copper salt in the hair (Person, 1985). Others also recommend shampooing twice per season with a copper chelating shampoo to deter the production of green hair (Goldschmidt, 1989). It is very important that the pH of the pool be properly maintained. The ideal pH is between 7.4 and 7.6.

Blonding and Drying of Hair

Epidemiology

Not uncommonly, avid swimmers who use chlorinated pools find their hair has been bleached and made much drier because of the chlorine. At-risk sports include diving, synchronized swimming, swimming, and water polo.

Clinical Presentation

Depending on the concentration of chlorine and the duration of time spent in the chlorinated pool, the swimmer's hair will become dry and bleached.

Diagnosis

Dry and bleached hair is self-evident.

Treatment and Prevention

Swimmers should use a conditioning shampoo or rinse immediately after swimming in pools.

Skin Bends

Epidemiology

This condition is also known as "nitrogen rash." It occurs when divers exceed their allowable time deep underwater. Nitrogen supersaturates the blood and dissolves in the subcutaneous tissue.

Clinical Presentation

Affected divers notice a pruritic, reticulated, cyanotic, purpuric eruption on the elbows and lateral abdomen.

Diagnosis

The diagnosis is straightforward after the history is obtained and is correlated with the clinical presentation.

Treatment and Prevention

Nitrogen rash self-subsides, but divers should not continue to dive until the eruption has cleared.

Bibliography

Basler RS, Basler GC, Palmer AH, et al. Special skin symptoms in swimmers. J Am Acad Dermatol 2000;43:299–305.

Goette DK. Swimmer's green hair. Arch Dermatol 1978;114:127–128.

Goldschmidt H. Green hair. Arch Dermatol 1979;115:1288.

Person JR. Green hair: treatment with a penicillamine shampoo. Arch Dermatol 1985; 121:717–718.

Sarnaik A, Vohra, Sturman SW, et al. Medical problems of the swimmer. Clin Sports Med 1986;5:47–64.

18. Anabolic Steroids

This second chapter in the section on sports-related conditions induced by the environment discusses the skin changes that occur as a result of an athlete's administration of anabolic steroids. Whereas the effects of copper on the athlete's hair (discussed in Chapter 17) are primarily cosmetic in nature, the effects of anabolic steroids have serious implications. Hepatic complications are among the most serious and include hepatitis and liver neoplasms. Anabolic steroids increase the athlete's risk for hypertension, atherosclerotic heart disease, and cerebrovascular accidents. Anabolic steroids affect mood by causing mania, neuroses, depression, irritability, sleep problems, and suicidal thoughts. Male users experience gynecomastia and testicular atrophy. Female users can develop amenorrhea, clitoral hypertrophy, hirsutism, and irregular menses. Human immunodeficiency virus infection has been transmitted through use of unsterilized needles (Scott and Scott, 1989a).

Clinicians who care for athletes are in a unique position to identify the cutaneous manifestations of anabolic steroid use. Upon discovery of these clues, the clinician must counsel the athlete on the deleterious effects of anabolic steroids.

Anabolic Steroid Use

Epidemiology

Anabolic steroids are synthetic derivatives of testosterone that quickly increase lean body mass. One very large study showed that 6.6% of 12th-grade male students had used anabolic steroids, and more than 67% of these students started using anabolic steroids before age 16 years. Sixty-five percent of anabolic steroid users participated in school-sponsored athletics. Of these athletes, approximately 40% played football and 15% each participated in wrestling, track and field, or baseball (or basketball) (Buckley et al., 1988).

Anabolic steroid use appears to increase further at the elite level. Some have estimated that more than 50% of the athletes at the 1988 Summer Olympic Games had used steroids at one time. The incidence of steroid use among professional players also has been estimated at approximately 50%. Finally, 90% to 100% of professional weightlifters and athletes who throw the discus, javelin, hammer, and shot put have used anabolic steroids (Scott and Scott, 1989a).

Athletes cycle their steroid use in part to evade detection by medical tests used by governing boards. In fact, elite athletes must inform officials about their exact location at all times because surprise testing can occur at a moment's notice.

Clinical Presentation

Striae distensae is one of the most common dermatologic manifestations of anabolic steroid use. One study of powerlifters at a championship revealed that athletes who used steroids developed acne (53%), increased body hair (47%), oily skin or hair (27%), and alopecia (20%) (Scott and Scott, 1989b). Other skin findings include cysts, folliculitis, hirsutism, jaundice, and pyoderma. Sebaceous gland size, the amount of dissolved skin surface lipids, and the number of acne-producing bacteria all significantly increase when athletes are exposed to high levels of anabolic steroids. Linear keloids have been noted in a hockey player and in bodybuilders (Scott et al., 1994).

Diagnosis

The diagnosis of anabolic steroid use can be suspected based upon the presence of the skin lesions listed under Clinical Presentation. Urinalysis is the typical method used to detect anabolic steroids.

Treatment

The treatment of striae distensae is difficult. Topical therapies have been mostly ineffective, but topical retinoids (tretinoin cream 0.1%) can be used. Laser therapy (585-nm, flash pump, pulsed-dye laser) also may be effective. Keloids can be injected with intralesional triamcinolone or treated topically with potent topical steroids under occlusion. Laser therapy also may be effective. The treatment of seborrheic dermatitis, acne, and alopecia related to anabolic steroids is difficult. Most of these side effects clear upon the discontinuation of anabolic steroid use, although alopecia often is irreversible.

Prevention

Although athletes may circumvent the testing for anabolic steroids by cycling their use, the only way to prevent the cutaneous manifestations of anabolic steroid use is to abstain from steroid use.

Bibliography

Buckley WE, Yesalis CE, Friedl KE, et al. Estimated prevalence of anabolic steroid use among male high school seniors. JAMA 1988;260:3441–3445.

Scott MJ, Scott MJ. Dermatologists and anabolic-androgenic drug abuse. Cutis 1989a;44: 30–35.

Scott MJ, Scott MJ. HIV infection associated with injections of anabolic steroids. JAMA 1989b;262:207–208.

Scott MJ, Scott MJ, Scott AM. Linear keloids resulting from abuse of anabolic steroid drugs. Cutis 1994;53:41–43.

19. Thermal Reactions

This next chapter in the section on sports-related conditions induced by the environment reviews the skin changes in athletes resulting from extreme temperatures. Athletes control nearly all variables that relate to their success or lack thereof during the practice of their sport. However, outdoor athletes cannot control the power of the environment.

Winter outdoor venues suffer not only from low temperatures but also from wind, which can significantly increase the amount of damage to the skin. Athletes whose activity occurs at high altitude, such as skiers and sledders, are exposed to even colder temperatures. The risk for frostbite in these athletes is discussed later in the chapter. Athletes exposed to cold yet nonfrigid weather, especially in the presence of moisture and water, endure separate skin conditions such as chilblains.

Reactions to extremely hot environments are reviewed in Chapter 7. The ultraviolet irradiation related to hot temperatures acutely creates sunburns and chronically can result in a variety of skin cancers. Athletes also are exposed to chronically and moderately hot temperatures while they are rehabbing sore muscles with heating pads. The unique skin condition related to use of this heat source is discussed first.

Erythema Ab Igne

Epidemiology

No studies have reviewed the epidemiology of erythema ab igne in athletes. Erythema ab igne results from chronic low-grade heat that is insufficient to actually create a burn.

Clinical Presentation

This heat source leads to characteristic well-defined, reticulated, brown patches on the exposed areas (Figure 19-1). Patients can develop nonmelanoma skin cancers, specifically squamous cell carcinoma. Actinic keratoses can appear in chronic lesions.

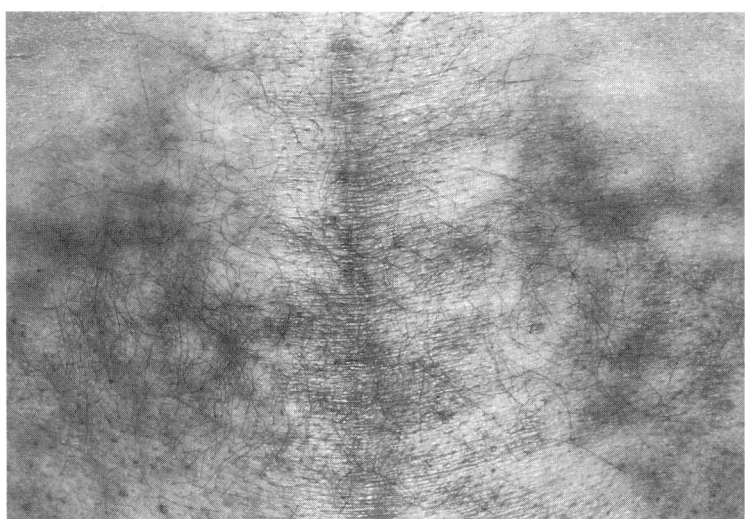

Figure 19-1. Erythema ab igne can develop beneath areas of heating pad use in the chronically exposed athlete.

Diagnosis

The diagnosis usually is straightforward and rarely is confused with other skin conditions. Reticulated erythema of livedo reticularis and cutis marmorata differ from erythema ab igne by the lack of pigmentary change.

Treatment

There is no known effective therapy. Once apparent, the area should be periodically observed for malignant change.

Prevention

Athletes should be careful not to chronically apply heat to their ailing muscles. Attention to the underlying problem is paramount.

Frostbite

Epidemiology

A National Ski Patrol study showed that 20% of all injuries were related to frostbite or cold. Any winter outdoor athlete is at risk for frostbite, but those athletes whose activity includes long periods of time outdoors or high rates of speed (e.g., cross-country skiers, cyclists, alpine skiers, ski jumpers, lugers, runners, snowmobilers, and speed skaters) are at greater risk. During the 1979 pre-Olympic trials, one race was canceled because 76 competitors developed superficial frostbite (frostnip). Male runners develop penile frostbite (Hershkowitz, 1977). Snowmobilers not infrequently develop frostbite on exposed areas on their face and neck. These enthusiasts often present with blisters, and some have dubbed the condition *polaris vulgaris* (Nissen et al., 1999). The cold temperatures combined with the wind chill factor created by the fast snowmobile result in optimal conditions for frostbite production. One case report discovered a snowmobiler experienced an effective temperature of −100°F for 1 to 2 hours.

Athletes with injuries often apply cold compresses and hold them in place with elastic bandages. If this procedure is prolonged, frostbite can occur beneath the cold compress (Cipollaro, 1992). Ethyl chloride sprays used as a cooling anesthetic also can result in frostbite. Another interesting observation was made during a National Football League championship held in frigid Green Bay, Wisconsin. Players on the Dallas football team developed cold injuries several times more frequently than members of the team from the colder climate.

Frostbite is related not only to the ambient temperature but also to wind, perspiration, protective clothing, and host factors. For instance, a temperature of 20°F with 45 mph winds is the same as −20°F. Downhill skiers experience extraordinary wind chills as they create their own wind while they attain high velocities. US ski team members have been noted to sweat even at subzero temperatures. The presence of sweat on any athlete increases heat loss through conduction.

Equipment influences frostbite development. For instance, the skintight downhill racing uniforms, required to maximize velocity, increase the risk of frostbite for the penis and breast (Hixson, 1981). Cross-country skiers experience constricted circulation due to the pole straps and the dorsal boot crease. In addition, their boots are not particularly insulated. Moreover, cross-country athletes are often exposed to very long periods outdoors.

Host factors also play a role. Certain medications and alcohol place the athlete at increased risk. Too frequent and thorough showering washes away protective skin oils, leaving the skin at greater risk for frostbite. Use of preshave and aftershave lotions may increase the risk of facial superficial frostbite (Stiles, 1971).

The four phases of frostbite are prefreeze, freeze/thaw, vascular stasis, and late ischemic (Kanzenbach and Dexter, 1999). The prefreeze phase can occur at nonfreezing temperatures from 37°F to 50°F and is characterized by slight numbness and swelling. The freeze/thaw phase occurs at temperatures between 5°F and 21°F as crystals form and then thaw inside and outside of cells. Numbness continues, as nerves are very sensitive to cold injury. During the vascular stasis phase, vasospasms occur and blood begins to coagulate. In the last phase, thrombosis, ischemia, and tissue destruction occur.

Clinical Presentation

Fifty-seven percent of all frostbite injuries include the lower extremities, specifically the foot and great toe, whereas 47% of the injuries include the hand. The face and ears account for only 17% of injuries (Sallis and Chassay, 1999).

The most likely anatomic areas for frostbite in athletes are the nose, ears, scrotum, and penis. Frostbite is categorized as either superficial (frostnip) or deep, and it can be graded in a manner similar to burns. First-degree and second-degree injuries are considered superficial, whereas third-degree and fourth-degree injuries encompass deep frostbite (Table 19–1). Clinically, frostbite appears as blue-white or waxy discoloration with numbness and swelling on the face or digit tips. Pain follows. Lack of pain in an area of obvious frostbite is of concern because it suggests a deep frostbite. In superficial frostbite the skin is somewhat pliable, but in deep frostbite the skin becomes firm (Figure 19–2).

After rewarming, vesicles or bulla may develop after 6 to 24 hours. Swelling occurs and may last for more than 1 month. Two to three days after rewarming, persistent throbbing and burning may occur in the affected area and last for several weeks. Ultimately a black scar develops in the first or second week, and autoamputation (if damage was severe) occurs 22 to 45 days after cold injury. One week after injury, ischemic neuritis may cause tingling, throbbing, and shooting pains for up to 6 months. The affected area may be highly sensitive for

Table 19-1. Frostbite Grading After Rewarming

Degree of Injury	Clinical Findings
First	Mottled and cyanotic
	Painful and burning
Second	Blistering
	Deeply erythematous
	Painful and burning
	Swollen
Third	Hemorrhagic blistering
	Necrotic skin and underlying tissue
	Severe aching and throbbing
	Swollen in entire area
Fourth	Anesthetic involved area
	Complete necrosis of skin and bone
	Not swollen in involved area

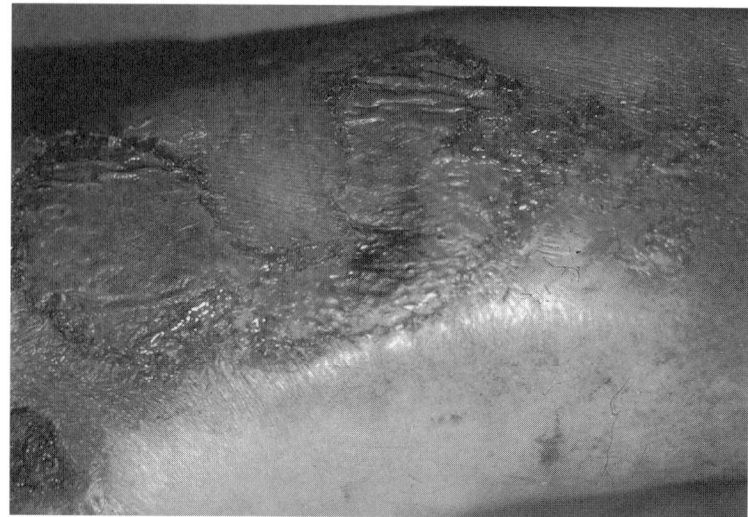

Figure 19-2. Frostbite can affect any winter outdoor athlete.

a long time. In general, most symptoms resolve in less than 1 month if no tissue was lost.

Diagnosis

The diagnosis is straightforward, but Doppler studies may be necessary to document the degree of vascular damage. Others have suggested triple-phase bone scan (scan of blood flow, blood pool, and bone blood uptake). The differential diagnosis includes trench foot, which differs from frostbite only in its etiology. In addition to cold temperatures, a wet environment is needed to induce trench foot.

Treatment

Protecting areas of frostbite from further freezing or trauma is essential. It is critical not to warm the area if it will later be reexposed to freezing risk. The freeze/thaw cycle causes a great deal of damage. The affected area must not be rubbed, and all wet clothing must be removed.

As soon as possible, the frostbitten skin must be rapidly immersed in 104°F to 108°F water for 15 to 30 minutes. The process is very painful, so affected

Table 19-2. Medical Approach to Frostbite

Stage	Action
Prewarming	No additional trauma
	No rubbing
	No transient thawing with mild heat
Warming	Rapid immersion in 104°F–108°F water for 15–30 minutes
Postwarming	Daily whirlpool
	Elevation
	Protection from trauma

athletes should be given an appropriate analgesic (e.g., morphine). Immediately after submersion, the athlete's skin will become erythematous, have increased sensation, and develop blisters. After submersion, the clinician can determine the depth (and degree) of damage (Table 19–2).

Continued pain management, elevation of the affected area, administration of nonsteroidal antiinflammatory drugs, and tetanus prophylaxis are mandatory. Most investigators' debride the clear blisters but not the hemorrhagic blisters. Antibiotics (intravenous penicillin G 500,000 U every 6 hours for 2–3 days) and surgical intervention may be required, depending on the extent and depth of damage. The athlete may use a whirlpool several times per day to help gently debride the affected area. Aloe vera should be applied thereafter (McCauley et al., 1983). Some have suggested that phenoxybenzamine may increase blood flow and decrease vasospasm (Christenson and Stewart, 1984). Not uncommonly, affected athletes later experience numbness, hypopigmented patches, nail changes, and hyperhidrosis.

Prevention

Skiers should not ski alone. Falling increases the risk of frostbite, so every attempt should be made not to fall. Athletes should dress appropriately for the duration of their practice or competition. Tight-fitting clothing may increase speed on downhill portions of the course, but these sleek outfits are not appropriate if the out door athlete is anticipating an extended period of time out in the cold. Male runners must wear snug-fitting underwear beneath their shorts or running tights; otherwise the penis may be at risk for frostbite. Athletes should wear clothing in layers, which aids in trapping warm air. The outerwear should be wind resistant. Synthetic moisture-wicking clothes are an integral part of layering and should be worn as the first layer. Gloves also should be layered. The innermost layer should be composed of synthetic moisture-wicking material, whereas the outermost layer should be waterproof.

Techniques other than clothing options can help prevent frostbite. Jewelry should not be worn because metal is an excellent heat conductor (Snowise and Dexter, 2004). Several commercially available warming packets are available. Athletes can insert these packets into their footwear (shoes or boots) or gloves, with or without adhesive. These devices are light and can stay warm for many hours. However, the packets can become very hot once activated, so athletes must be careful about burns. If fingers become cold in the very early stages, athletes should place their fingers in their axillae, where the temperature is much higher.

Skier's Cold Purpura

Epidemiology

One single case report noted this condition. Precipitation of normal globulins or other proteins at extremely cold temperatures is believed to cause the condition.

Clinical Presentation

A young male cross-country skier developed well-defined purpura over his shins. He did not have any trauma to the area, nor did he have any other medical problems. He had competed in a competition where the temperature (without wind chill factor) was −25°C. He noted cold areas on the shins, but he did not develop immediate local cold injuries (Nordlind et al., 1983).

Diagnosis

Biopsy is necessary to make the diagnosis. It is important to differentiate this condition from traumatic purpura and skin disorders related to cryoglobulins or cryofibrinogen. History of trauma and serologic tests exclude those diagnoses, respectively. In order to make the correct diagnosis of skier's cold purpura, the clinician must obtain a history of cold exposure.

Treatment

No treatment is necessary.

Prevention

Skiers should not ski alone. Falling increases the risk of cold exposure, so every attempt should be made not to fall. Cross-country skiers who will spend considerable time outside in subzero temperatures must dress and protect themselves appropriately.

Chilblains

Epidemiology

The epidemiology of chilblains in athletes is not well studied, but the condition usually is seen in athletes who participate in cold and wet sports, such as tobogganing and fishing (Long and Holt, 1992). Women seem to be more at risk than men (Snowise and Dexter, 2004). After prolonged exposure to cold [but not to freezing temperatures (32°F–50°F)] and damp environments, athletes develop a chronic vasculitis.

Clinical Presentation

Chilblains presents clinically with violaceous to erythematous, well-defined, tender papules, plaques, nodules, bulla, and ulcers. The lesions typically are distributed over the ears, nose, dorsal aspects of the proximal digits on the toes and fingers, and plantar surfaces of the toes (Figure 19–3). Tobogganers, whose pants often become wet, develop lesions on the thighs.

Diagnosis

Biopsy reveals papillary dermal edema and a superficial and deep vasculitis. The differential diagnosis includes other vasculitides, erythema elevatum diutinum, palmoplantar eccrine hidradenitis, and pulling boat hands.

Treatment

The key therapy is warming the affected area. Nifedipine and other calcium channel blockers decrease pain and time to clearance.

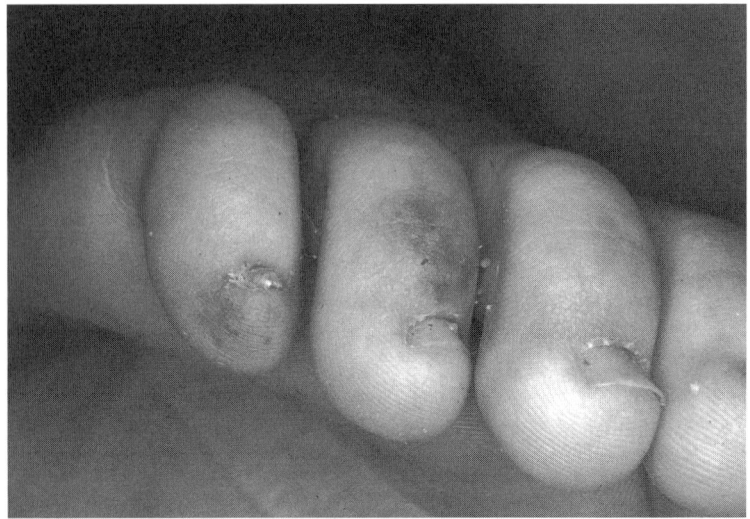

Figure 19-3. Erythematous to violaceous papules typify chilblains.

Prevention

The key to preventing chilblains is to keep the affected area not only warm but also dry. Prone athletes should wear layers of clothing, and the layer closest to the skin should be synthetic and moisture wicking. Some have suggested using aluminum chloride solution to decrease sweating. Commercially available warm packets keep the inside of boots or athletic wear at comfortable temperatures for many hours (Figure 19–4).

Equestrian Panniculitis (Equestrian Perniosis)

Epidemiology

The epidemiology has not been studied, although several small case series of females are reported (Beacham et al., 1980; De Silva et al., 2000).

Clinical Presentation

After prolonged exposure to cold temperatures and wind (atmospheric and gallop related) while horse riding, equestrians develop lesions on the superior lateral aspects of the thighs. Wearing tight-fitting, noninsulated pants increases the risk for disease by decreasing blood flow to the thigh. Morphologically, the lesions of equestrian panniculitis initially appear as multiple, erythematous, small, pruritic papules that eventually evolve into multiple, erythematous to violaceous, tender nodules. The reports note yearlong, persistent, dusky, tender plaques in the same locations.

Diagnosis

Biopsy of the nodular type reveals findings consistent with cold panniculitis. Typically only the fat of children reveals cold susceptibility. Lateral thigh fat in women may possess similar sensitivity. Serum cryoglobulins and cryofibrinogens are negative.

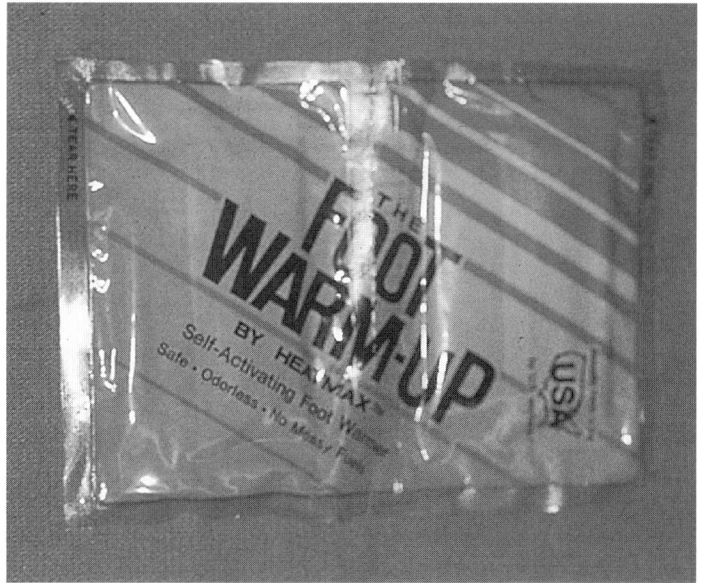

Figure 19-4. Commercially available shoe or boot warmers create exothermic reactions that can prevent frostbite and chilblains.

The clinical presentation of plaques has different histopathologic findings characterized by perniosis with no panniculitis. Serum cryoglobulins and cryofibrinogens are negative, but monoclonal cold agglutinins have been positive. The clinical differential diagnosis for the two lesions includes other types of panniculitis and perniosis.

Treatment

Nifedipine has been used without success. Heating pads improved the eruption significantly.

Prevention

Female equestrians can significantly improve lesions by wearing loose, insulated pants.

Bibliography

Beacham BE, Cooper PH, Buchanan CS, et al. Equestrian cold panniculitis in women. Arch Dermatol 1980;116:1025–1027.

Christenson C, Stewart C. Frostbite. Am Fam Pract 1984;30:111–122.

Cipollaro VA. Cryogenic injury due to local application of a reusable cold compress. Cutis 1992;50:111–112.

De Silva BD, McLaren K, Doherty VR. Equestrian perniosis associated with cold agglutinins: a novel finding. Clin Dermatol 2000;25:285–288.

Hershkowitz M. Penile frostbite: an unforeseen hazard of jogging. N Engl J Med 1977; 296:178.

Hixson EG. Injury patterns in cross-country skiing. Phys Sportsmed 1981;8:45–53.

Kanzenbach TL, Dexter WW. Cold injuries. Postgrad Med 1999;105:72–78.

Long CC, Holt PJC. Tobogganer's thighs. Clin Exp Dermatol 1992;17:466–467.

McCauley RL, Hing DN, Robson MC, et al. Frostbite injuries: a rational approach based on the pathophysiology. J Trauma 1983;23:1437.

Nissen ER, Melchert PJ, Lewis EJ. A case of bullous frostbite following recreational snowmobiling. Cutis 1999;63:21–23.

Nordlind K, Bondesson L, Johansson SG, et al. Purpura provoked by cold exposure in a skier. Dermatologica 1983;167:101–103.

Sallis R, Chassay CM. Recognizing and treating common cold-induced injury in outdoor sports. Med Sci Sports Exerc 1999;31:1367–1373.

Snowise M, Dexter WW. Cold, wind, and sun exposure. Phys Sportsmed 2004;32:26–32.

Stiles MH. Medical aspects of skiing. J Maine Med Assoc 1971;June:136–138.

20. Encounters with Animals

This is the last chapter in the section on sports-related conditions induced by the environment and the last chapter of this book. This chapter discusses the myriad skin reactions to members of the animal kingdom encountered in the athlete's venue. The type of skin eruption is largely related to the specific organism involved. Athletes whose competition take them to the outdoor turf or surf risk involvement. Although the overall incidence of skin reactions likely is greater in the grounded athlete, the variety of skin conditions experienced by the aquatic athlete is vast.

Seabather's Eruption

Epidemiology

Many epidemics of seabather's eruption, also termed *sea lice*, have occurred. In 1980 on the south shore of Long Island, several thousand swimmers developed the condition. In 1992 along the coast of South Florida, at least 10,000 swimmers were affected. Seabather's eruption typically creates havoc in the ocean along the Atlantic coast, Bermuda, Bahamas, and other Caribbean islands. Outbreaks occur between March and August but peak in May. Snorkelers and swimmers, but not deep-sea divers, develop the condition. The organisms causing seabather's eruption do not live at deep-sea depths.

It is widely believed that Cnidaria larvae cause seabather's eruption. Cnidaria is a phylum consisting of jellyfish, corals, sea anemones, and hydroids. Investigators have identified the larvae (planula) of *Linuche unguiculata* as the cause of epidemics in Florida and the Caribbean (Tomchik et al., 1993). However, the larvae of *Edwardsiella lineata* cause seabather's eruption on the coast of New York. Observations suggest that in addition to the larval forms of Cnidaria, adult medusa and immature medusa (ephyra) can cause seabather's eruption (Segura-Puertas et al., 2001).

The ephyra range in size from 0.5 to 6mm and prevail during January and March. Adult medusas are small jellyfish and grow to 2.5cm; they predominate from March to May. The planula predominate from May to June. These organisms are 0.5mm in size and are barely visible with the naked eye. The finding that all forms of *L. unguiculata* can cause seabather's eruption explains how a swimmer can develop seabather's eruption in the early spring when mature medusas exist. It is thought that the small-sized organisms flow through bathing suits, become trapped, and discharge their nematocysts onto the swimmer's skin.

Several factors impact the probability of disease. First, host factors are necessary, as not all exposed swimmers develop seabather's eruption. A swimmer's skin not only responds to the toxic effect of the nematocysts but also may develop an immunologic response to the antigen. The cell-mediated immunity is critical. The organisms are not distributed evenly in the water and can appear as cloudy areas. Finally, longer water exposure and swimsuits that cover greater areas of the body increase the likelihood of disease.

Clinical Presentation

Swimmers may experience a prickling sensation while they are still in the water. The skin lesions typically develop 4 to 24 hours after exposure, but may take up to four days to appear. One study showed that swimmers who had seabather's eruption in the past were statistically more likely to experience the prickling sensation while they were in the water (Tomchik et al., 1993).

The distribution of seabather's eruption is distinctive. Swimmers develop lesions concentrated beneath the swimming suit or on uncovered areas of the body that experience a great deal of friction (e.g., axillae and thighs). Lesions also occur under bathing caps and swimming fins. Surfers develop lesions on their chest and abdomen that result from trapping the stinging organisms as the surfers lie on the board heading out to catch a wave. Morphologically, the lesions of seabather's eruption appear as well-defined, discrete macules and papules; vesicles may be seen (Figure 20-1). The lesions can be painful or pruritic. In general the eruption clears within 1 to 2 weeks; most clear in 1 week.

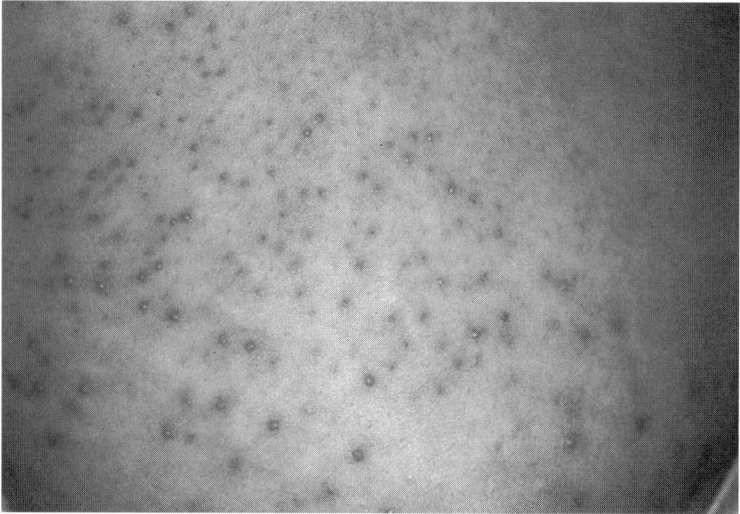

Figure 20-1. In seabather's eruption, athletes develop erythematous papules and vesicles beneath swim wear.

Investigators have documented persistent vesicular eruptions even 1 year after initial exposure. It is important to note that although the larva die in the bathing suit, the nematocysts persist and can continue to discharge their toxin. Associated systemic findings include fever, chills, headache, malaise, arthralgia, myalgias, and diarrhea. Complications include conjunctivitis, hyperpigmentation, keloidal formation, and atrophy.

Diagnosis

The distinctive distribution of seabather's eruption should alert the clinician. If the swimmer has been stung by the adult medusa, bell-shaped erythema may be noticed. The differential diagnosis is vast and includes swimmer's itch, insect bite reaction, urticaria (unrelated to sea creatures), sponge-diver's disease (ghost anemone), and viral or drug eruptions. Biopsy reveals a hypersensitivity reaction and is not particularly helpful in delineating the diagnosis. Some investigators have suggested ELISA may be a useful serologic test to confirm the diagnosis (Burnett et al., 1995).

Treatment

The most important treatment is removal of the swimming suit as soon as possible after the swimmer gets out of the sea water. Swimmers should not remove the suit while taking a shower because tap water may actually cause nematocyst activation. Many agents have been used to deactivate the nematocysts before they fire and include vinegar, baking soda, and isopropyl alcohol. Unfortunately, these compounds occasionally can conversely cause nematocysts to activate. No studies support the use of any particular therapy.

Once injected by the nematocysts, the swimmer should take antihistamines throughout the day. Topical steroids may benefit the swimmer. Some authors have used oral thiabendazole 1.5 g twice per day for 2 days (Burnett, 1992). Systemic steroids may be necessary in severe cases. The affected swimming suit should not be worn until it has been laundered (Table 20-1).

Table 20-1. Treatment of Seabather's Eruption

Immediate removal of swimming suit (not in tap water)
Application of vinegar or baking soda
Oral antihistamines
Topical steroids
Oral steroids (if severe)
Oral thiabendazole

Prevention

Swimmers should avoid cloudy areas (representing groups of organisms) in the ocean and areas with high density of adult medusa. Swimmers should avoid wearing T-shirts (they should wear water-resistant sunscreen instead), and women should consider wearing a two-piece suit. Because a swimmer's suit traps the nematocysts, decreasing the area covered by clothing is critical. Surfers and divers can wear wets suits with restrictive cuffs. A topical product that reduces the incidence of dermatitis from firing nematocysts is available and should be worn in oceans with high infestations. Finally, a sure method to prevent seabather's eruption is to avoid swimming along the eastern seaboard during peak months. It is interesting to note that some swimmers develop antibodies that may protect certain chronically exposed individuals.

Swimmer's Itch

Epidemiology

Several authors have noted epidemics of swimmer's itch, sometimes termed *schistosome dermatitis*, *cercarial dermatitis*, or *clam digger's itch* (Hoeffler, 1997). Fifty-six percent of snorkelers in one series developed swimmer's itch as did 250 swimmers in England in June and July 1970. An epidemiologic study in Quebec noted a 12% incidence of swimmer's itch. Sixty-nine percent of all cases were related to exposure to one specific beach (Levesque et al., 2002). In contrast to seabather's eruption, this condition occurs in fresh water. It occurs primarily in the northern United States and Canada, but it also is seen in California, Louisiana, Texas, and Washington. It has been noted on all continents except Antarctica.

The peak density of schistosomes in the northern United States correlates with mid-summer. Cercarial shedding from snails increases with increasing light and warm water temperatures. Shedding still occurs, albeit at a much lower rate, during the fall and early spring.

Cercariae of schistosomes cause swimmer's itch. Ducks and rodents, not humans, are the normal hosts for these microorganisms. Cercariae typically invade the feet of the normal host and reproduce in the mesenteric veins. The schistosomes' eggs are deposited in the host's feces, which infect intermediately aquatic snails. Once the cercariae emerge, they attempt to complete their life cycle by penetrating the feet of ducks or rodents. The cercariae must find their next host within 12 to 24 hours or face death. The cercariae may, at this point, unintentionally invade the human skin. The penetration results in a cutaneous hypersensitivity reaction. Snails particularly like shallow water, so, not surprisingly, most swimmers develop swimmer's itch while swimming in shallow water (Levesque et al., 2002).

Clinical Presentation

The swimmer develops pruritus approximately 1 hour after cercarial penetration. Within 24 hours, the athlete develops intensely pruritic, well-defined, erythematous, small (<0.5 cm) papules, macules, and occasionally vesicles on all exposed skin. Development of lesions on the face is very unusual. Most swimmers have more than 20 lesions, 23% of swimmers have between five and 20 lesions, and less than 10% of swimmers have fewer than five lesions. The lesions resolve without therapy in 1 to 2 weeks. Lengthy exposures to infested water and lack of extensive swimming suit coverage increase the severity of disease.

Systemic symptoms such as fever, chills, and lymphadenopathy are reported (Levesque et al., 2002). Postinflammatory hyperpigmentation is an occasional complication.

Diagnosis

The clinician should make the diagnosis of swimmer's itch based on the findings of temporal association with swimming and typical distribution of lesions. The differential diagnosis includes arthropod bite reaction, seabather's eruption, urticaria (unrelated to sea creatures), sponge-diver's disease (ghost anemore), and viral or drug eruptions (Table 20-2).

Treatment

Athletes who swim in infested waters should rigorously dry off with a towel. This method may dislodge some schistosomes before they penetrate the

Table 20-2. Comparison of Seabather's Eruption and Swimmer's Itch

	Seabather's Eruption	**Swimmer's Itch**
Epidemiology	Atlantic and Caribbean Oceans	Fresh water
Etiology	Cnidaria larvae	Schistosomes
Distribution	Beneath swimming suit	Spares the swimming suit area

skin. Some evidence indicates that this procedure is not effective. Athletes who air-dry develop worse disease (Baird and Wear, 1987). Treatment is directed at relieving symptoms because the condition is self-limited. Symptomatic swimmers should take antihistamines throughout the day. Topical steroids may benefit the swimmer. Systemic steroids may be necessary in severe cases.

Prevention

Swimmers should avoid highly snail-infested areas. Dense water vegetation promotes the growth of snails and indirectly promotes the growth of schistosomes. Investigators have shown that removing an overgrowth of snails and discouraging people from feeding water fowl decrease the incidence of swimmer's itch (from 12% before intervention to 0% afterward). Application of granular niclosamide to the exposed skin may help prevent swimmer's itch. In contrast to seabather's eruption, it is in the best interest of the swimmer to have as much clothing as possible covering the body.

Arthropod Bite Reactions

Epidemiology

All outdoor athletes experience arthropod bite reactions (bug bites), although no studies describe its epidemiology. Mosquitoes and flies bite humans because the insects need blood to live. The insect cuts through the skin and injects enzymes that allow easier suction of blood. The host's cell-mediated immunity then reacts to the foreign substances injected by the biting insect.

Mosquitoes of the *Aedes* genus most commonly bite humans, and only the females do the blood sucking. These insects breed well in standing water and increase activity near dusk and into the night. During the day, they prefer wooded, shaded, and cooler areas. They can be particularly dense where golfers search the woods for their errant balls. Some athletes (e.g., those with sweat, dark-colored skin, or perfumes) appear more likely to attract mosquitoes (Frazier, 1977).

Blackflies are repelled to some degree by cigarette smoke, but they are attracted to carbon dioxide given off by the performing athlete. These particular flies are most active during the daytime and can plague the golfer or tennis player. Biting midges become active around dusk. Deerflies are found more often in wooded areas.

Clinical Presentation

Most often the resulting eruptions are located on the exposed skin, although some insects bite through thin clothing. The clinical presentation may differ depending on the type of biting insect.

Mosquitoes

Clinically two main types of reactions occur: immediate and delayed. The immediate-type reaction leads to multiple, scattered, intensely pruritic, erythematous wheals. The delayed-typed reaction occurs several hours after insect bites and presents as pruritic, edematous, erythematous papules. Some athletes develop very brisk and intense inflammatory reactions characterized by significant swelling, heat, and erythema. Because of their size, color, and intense erythema, these lesions may be clinically confused with cutaneous infections; this reaction has been termed *skeeter syndrome* (Figure 20-2) (Simons and Peng, 1999). Systemic symptoms include fever, malaise, nausea, and vomiting. Anaphylaxis rarely occurs.

Biting Flies

Black Flies

During epidemics, outdoor sports may be limited. Clinically, the bitten athlete develops painful lesions. Unfortunately, the black fly injects an anesthetic at the time of the bite so that the pain is felt only after the insect is long gone. Two morphologies occur on the skin. The most common reaction is a well-defined, erythematous, scaling plaque that may develop vesicles. In rare cases, athletes develop pruritic, firm, brown nodules. Anaphylaxis can occur.

Biting Midges

These insects do not inject an anesthetic when they puncture the human skin. As a result, the intensely painful bite is felt immediately. Most species of these flies cause mildly pruritic and erythematous papules; however, on occasion specific species create urticarial, pruritic wheals. The severity of urticarial plaques varies; some resolve in a few days whereas others persist for weeks.

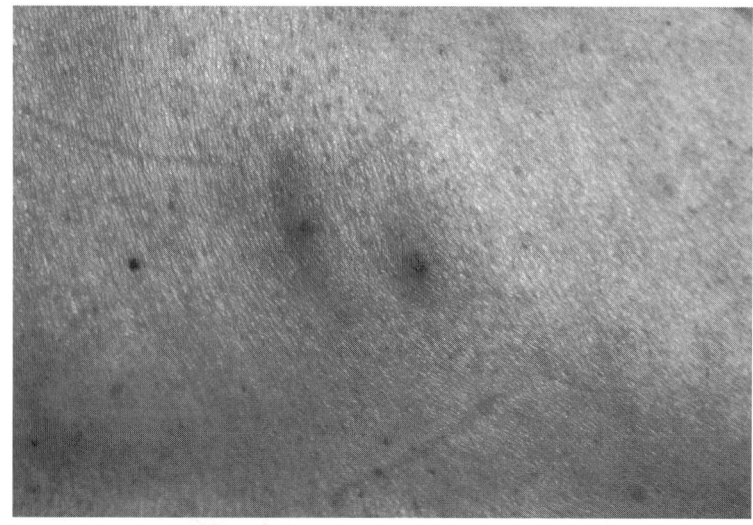

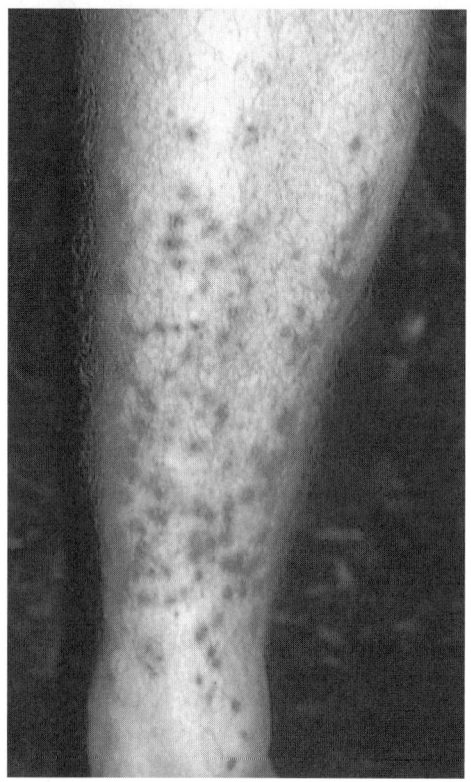

Figure 20-2. **A**: Arthropod bite reactions most often are nonspecific, erythematous, edematous papules. The punctum from the bite or sting may be visible. **B**: Occasionally there are hundreds of bites.

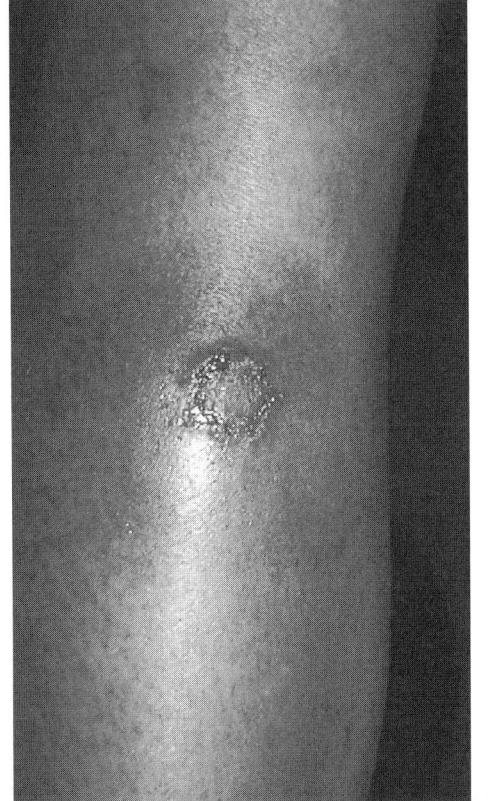

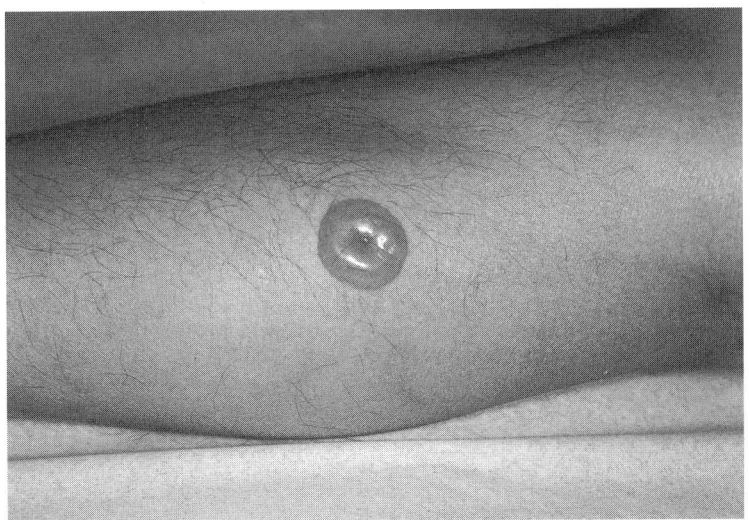

Figure 20-2 *Continued* **C**: Not uncommonly the bites become centrally crusted and peripherally very erythematous and edematous. **D**: Unique skin reactions to arthropods include development of a pure blister.

Deerflies

Deerflies are persistent biters and are not deterred by waving hands, arms, or hats. The bite is painful and results in wheals. Athletes may suffer from systemic symptoms such as respiratory difficulty, dizziness, and weakness. Anaphylaxis can occur.

Diagnosis

In general, the diagnosis can be made based on the typical distribution and morphology. Not all bites are felt initially, so the history of timing of bites may not be known. Biopsy specimens reveal a superficial and deep, perivascular, moderately dense lymphocytic infiltrate. The differential diagnosis includes viral or drug eruptions, prurigo simplex, scabies, and folliculitis.

Treatment

Affected athletes may require oral antipruritic agents such as hydroxyzine, cetirizine, and doxepin. Moderate-potency topical steroids should be used for nonfacial lesions; nonsteroidal topical drugs include pimecrolimus, tacrolimus, and doxepin. For very rare and severe cases, systemic steroids may be necessary. The lesions most likely resolve in a few days; uncommonly, athletes develop persistent arthropod bite reactions that persist for weeks.

It is important to be wary of lesions that develop secondary bacterial infections. Most of these lesions are keenly pruritic, and bacterial infection can be introduced through the athlete's scratching. Athletes or their clinicians should apply warm, moist washcloths to affected areas. Topical antibiotics may be necessary.

Prevention

To prevent these bites, athletes should decrease the amount of exposed skin. If the weather is particularly warm during their activities, athletes can wear long-sleeved, cooling, moisture-wicking clothing. Light-colored clothing is recommended because dark-colored clothing attracts the pests (Frazier, 1977). Athletes should avoid wearing perfumes at their outdoor venues. If an area has an epidemic of mosquitoes or flies, athletes should try to avoid the hours during which the specific pest is most plentiful. Products containing 20% DEET (N, N-diethyl-meta-toluamide) best deter insects from biting. Clinicians should use DEET carefully in children. Not uncommonly, habitually bitten sport enthusiasts develop tolerance to the antigen causing hypersensitivity. In cases of severe reactions, referral to an allergy specialist may be necessary to evaluate for desensitization therapy.

Arthropod Stings

Epidemiology

All outdoor enthusiasts risk encounters with Hymenoptera. These are stinging insects, and up to 20% of the normal population is allergic to the substances found in their venom. The types of insects in this pesky group include bees, hornets, wasps, yellow jackets, and fire ants.

Clinical Presentation

The stings from all of the stinging insects except the fire ant can create lesions that appear similar. A solitary sting spawns a painful (and subsequently pruritic), centrally erythematous, peripherally pale papule or nodule within a few short minutes to hours. A moderate amount of swelling is to be expected, but persistent swelling should caution the clinician to inquire about systemic symptoms. Sensitive athletes may develop periorbital and perioral swelling, wheezing, and generalized wheals; most of these athletes will not progress any further. Some athletes require immediate intensive medical attention because they may develop respiratory and vascular collapse. Signs and symptoms of this syndrome include hoarseness, dyspnea, intense nausea and vomiting, dizziness, tachycardia, and confusion. Frank severe anaphylaxis may occur rapidly within minutes and can be fatal in less than 30 minutes.

Unlike other stinging insects, fire ants sting multiple times. The pain is immediate but subsides in minutes. Within the first day after the sting, the lesions become pustules surrounded by edema and erythema. The lesions resolve, perhaps with scarring, after several days.

Diagnosis

Because the pain of the sting and the cutaneous response are so temporally associated, the diagnosis is rarely in question. The clinician should carefully monitor the athlete to ensure that early anaphylaxis has not started. Auscultation of the lungs and assessment of the circulatory system are required.

Treatment

For mild cases of arthropod stings, the most important initial therapy is application of ice. A tourniquet decreases the absorption of toxin; stingers should be removed. Subsequently, athletes should apply a warm, damp washcloth on the lesion for 10 minutes three or four times per day. Regularly scheduled oral antihistamines should be given.

For athletes with systemic symptoms, the airway and circulatory status must be stabilized and maintained. These athletes require immediate subcutaneous injection with epinephrine 1:1000 (0.3–0.5 ml), and a repeat dose may be needed after 10 to 20 minutes. Affected athletes may also require intramuscular antihistamines or intravenous steroids; immediate transfer to the nearest hospital must occur.

It is important to be wary of lesions that develop secondary bacterial infections. Most of these lesions are keenly pruritic, and bacterial infection can be introduced through the athlete's scratching. Athletes or their clinicians should apply warm, moist washcloths to affected areas. Topical antibiotics may be necessary.

Prevention

Athletes must take care to follow simple rules when they are in outdoor arenas. They should not wear bright-colored clothing (e.g., yellow) because bright colors attract many stinging insects. Athletes should not wear scented products (e.g., perfumes) or shiny jewelry, which further serve to attract the insects. Athletes should not wear sandals or go barefoot in the grass, lest they unknowingly step on one of these insects. It is not safe to position garbage containers near areas of congregation; athletes should avoid these open containers. I have attended several national cross-country meets where the posted team and individual results were juxtaposed to multiple open garbage cans containing and overflowing with hundreds of bees. Officials should be cognizant of receptacle placement, especially during the warm months.

Athletes should not confront these insects or attempt to squash offenders. Yellow jackets, for example, are social insects and live in nests with thousands of others. When destroyed, yellow jackets release a pheromone that incites all of the nest's insects within 15 feet to come to its aid; this process may take less than 15 seconds. The athlete who crushed the yellow jacket can be swarmed by the nests' contents.

In cases of severe reactions, referral to an allergy specialist may be necessary to evaluate for potential desensitization therapy. These athletes should always carry an EpiPen (epinephrine auto-injector) with them. Athletic venues (e.g., cross-country meets, tennis matches, and golf tournaments) should always have available a medical kit containing alcohol swabs, tourniquets, ice packs, and epinephrine.

Sea Creature Stings

Coelenterates

Epidemiology

There are several subtypes of Coelenterates, all containing nematocysts that are triggered to puncture and release a toxin when brushed upon skin. The components of the venom include histamine, catecholamines, and serotonin (Manowitz and Rosenthal, 1979). The organisms in this group include the Portuguese man-of-war, fire coral (which is not a true coral), jellyfish, and sea anemone. One study revealed that 26% of windsurfers experience jellyfish stings (Rosenbaum and Dietz, 2002). Other at-risk sports include swimming, scuba diving, boating, waterskiing, water tubing, sailing, surfing, kayaking, snorkeling, and jet skiing.

The stings of Coelenterates generally create similar clinical presentations that differ slightly in extent relative to the creature's size.

Portuguese Man-of-War

Epidemiology

This organism floats on top of the sea and hangs long dangling tentacles. Some of these tentacles may be up to 100 feet long.

Clinical Presentation

Portuguese man-of-war stings produce pruritic, erythematous, patterned, urticarial plaques that resolve in 3 to 7 days. Occasionally the area becomes violaceous and develops vesicles or necrosis. Conjunctivitis has been noted. Rarely, the swimmer suffers dizziness, nausea, weakness, and even death.

Diagnosis

The diagnosis is based on the history and cutaneous findings.

Treatment

Vinegar should be applied to the wound in most cases. Some authors recommend rubbing sand on the affected area to remove any unfired nematocysts. Oral antihistamines, topical steroids, and warm compresses applied several times per day may speed healing. Systemic symptoms require immediate attention, with maintenance of the circulatory and respiratory systems. Epinephrine may be required. Pain management and tetanus prophylaxis are necessary. It is important to realize the potential for superinfection.

Prevention

Swimmers who plan on being in high-risk waters should consider wearing a diving suit.

Fire Coral

Epidemiology

Fire coral prospers in tropical waters. It varies in height from a few inches to several feet. Fire coral is a blandly colored, stinging organism that gets its name from the reaction that occurs in the unsuspecting transgressing swimmer (Manowitz and Rosenthal, 1979; Rosco, 1977).

Clinical Presentation

The affected swimmer notes a deeply erythematous, burning lesion upon contact that results from the formic acid on the fire coral's outer shell.

Diagnosis

The diagnosis is based on the history and cutaneous findings.

Treatment

Ammonium neutralizes the formic acid. Oral antihistamines, topical steroids, and warm compresses applied several times per day may speed healing.

Systemic symptoms require immediate attention, with maintenance of the circulatory and respiratory systems. Pain management and tetanus prophylaxis are necessary. It is important to realize the potential for superinfection.

Prevention

Swimmers who plan on being in high-risk waters should consider wearing a diving suit.

Jellyfish

Epidemiology

Many different types of jellyfish are found throughout the world's seas.

Clinical Presentation

Exposure to the tentacles (which may be found tangled in seaweed, apart from the organism) produces painful, linear, erythematous plaques. Urticaria, vesicles, pustules, and hemorrhage can occur (Figure 20-3). Systemic complications are unusual and occur with box jellyfish stings found in the South Pacific (Soppe, 1989). Systemic findings include fever, headache, nausea, vomiting, malaise, weakness, and cardiac and respiratory depression leading to death. Subsequent complications include scars, hypopigmentation, hyperpigmentation, and subcutaneous atrophy.

Diagnosis

The diagnosis is based on the history and cutaneous findings.

Treatment

Vinegar should be applied to the wound in most cases. Alcohol and human urine should not be used because these agents induce the firing of nematocysts. Some authors recommend rubbing sand on the affected area to remove any unfired nematocysts. Swimmers should not immerse their skin in fresh water because this will result in nematocyst firing. Oral antihistamines, topical

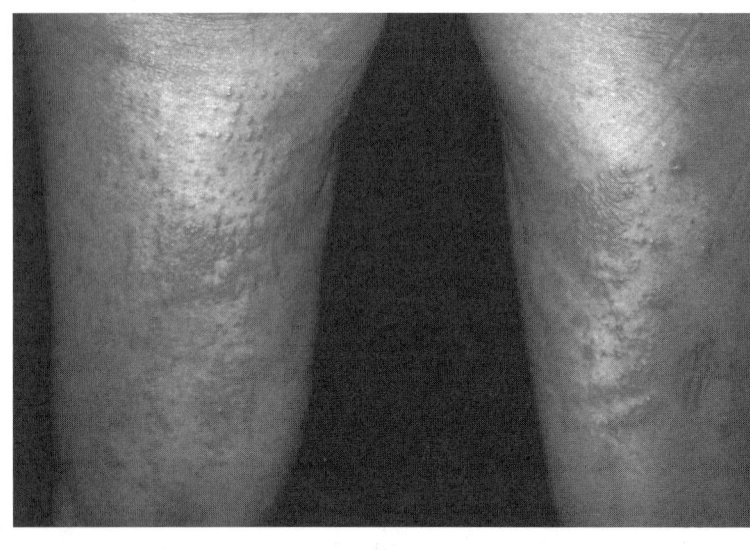

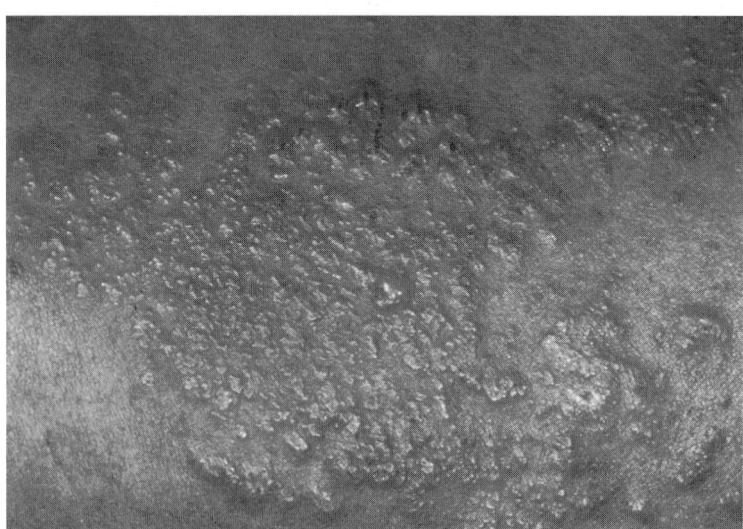

Figure 20-3. **A**: The extremities most often suffer the consequences of an encounter with a jellyfish. The linear erythematous plaques should alert the clinician that an outside force created the eruption. **B**: Closer view of the eruption shows the vesicular nature of the skin eruption caused by jellyfish.

steroids, and warm compresses applied several times per day may speed healing. Systemic symptoms require immediate attention, with maintenance of the circulatory and respiratory systems. Epinephrine may be required. Pain management and tetanus prophylaxis are necessary (Halstead, 1987).

Prevention

Swimmers who plan on being in high-risk waters should consider wearing a diving suit. Snorkelers should not enter areas with high densities of jellyfish. Dead or beached jellyfish cause stings and should be avoided. After sea storms, jellyfish tentacles become dislodged and float freely in the ocean. In these scenarios, great caution is needed when entering the ocean.

Once stung, aquatic enthusiasts must get out of the ocean to avoid drowning if systemic complications occur or panic ensues. Scuba divers must examine their regulators to ensure that tentacles have not become entangled.

Sea Anemone

Epidemiology

The sea anemone contains several long cylindrical projections. Sea anemones often reside among sponges, and poisoned swimmers develop what has been termed *sponge-diver's disease*. One epidemic of more than 100 cases in Long Island occurred after swimmers were exposed to a burrowing sea anemone in the sediment (so-called *ghost anemone*) (Freudenthal and Barbagallo, 2002). Some anemones release a thalassin-containing toxin that can induce bronchospasm.

Clinical Presentation

The stung swimmer develops painful, erythematous, edematous, necrotic plaques at points of contact. Fever, chills, nausea, vomiting, and headache can occur. The resultant ulcers are recalcitrant to therapy.

Exposure to the ghost anemone causes pruritic, erythematous, vesicular plaques (Freudenthal and Barbagallo, 2002). The pruritus and pain may last for weeks. The toxin is a mixture of low-molecular-weight substances composed of histamine and serotonin.

Diagnosis

The diagnosis is based on the history and cutaneous findings. It is documented that physicians do not often correctly make the diagnosis. The differential diagnosis includes seabather's eruption and swimmer's itch.

Treatment

The area should be rinsed with vinegar, baking soda, or warm sea water. Pain management and tetanus prophylaxis are necessary. It is important to realize the potential for superinfection.

Prevention

Swimmers who plan on being in high-risk waters should consider wearing a diving suit. Fresh water should not be used to rinse the area.

Mollusks

Epidemiology

These organisms are the marine snails. The typical example is the cone shell. Some of the most deadly cone shells are found in California and Australia. The octopus is also a mollusk.

Cone Shell

Clinical Presentation

Cone shells are 4 inches long, typically are located in Australia and California, and are nocturnal inhabitants of sandy areas. These mollusks possess beautifully colored shells, and swimmers may make the mistake of collecting them. Most encounters with cone shells produce an erythematous, edematous plaque much like a sharp burning sting from a land arthropod. On occasion, the venom results in numbness, muscle weakness, blurred vision, and respiratory and circulatory collapse. The mortality rate is 15% to 20%, and the cause of death generally is respiratory failure (Rosco, 1977; Williamson, 1987).

Diagnosis

The diagnosis is based on the history and cutaneous findings.

Treatment

Application of heat to the affected area may be helpful. The heat is generally recommended in the form of 50°C sea water immersion for 30 to 60 minutes. Pain management and tetanus prophylaxis are necessary. Supportive care in the scenario of respiratory and vascular failure is mandatory (Mandojana and Sims, 1987). Epinephrine may be required.

Prevention

Swimmers must avoid these creatures and must wear gloves if they choose to pick up the cone shells.

Australian Blue-Ringed Octopus

Epidemiology

This type of octopus is only 4 inches long, would fit in a swimmer's palm, and typically is found along the Australian coastline. Its venom contains tetrodotoxin that is one of the most potent neuromuscular toxins in the world.

Clinical Presentation

The sting usually is painless and leaves very little evidence on the skin. Rarely the clinician notices a stinging area of edema at the bite site. Within 10 to 15 minutes, the face becomes numb. Nausea, vomiting, dyspnea, muscle weakness, and respiratory failure can follow. The severity of disease relates to the dose of venom. The mortality rate is 20% (Rosco, 1977; Williamson, 1987).

Diagnosis

The diagnosis is based on the history and systemic findings.

Treatment

Clinicians must immediately immobilize and apply compression to the affected limb. Some recommend immediate surgical excision. Pain management and tetanus prophylaxis are necessary. Epinephrine may be required. The affected swimmer must be transported as soon as possible to a hospital setting where respiratory and vascular support can be instituted.

Prevention

Swimmers must avoid these small but deadly creatures and be cognizant of areas in which they populate.

Arthropods

Epidemiology

Horseshoe crabs possess a tail with a very sharp point and numerous spicules. They are found along the Atlantic coast as well as Asian Pacific coasts.

Clinical Presentation

The puncture of the sharp tail causes the major damage to beachgoers, who experience immediate pain, bleeding, and erythema. The sharp tail may remain in the skin.

Diagnosis

The diagnosis is based on the history and cutaneous findings. Radiographic examination may be necessary to identify the spine.

Treatment

The injured site should receive warm-water soaks for 5 to 10 minutes three or four times per day. The spine should be removed surgically. Pain management and tetanus prophylaxis are necessary. It is important to realize the potential for superinfection. One case report noted a resultant infection with *Vibrio alginolyticus* and *Enterobacter cloacae* that was treated with ceftriaxone and doxycycline (Lutz et al., 2000).

Prevention

Beachgoers must be careful of scurrying arthropods on the beach near the water and in the shallow portions of the sea.

Echinoderms

Epidemiology

Echinoderms that cause skin problems in seafarers include the brittle stars, sea cucumber, sea urchin, and starfish. The venom from these organisms often consists of acetylcholine and serotonin-like substances.

Sea Cucumber

Epidemiology

This sausage-shaped animal looks like a piece of old tire from which white milky tangles extend.

Clinical Presentation

This organism produces holothurin on its surface that, when handled by divers or swimmers, causes an acute dermatitis. Conjunctivitis has been reported (Soppe, 1989).

Diagnosis

The diagnosis is based on the history and clinical findings.

Treatment

The exuded holothurin should be rinsed off immediately with warm water.

Prevention

Swimmers and divers should not handle the sea cucumber without wearing gloves. The milky extensions should not be touched.

Sea Urchin

Epidemiology

Sea urchins are spherical creatures with spines of varying lengths protruding from the body. They can be found in shallow areas of the sea. Most are nonvenomous.

Clinical Presentation

After stepping on a sea urchin, the swimmer notes immediate pain, swelling, bleeding, and a curious black color around the puncture sites. Punctures over joints can cause synovitis. On occasion, the spines remain in the deep dermis and produce a granulomatous foreign body reaction (Baden, 1987).

Diagnosis

The diagnosis is based on the history and clinical findings. Radiographic evaluation of joints may reveal spines in or around joints or tendons.

Treatment

The swimmer should apply warm-water soaks to the injury. The spines are somewhat fragile and may not be easily removed. Other treatments include rubbing a stone on the puncture site to break the spines into smaller pieces and applying salicylic acid paste or vinegar to the site. The lesions of foreign body reaction may require excision. Pain management and tetanus prophylaxis are necessary.

Prevention

In high-risk areas, swimmers and divers must wear puncture resistant boots or avoid these animals altogether.

Starfish

Clinical Presentation

Some starfish (namely, the "crown of thorns starfish" found off the Great Barrier Reef) have thorns that puncture the skin and inject a venom causing an erythematous, edematous plaque. Occasionally the hard spine remains in the skin, resulting in a foreign body skin reaction.

Diagnosis

The diagnosis is based on the history and clinical findings.

Treatment

The affected area must be washed with vinegar or normal saline, and heat should be applied immediately to the wound. This heat is generally recommended in the form of 50°C sea water immersion for 30 to 60 minutes. Pain management and tetanus prophylaxis are necessary.

Prevention

Because these organisms hide in the sandy bottom of the ocean, swimmers and divers must wear puncture-resistant boots in high-risk areas.

Poisonous Fish

Scorpion Fish

Epidemiology

This general term of fish refers to the stonefish and the lionfish. These fish fatally (or nearly so) injure 300 people each year. Scuba divers and fishermen along the United States coast suffer significantly. Stonefish prefer the shallow sea in the sand or in coral reefs. The multicolored lionfish can be found in the Indo-Pacific seas.

Clinical Presentation

The scorpion fish inflicts its damage by injecting a polypeptide venom using its dorsal spine. The puncture site may be exquisitely tender and can cause the victim to thrash about and lose consciousness. The affected individual develops a painful, edematous, ecchymotic plaque that eventually may blister and become necrotic. Some injection sites become numb. Nausea, vomiting, fever, chills, muscle paralysis, respiratory and circulatory collapse, and death can occur. No fatalities from lionfish are reported.

Diagnosis

The diagnosis is based on the history and clinical findings.

Treatment

Antivenom is available in Australia, and the dose in ampules is related to the number of punctures a diver or swimmer has received. Clinicians must apply heat to the affected area as soon as possible in an attempt to denature the venom. This heat is generally recommended in the form of 50°C sea water immersion for 30 to 60 minutes. Pain management and tetanus prophylaxis are necessary.

Prevention

Swimmers and divers in high-risk areas must recognize and avoid these fish. If the fish must be handled, the individual should wear arm and hand protection.

Sea Snake

Epidemiology

The tropical sea waters of the Indian and Pacific Oceans contain sea snakes. The poison of sea snakes is over 300 times more potent than the poison of land snakes, but fortunately these snakes have very small mouths and cannot bite humans effectively. Furthermore, the animal is not particularly aggressive. It will wrap itself around a swimmer's extremity and may bite only when it becomes entangled in a surge of the surf (Tu and Fulde, 1987). The systemic manifestations of encounters with the sea snake relate to its neurotoxin, which resembles that of the cobra.

Clinical Presentation

Pain at the bite site is nonexistent. Cutaneous signs are rare and may include only a fang remnant or two very small puncture wounds (Tu and Fulde, 1987). The main symptoms include very tender lymphadenopathy, muscle spasms, weakness, and paralysis.

Diagnosis

The diagnosis is based on the history and clinical findings. The lack of skin findings helps differentiate this bite from stings of other aquatic organisms. Seventy percent of patients will develop myoglobinuria.

Treatment

Immobilization and firm pressure first at the bite site and then along the affected limb are mandatory. The area should not be incised because this procedure can enhance venom absorption. Pain management and tetanus prophylaxis are necessary. The patient should be transferred to a medical facility as soon as possible and given antivenom. Respiratory and circulatory support are needed for the individual in shock.

Prevention

Divers should not provoke sea snakes. Divers should wear thick diving suits in high-risk areas.

Stingrays

Epidemiology

More than 1500 cases of stingray injuries are reported each year in the United States (Halstead and Vinci, 1987). Stingrays populate the coast and often reside in the sandy ocean bottom and warm lakes and rivers.

Clinical Presentation

The stung swimmer receives a venomous dose from the razor-sharp tail, typically when the swimmer inadvertently steps on the animal. Immediate throbbing and sharp pain occurs. In addition to the injected venom, the swimmer receives a laceration. The spine may even penetrate to the bone (Rosco, 1977). The tail has reverse serrated edges, and most cutaneous damage occurs when the spine is withdrawn. The lesion becomes erythematous, edematous, and purpuric. Eventually necrosis may ensue. Systemic complications are not typical but include nausea, vomiting, respiratory collapse, and cardiac arrhythmias. Chest wounds have resulted in death.

Diagnosis

The diagnosis is based on the history and clinical findings.

Treatment

No antivenom is available, but vinegar should be applied to the wound. Clinicians should remove all spinal parts from the skin and immerse the affected area (usually a limb) in 50°C sea water for 30 to 60 minutes. Pain management and tetanus prophylaxis are necessary.

Prevention

If the sandy ocean floor is known to have stingrays, the swimmer should shuffle their feet through the sand upon entering the ocean. This entry method warns the stingray of the swimmer's presence, and it will swim away without using its barbed tail as a defense mechanism (Soppe, 1989).

Sea Creature Abrasions

Coral

Epidemiology

Aquatic enthusiasts may mistake the beauty of coral for safety. At-risk sports include swimming, scuba diving, boating, waterskiing, water tubing, sailing, surfing, windsurfing, kayaking, snorkeling, and jet skiing.

Clinical Presentation

Water athletes who rub against the coral develop irregularly shaped lacerations. The abrasion with coral may introduce foreign bodies or microorganisms into the wound.

Diagnosis

The diagnosis is based on the history and clinical findings.

Treatment

Therapy consists of warm-water soaks three times per day, debridement, and application of topical antibiotics. Occasionally, systemic antibiotics are necessary.

Prevention

Snorkelers, swimmers, and surfers should avoid contact with coral reefs. Although snorkeling can be a beautiful exercise, coral should not be touched.

Sponges

(See Chapter 9: Irritant Contact Dermatitis)

Bibliography

Baden HP. Injuries from sea urchins. Clin Dermatol 1987;5:112–117.
Baird JK, Wear DJ. Cercarial dermatitis: the swimmer's itch. Clin Dermatol 1987;5:88–91.
Burnett JW, Kumar S, Malecki JM. The antibody response in seabather's eruption. Toxicon 1995;33:99–104.
Burnett JW. Seabather's eruption. Cutis 1992;50:98.
Frazier CA. Insect reactions related to sports. Cutis 1977;19:439–444.
Freudenthal AR, Barbagallo JS. Ghost anemone dermatitis. J Am Acad Dermatol 2002; 47:722–726.
Halstead BW. Coelenterate stings and wounds. Clin Dermatol 1987;5:8–13.
Halstead BW, Vinci JM. Venomous fish stings. Clin Dermatol 1987;5:29–35.
Hoeffler DF. Swimmer's itch (Cercarial dermatitis). Cutis 1977;19:461–467.
Levesque B, Giovenazzo P, Guerrier P, et al. Investigation of cercarial dermatitis. Epidemiol Infect 2002;129:379–386.
Lutz LL, Goldner R, Burnett JW. Penetrating injury from horseshoe crab tail. Cutis 2000;66:13–14.
Mandojana RM, Sims JK. Miscellaneous dermatoses associated with the aquatic environment. Clin Dermatol 1987;5:134–145.
Manowitz NR, Rosenthal RR. Cutaneous-systemic reactions to toxins and venoms of common marine organisms. Cutis 1979;23:450–454.
Rosco MD. Cutaneous manifestations of marine animal injuries. Cutis 1977;19:507–510.
Rosenbaum DA, Dietz TE. Windsurfing injuries. Phys Sportsmed 2002;30:15–24.
Segura-Puertas L, Ramos ME, Aramburo C. One *Linuche* mystery solved: all 3 stages of the cornate scyphomedusa *Linuche unguiculata* cause seabather's eruption. J Am Acad Dermatol 2001;44:624–628.
Simons FER, Peng Z. Skeeter syndrome. J Allergy Clin Immunol 1999;104:705–707.
Soppe GG. Marine envenomations and aquatic dermatology. Am Fam Pract 1989;40: 97–106.
Tomchik RS, Russell MT, Szmant AM, et al. Clinical perspectives on seabather's eruption, also known as "sea lice." JAMA 1993;269:1669–1672.
Tu AT, Fulde G. Sea snake bites. Clin Dermatol 1987;5:118–126.
Williamson JAH. The blue-ringed octopus bite and envenomation syndrome. Clin Dermatol 1987;5:127–133.

Index

A

Abrasions and chafing, 203–207
 Curvularia lunata infections of, 78
 as impetigo risk factor, 4
 sea creature-related, 337
 track bites, 237
Accessories. *See also* Sports equipment
 as contact dermatitis cause, 145–147
Acne keloidalis nuchae, 287–288
Acne mechanica, 282–285, color plate VIII
Acne vulgaris, differential diagnosis of, 5, 15, 43
Allergic reactions
 contact dermatitis, 127–163
  accessories-related, 145–147
  athletic shoes-related, 135–137
  balls-related, 143–145
  exercise-induced anaphylaxis, 127, 183, 195–199
  handles-related, 140–143
  helmets and face masks-related, 138–139
  manual implements-related, 139–140
  medical supplies-related, 148–154
  nose clips and earplugs-related, 134–135
  photolichenoid, 156–157
  Rhus (poison ivy)-related, 154–155
  shin and knee guard-related, 137–138
  swim fins-related, 131–132
  swim goggles-related, 127–130
  swimming cap-related, 133–134
  underwater masks-related, 132–133
  wet suit-related, 130–131
 pruritus and urticaria, 180–194
Alopecia
 aquaslide, 241–243
 balance beam, 243
 jogger's, 244
Anabolic steroids, 297–299
Anaphylaxis
 arthropod stings-related, 321, 322
 exercise-related, 127, 183, 195–199
Ancylostoma braziliense, 84
Anesthetics, topical, as contact dermatitis cause, 150–151
Angioedema. *See also* Exercise-induced angioedema/anaphylaxis
 vibratory, 197

Animals, encounters with, as skin disorders cause, 311–338
Antibiotics
 photosensitizing effects of, 108
 topical, as contact dermatitis cause, 152
Anti-inflammatory agents, topical, as contact dermatitis cause, 149–150
Aquaslide alopecia, 241–243
Archers
 archery arms in, 207–208
 callosities (calluses) in, 216–219
Arthropod bite reactions, 24, 26, 316–321
Arthropod stings, 321–323
Athlete's foot. *See* Tinea pedis
Athletic shoes. *See* Footwear

B

Bacterial skin infections, 3–34. *See also* names of specific bacteria
 gram-negative, 3–4, 22–30
 gram-positive, 3, 4–22
Badminton players
 callosities (calluses) in, 218
 racquet-related allergic contact dermatitis in, 141–143
 stringer's fingers in, 235–236
Balance beam alopecia, 243
Ballet dancers, subungual exostosis in, 279–280
Balls, as contact dermatitis cause, 143–144, 171–172
Basal cell carcinoma, 106, 115–118
Baseball pitcher's friction dermatitis, 177–178
Baseball players. *See also* Outdoor sports athletes
 allergic contact dermatitis in, 138–139
 baseball pitcher's friction dermatitis, 165, 177–178
 bullae (blisters) in, 209
 callosities (calluses) in, 216–219
 molluscum contagiosum in, 50
 pads in, 103–104
 palmoplantar eccrine hidradenitis in, 248
 traumatic plantar urticaria, 193
Basketball pebble fingers, 165, 171–172

Basketball players
  allergic contact dermatitis in, 143–144,
      147, 171–172
    athletic tape-related, 148
    basketballs-related, 143–144
    shin and knee guard-related, 137–138
  basketball pebble fingers in, 165, 171–172
  black heel in, 245–246
  Center's callosities in, 272–273
  exercise-induced angioedema/anaphylaxis
      in, 195–198
  folliculitis in, 13
  furunculosis in, 11, 13
  gram-negative infections in, 22–23
  green foot in, 22–23
  irritant contact dermatitis in, 165,
      171–172
  onychocryptosis (ingrown toenail) in,
      266–268
  pitted keratolysis in, 18
  tinea pedis in, 57, 58
  traumatic plantar urticaria in, 192–193
Basketballs, as contact dermatitis cause,
    171–172
Bee stings, 321–322
Bicycle spoke injuries, 228
Bicyclists. *See* Cyclists
Bicyclists' nipples, 208–209
Bikini bottom, 20–21
Billiard cues, as contact dermatitis cause,
    146
Billiard players
  billiard cue-related contact dermatitis in,
      146–147
  callosities (calluses) in, 216–219
"Black dots," 49, 53, 217, 220, 221, color
    plate VI
Black fly bites, 316, 317
Black heel (talon noire), 245–246, color
    plate VI
Black palm, 247–248
Bleached swimmer syndrome, 158–159
Blisters. *See* Bullae
Blister shield, 216
Blubber finger (erysipeloid), 21–22
Boaters. *See also* Outdoor sports athletes
  aquagenic urticaria in, 190–191
  atypical mycobacterial skin infections in,
      81–83
  bikini bottom, 20–21
  canyoning hands in, 164–165
  cold urticaria in, 184–186
  contact urticaria in, 191–192
  gram-positive infections in, 4

  irritant contact dermatitis in
    red tide dermatitis, 168–169
    sea water dermatitis, 169
    seaweed dermatitis, 169–170
  otitis externa, 28–30
  pulling boat hands in, 286–287
  seabather's eruption in, 311–314
  sea creature-related abrasions in, 337
  sea creature-related stings in, 323–336
  seaweed dermatitis in, 169
  sponge dermatitis in, 170–171
  swimmer's itch in, 314–316
  swimming pool granuloma in, 81–83
Boogie boards, as contact dermatitis cause,
    174–175
Bowlers
  allergic contact dermatitis in, 139–140
  bowler's fingernail in, 268–269
  callosities (calluses) in, 216–219
  lawn, allergic contact dermatitis in,
      139–140
Bowler's fingernail, 268–269
Bowls grip, 139–140
Boxers
  nodules in, 95, 103–104
  pads in, 95, 103–104
  smallpox in, 35
Braces, knee and ankle, as contact dermatitis
    cause, 153
Bug bites. *See* Arthropod bite reactions
Bullae (blisters), 209–216, 217, 222, 223

C

Calcium oxide, as contact dermatitis cause,
    165–167
Callosities (calluses), 216–219, color plate V
  Center's, 272–273
  differentiated from warts (verrucae), 53,
      217
  as protection against bullae (blisters), 216
Candida/candidiasis, 17, 59, 71, 72–72
Canoeists. *See also* Boaters
  callosities (calluses) in, 216–219
  furunculosis/furuncles in, 4, 11, 13–14
  impetigo in, 4
  nodules in, 95, 96
  "soft skin" in, 209
Canyoning hands, 164–165
Catchers, traumatic plantar urticaria in, 193
Cellulitis, differential diagnosis of, 22
Cement burns, 165–167
Center's callosities, 272–273
Cercariae, 314–316
Cercarial dermatitis, 314

Chafing. *See* Abrasions and chafing
Chalk
 as allergic contact dermatitis cause, 145
 as irritant contact dermatitis cause, 176–177
Cheilitis, actinic, 119
Chemical deposition, 293–296
Chilblains, 286, 307–308
Chlorine, effect on hair, 293, 295
Cicatrices, karate, 226–227
Clam digger's itch, 314. *See also* Swimmer's itch
Coelenterate-related injuries, 323–328
Cold injuries
 canyoning hands, 164–165
 chilblains, 307–308
 cold urticaria, 181, 184–186
 frostbite, 302–306
 skier's cold purpura, 306–307
Cold urticaria, 181, 184–186
Cone shell, 328–329
Conjunctivitis, herpes, 41
Copper deposits, in swimming pools, 293–294, 297
Coral, as abrasion cause, 337
Corneocytes, color plate IV
Corns, 220–222, color plate V
 differentiated from
  callosities (calluses), 217
  warts (verrucae), 53
Corynebacterium, 18
Corynebacterium minutissimum, 17
Crab poisoning (erysipeloid), 21–22
Crew members. *See* Rowers
Cricket players, port-wine stains in, 254–255
Curvularia lunata, 78–79
Cutaneous larva migrans, 84–85
Cutaneous myiasis, 85–86
Cutis marmorata, 301
Cycler's nodules, 95, 100–102
Cyclists. *See also* Outdoor sports athletes
 abrasions and chafing in, 203–207
 allergic contact dermatitis in, 150
 bicyclists' nipples, 208–209
 callosities (calluses) in, 216–219
 cholinergic urticaria in, 182–184
 exercise-induced angioedema/anaphylaxis in, 195–198
 friction injuries to the skin in, 203–207
 frostbite in, 302–306
 lacerations in, 204, 228
 nodules in, 95, 100–102
 saddle sores in, 233–235
 subungual exostosis in, 279–280

Cyclists' nipples, 208–209
Cysts, epidermoid, 15

D

Dancers
 acne mechanica in, 282, 284
 callosities (calluses) in, 216–219
 jazz ballet bottom in, 224–225
 onychocryptosis (ingrown toenail) in, 266–268
 palmoplantar eccrine hidradenitis in, 248
 subungual exostosis in, 279–280
Debromoaplysiatoxin, 169
Deerflies bites, 320–321
Dermatitis
 allergic contact, 127–163
  athletic equipment-related, 127–147
  environment-related, 154–160
  medical supplies-related, 147–153
 atopic, 6
  differential diagnosis of, 43
 chronic lichenified, 234
 diving suit, 23–24
 irritant contact, 127, 164–179
  athlete's implements-related, 164, 171–177
  playing fields-related, 164–171
  red tide dermatitis, 168–169
  seawater-related, 168–171, 337
  seaweed-related, 169–170
 seborrheic, differential diagnosis of, 17
Dermatographism, 186–187
Dermatophyte infections, 3, 57–80
 as basis for athletic disqualification, 57
Discus throwers, anabolic steroid use in, 297
Divers (platform). *See also* Scuba divers
 abrasions and chafing in, 203–207
 aquagenic urticaria in, 190–191
 atypical mycobacterial skin infections in, 81
 cold urticaria in, 184–186
 contact urticaria in, 191–192
 dried or discolored hair in, 293–295
 friction injuries to the skin in, 203–207
 green hair in, 293–294
 molluscum contagiosum, 8, 47–51
 otitis externa (swimmer's ear) in, 29
 pool water irritant contact dermatitis in, 158–160, 167–168
 pruritus in, 180–182
 purpura in, 253–254
 swimming pool granuloma, 81–83
 warts (verruca), 36, 50, 51–54

Index

Diving suit dermatitis, 23–24
Dry skin. *See* Xerosis

E

Earplugs, as allergic contact dermatitis cause, 134–135
Echinoderms, 331–333
Eczema, 127. *See also* Dermatitis
Environment-induced skin disorders
 allergic contact dermatitis, 154–160
 anabolic steroids-related, 297–299
 animal-related, 311–338
 chemical deposition-related, 293–296
Epidermolysis bullosa simplex, 210
Epidermophyton, 60, 65
Equestrians
 callosities (calluses) in, 216–219
 panniculitis (perniosis) in, 308–310
Erysipeloid, 21–22
Erythema
 perianal, 234
 reticulated, of livedo reticularis, 301
Erythema ab igne, 300–301
Erythrasma, 17–18
Exercise-induced angioedema/anaphylaxis (EIA), 127, 183, 195–199
Exostosis, subungual, 279–280

F

Face masks, as contact dermatitis cause, 138–139
Fencers
 furunculosis in, 11, 12
 molluscum contagiosum in, 50
Fever blisters. *See* Herpes simplex virus infections
Fire ant stings, 321
Fire coral, 324–325
Fish, poisonous, 334–336
Fishermen. *See also* Outdoor sports athletes
 allergic contact dermatitis in, 146–147
  fishing bait-related, 147
  fishing rod-related, 142–143
 basal cell carcinoma in, 115–122
 callosities (calluses) in, 216–219
 chilblains in, 307–308
 erysipeloid in, 21, 22
 squamous cell carcinoma in, 118
 Vibrio infections in, 30–31
Fish handler's disease (erysipeloid), 21–22
Fishing bait, as contact dermatitis cause, 146–147

Fishing rods, as contact dermatitis cause, 142–143
Fly bites, 316, 317–321
Folliculitis, 6, 8–11, 15
 hot-tub, 8, 24–27
Fomites, 9
Foosball finger, 222–224
Football players. *See also* Outdoor sports athletes
 acne keloidalis nuchae in, 287–288
 acne mechanica in, 282, 283, 284
 allergic contact dermatitis in, 150
  helmets and face masks-related, 138–139
 black heel in, 245–247
 cholinergic urticaria in, 182–184
 curvularia lunata in, 78–79
 dermatographism in, 186–187
 football toenail in, 274–275
 frostbite in, 302–306
 folliculitis in, 12–13, 14, 15
 furunculosis in, 11, 12–13, 16
 gram-positive infections in, 4
 hot-tub folliculitis in, 24, 25
 impetigo in, 4, 5
 nodules in, 95–96
 onychocryptosis (ingrown toenail) in, 266–268
 tinea cruris in, 71, 72–73
 warts (verrucae) in, 51
Football toenail, 274–275
Footwear
 as allergic contact dermatitis cause, 135–137
 as bullae cause, 210, 213–214, 215
Freckles, sun damage-related, 119
Frisbee nail, 269–270
Frostbite, 302–306
Frostnip, 302
Fungal skin infections. *See* Dermatophyte infections
Furunculosis/furuncles, 4, 11–16
Fusobacterium ulcerans, 311

G

Ghost anemone, 327
Goggles
 as allergic contact dermatitis cause, 127–130
 as purpura cause, 257–258
Golfers. *See also* Outdoor sport athletes
 acne mechanica in, 282, 283, 284
 callosities (calluses) in, 216–219
 golfer's nail in, 270

Index 343

Golfer's nail, 270
Granuloma, swimming pool, 81–83
Green foot, 22–23
Green hair, 293–294
Green nails, 66
Gymnasts
 abrasions and chafing in, 203–207
 alopecia in, 243
 balance beam alopecia in, 243
 callosities (calluses) in, 216–219
 friction injuries in
  to the hair, 242–243
  to the skin, 203–207
 irritant contact dermatitis in, 176–177
 molluscum contagiosum in, 47
 warts (verrucae) in, 51

H
Hair
 blonding (bleaching) or drying of, 158–159, 295
 friction injuries to, 241–244
 green, 293–294
Hammer throwers, anabolic steroid use by, 297
Hammertoe deformity, 210
Handball players, exercise-induced angioedema/anaphylaxis in, 195–198
Handles, as allergic contact dermatitis cause, 140–143
Hand protection, for karate practitioners, 227
Heating pads, 300–301
Helmets
 as acne keloidalis nuchae cause, 287, 288
 as acne mechanica cause, 282, 284
 as allergic contact dermatitis cause, 138–139
Hematomas, subungual, 263, 264, 272, 275, 276, 277, 278
Herpes gladiatorum, 6, 37, 39–41, 42, 43, 44, 46, 285, color plate II
 designated as herpes luctator, 39
 return-to-play guidelines for, 45, 46
Herpes labialis, 35–38
Herpes luctator, 39. *See also* Herpes gladiatorum
Herpes rugbeiorum, 37, 39, 40–41, 43, 44, 46, color plate II
Herpes simplex virus infections, 35, 38–47
 prevention of, 44–47
Hidradenitis, idiopathic palmoplantar, 28, 248–249, color plate VI
High-altitude exposure, 300
Hives. *See* Urticaria

Hockey dermatitis, 165
Hockey players
 abrasions and chafing in, 203–207
 acne mechanica in, 282, 284
 allergic contact dermatitis in, 138–139
 cold urticaria 181, 184–186
 friction injuries to the skin in, 203–207
 hockey dermatitis, 165
 irritant contact dermatitis in, 172–173
 lacerations in, 204
 molluscum contagiosum in, 50
 nodules in, 95
 pseudonodules in, 102
 skater's toenail in, 278–279
 skier's cold purpura, 306–307
 tinea pedis in, 60
Hockey sticks, as contact dermatitis cause, 172–173
Horseback riders. *See* Equestrians
Horseshoe crab stings, 330–331
Hot-foot syndrome, 27–28
"Hot spots," 210, 211, 214, 216
Hot-tub folliculitis, 8, 24–27
Hot tubs, sanitation equipment for, 7, 11
Human papilloma virus, 52
Hurdlers, abrasions in, 203
Hymenoptera stings, 321–322
Hyperkeratosis, subungual, 264

I
Ice packs, as contact dermatitis cause, 173–174
Ice skaters. *See also* Hockey players
 abrasions and chafing in, 203–207
 friction injuries to the skin in, 203–207
 lacerations in, 204
 skate bite, 102
 skater's toenail in, 278–279
 speed skaters, frostbite in, 302–306
Impetigo, 4–8, 285, color plate I
 differential diagnosis of, 43
Ingrown toenails (onychocryptosis), 262–263
Injured athletes. *See also* Trauma-related skin conditions
 allergic contact dermatitis in
  athletic tape-related, 148
  elbow splints-related, 153–154
  hot tub folliculitis, 8, 24–27
  jogging cream-related, 149
  knee and ankle braces-related, 153–154
  topical anesthetics-related, 151
  topical antibiotics-related, 152–153
  topical anti-inflammatory agents-related, 150

Injured athletes (*cont.*)
  cholinergic urticaria in, 182–184
  erythema ab igne in, 300–301
  herpes simplex virus infections in, 38–47
  ice pack-related irritant contact dermatitis in, 173–174
  verrucous squamous cell carcinoma in, 82
  warts (verrucae) in, 52
Insect bites. *See* Arthropod bite reactions
Insect stings, 321–322. *See also* Arthropod bite reactions
Intertrigo
  Candida-related, 71, 72–73
  maceration, differential diagnosis of, 17
Itching. *See* Pruritus

J
Javelin throwers, anabolic steroid use by, 297
Jazz ballet bottom, 224
Jellyfish stings, 323–324, 325–327
Jet skiers. *See also* Boaters
  wet suit-related dermatitis in, 130
Jock itch. *See* Tinea cruris
Joggers. *See also* Runners
  alopecia in, 244
  jogging cream-related contact dermatitis in, 149
Jogger's nipples, 225–226
Jogger's toenail, 262
Jogging cream, as contact dermatitis cause, 148–149
Judo carpet, as contact dermatitis cause, 160
Judo practitioners
  callosities (calluses) in, 216–219
  contact dermatitis in, 160
  tinea pedis in, 58, 60, 62

K
Karate cicatrices, 226–227
Karate nail, 271
Karate practitioners
  callosities (calluses) in, 216–219
  karate cicatrices in, 226–227
  karate nail in, 271
Kayakers. *See also* Boaters
  callosities (calluses) in, 216–219
  pulling boat hands in, 285–287
  "soft skin" in, 209
Keratolysis, pitted, 18–20
Keratoses
  actinic, 118–120, 300
  hyperkeratotic, 53

Knee and shin guards
  as allergic contact dermatitis cause, 137–138
  as folliculitis cause, color plate I
Knuckle pads, 103–104

L
Lacerations, 204, 226–229
Lacrosse players
  allergic contact dermatitis in, 138–139
  black heel in, 245–246
Lawn bowlers, allergic contact dermatitis in, 139–140
Leukoderma, raccoonlike periorbital, 128–129
Lice, 84, 86–88. *See also* Pediculosis
  sea lice (seabather's eruption), 311–314, 315
Lichen simplex chronicus, 234
Line markers, as irritant contact dermatitis cause, 165–167
Livedo reticularis, reticulated erythema of, 301
Lugers. *See also* Outdoor sports athletes
  chilblains, 286, 307–308
  cold urticaria in, 184–186
  frostbite in, 302–306
  skier's cold purpura, 306–307
Lyngbya majuscula, 169
Lyngbyatoxin, 169

M
Manual implements, as contact dermatitis cause, 139–140
Mask burn, 132
Masks, as allergic contact dermatitis cause, 132–133, 138–139
Medical supplies, as allergic contact dermatitis cause, 147–153
Medications
  as contact dermatitis cause, 149–153
  photosensitizing, 108, 109
Melanoma, 106, 111–115 color plate VI
  amelanotic, 112
  differentiated from
    black heel, 245, 246
    center's callosities, 272–273
    football toenail, 274
    jogger's toenail, 262
    skater's toenail, 278–279
    skier's toenail, 275–277
    soccer toenail, 277–278
    tennis toe, 262–264
    windsurfer's nail, 280–281

Methicillin resistance, in *Staphylococcus aureus*, 6, 7, 9, 10, 11–16
Micrococcus, 18
Microsporum, 65
Midge bites, 317
Military personnel, bullae (blisters) in, 209
Molluscum contagiosum, 8, 47–51, color plates II, III
Mollusk-related injuries, 328–329
Mosquito bites, 316, 317, 320
Mountaineers. *See also* Outdoor sports athletes
  canyoning hands in, 164–165
  palmoplantar eccrine hidradenitis in, 248
Mouth guards, for karate practitioners, 227
Mupirocin, 7, 10
Mycobacterial infections, in swimmers, 3
  atypical, 81–83
Mycobacterium marinum infections, 81–83
Mycobacterium scrofulaceum infections, 81
Myiasis, cutaneous, 85–86

N
Nails, traumatic injuries to, 262–289
National Collegiate Athletic Association
  injury surveillance system of, 39, 86, 88
  skin infection guidelines of, 64, 68
    for furunulosis, 16
    for herpes gladiatorum, 45, 46
    for impetigo, 7
    for lice, 87–88
    for molluscum, 50
    for scabies, 91
    for tinea corporis gladiatorum, 75
    for tinea pedia, 64
    for verruca, 54
    for wrestlers, 7, 10–11, 16, 50, 54, 75, 88
National Federation of State High School Associations, 47
National Football League, 287–288, 302
Neosporin, allergic reactions to, 151–152
Nike nodules, 102
Nipple injuries
  in cyclists, 208–209
  in joggers, 208
Nitrogen bends, 295–296
Nodules
  athlete's, 95–105
  Nike, 102
Noncontact sports athletes. *See also specific noncontact sports*
  herpes labialis in, 35–38
Nose clips, as contact dermatitis cause, 134–135

O
Octopus stings, 329–330
Olympic athletes, anabolic steroid use by, 297
Onychauxis, 278
Onychocryptosis (ingrown toenail), 262–263
Onycholysis, 264, 265, 278, 279
Onychomycosis (tinea unguium), 64, 65–68
  confused with center's callosities, football toenail, jogger's toenail, skater's toenail, soccer toenail, skier's toenail, tennis toe, windsurfer's nail, 262–264
Onychoptosis defluvium, 272
Orthotics, for callosities (calluses) prevention, 219, 222
Otitis externa (swimmer's ear), 28–30
Outdoor sports athletes. *See also* names of specific outdoor sports
  arthropod bite reactions in, 316–322
  arthropod stings in, 322–323
  basal cell carcinoma in, 115–118
  herpes labialis in, 35, 37
  melanoma in, 111–115
  poison ivy in, 154–155
  solar urticaria in, 187–190
  squamous cell carcinoma, 82, 106, 118–122, 300
  sunburn in, 106–111
  ultraviolet radiation in, 300

P
Pack dermatitis, 165
Pads, sports-related, 103–104
Paintball purpura, 249–250
Palmoplantar eccrine hidradenitis, 28, 248–249, color plate VI
Panniculitis, equestrian, 308–310
Papillomatosis, confluent and reticulated, 69–70
Parasitic skin infections, 3, 84–92
"Pebble in shoe" sensation, 220
Pediculosis, 86–88
Perniosis, equestrian, 308–310
Photolichenoid dermatitis, 155–157
Photosensitization, medication-induced, 108, 109
Piezogenic pedal papules, 250–252, color plate VII
Ping-pong patches, 252–253
Pityrosporum infections, 8, 24, 26, 69
Plants, as contact dermatitis cause, 154–157
Platform purpura, 253–254
Playing fields, as contact dermatitis cause, 164–171

Poison ivy, 154–155
Polaris vulgaris, 302
Pool dermatitis, 165, 167–168
Pool palms, 229–230
Pool water dermatitis, 158–159, 167–168
Portuguese man-of-war stings, 323–324
Port-wine stains, 254–255
Powerlifter's patches, 230–231
Powerlifter's purpura, 255–256
Prodrome, herpes labialis-related, 36
Protective equipment. *See also* Helmets
  as allergic contact dermatitis cause, 137–139
Pruritus, 180–182. *See also* Urticaria
  aquagenic, 180, 181
  exercise-induced angioedema/anaphylaxis (EIA)-related, 195
Pseudomonas infections, 3–4
  diving suit dermatitis, 23–24
  green foot, 22–23
  green nails, 66
  hot-foot syndrome, 27–28
  hot-tub folliculitis, 25
  otitis externa (swimmer's ear), 29
  onychomycosis (tinea unguium)-associated, 66
  tinea pedis-associated, 62
Pseudonodules, 102–103
Psoriasis
  differential diagnosis of, 17, 64, 65–68, 141, 262–263
  inverse, differential diagnosis of, 17
Pulling boat hands, 286–287
Purpura
  gogglorum, 257–258
  paintball, 249–250
  platform, 253–254
  powerlifter's, 255–256
  of prolonged running, 256–257
  skier's cold, 306–307

R

Race walkers, jogger's toenail in, 264–266
Racquetball players
  black palm in, 247–248
  callosities (calluses) in, 218
  exercise-induced angioedema/anaphylaxis in, 195–198
  hot-tub folliculitis in, 24
  racquet-related allergic contact dermatitis in, 141–143
  racquet sport patches in, 258–260
  stringer's fingers in, 235–236
Racquets, as contact dermatitis cause, 141–142

Racquet sport athletes. *See also* Badminton players; Racquetball players; Squash players; Tennis players
  contact dermatitis in, 141–142
Racquet sport patches, 258–259, color plate VII
Rafters. *See also* Outdoor sports athletes
  contact dermatitis in, 174–175
  furunculosis in, 11, 13–14, 15
Raspberry (abrasion), 205
Red tide dermatitis, 168–169
Rehabilitation, hot-tub folliculitis transmission during, 24
Rhus dermatitis (poison ivy), 154–155
River rafting guides, furunculosis in, 13–14
Rollerbladers. *See also* Outdoor sports athletes
  abrasions and chafing in, 203–207
  callosities (calluses) in, 216–219
  friction injuries to the skin in, 203–207
  palmoplantar eccrine hidradenitis in, 248
  protective equipment use by, 207
  skate bite, 102
  skater's toenail, 278–279
Rowers. *See also* Boaters
  callosities (calluses) in, 216–219
  rower's rump in, 231–232
  track bites in, 237
  warts (verrucae) in, 36, 51–52
Rower's rump, 231–232
Rubber allergy, 130–131
Rugby players. *See also* Outdoor sports athletes
  furunculosis in, 11, 12
  gram-positive infections in, 4
  herpes rugbeiorum in, 39, 40, 41
  herpes simplex virus infections in, 36, 38, 39, 40, 41, 46
  impetigo in, 4, 5
  lacerations in, 227–228
  molluscum contagiosum in, 47
  tinea corporis in, 3, 6, 73–77, 285
  tropical ulcers in, 31
Runners. *See also* Outdoor sports athletes
  allergic contact dermatitis in, 150
    athletic shoes-related, 135–137
    jogging cream-related, 149
  callosities (calluses) in, 216–218
  cholinergic urticaria in, 182–184
  cross-country
    molluscum contagiosum in, 36, 49
    sunscreen use by, 110, 117, 121
  exercise-induced angioedema/anaphylaxis (EIA) in, 195–198

footwear for, 213–214
  as abrasion and chafing cause, 135–137
frostbite in, 302–306, 305
jogger's alopecia in, 243–244
jogger's nipples in, 225–226
long-distance, jogger's toenail in, 264–266
marathon
  bullae (blisters) in, 209
  chafing and abrasions in, 203
  jogger's nipples in, 225–226
  jogger's toenail in, 264
  tinea pedis in, 59, 60, 62
molluscum contagiosum in, 36, 47, 49
"Nike" nodules, 102
nodules in, 95
onychomycosis (tinea unguium) in, 65
palmoplantar eccrine hidradenitis in, 248
piezogenic pedal papules in, 250–252
pitted keratolysis in, 18
pseudonodules in, 102
purpura of prolonged running in, 256–257
runner's rubrum in, 77–78
runner's rump, 233
runner's toe, 265–266
steeplechase, abrasions in, 203
tinea pedis in, 57, 58–59
tinea unguium (onychomycosis) in, 65
traumatic plantar urticaria in, 192–193
treadmill tracks in, 237–238
vibratory angioedema in, 197
Runner's rubrum, 77–78
Runner's rump, 233
Runner's toe, 265–266. *See also* Tinea unguium (onychomycosis)

S
Saddle sores, 233–235
Sailors. *See* Boaters
Scabies, 24, 26, 84, 88–92
Schistosome dermatitis, 314
Scorpion fish, 334
Scrum kidney, 6
Scrum pox, 39
Scrum strep, 4
Scuba divers. *See also* Boaters
  abrasions and chafing in, 203–207
  allergic contact dermatitis in, 131, 132–133
    diving suit dermatitis in, 23–24
    sea water dermatitis, 157–158
    swim fin-related, 131–132
    underwater mask-related, 132–133
    wet suit-related, 130
  chafing in, 203

friction injuries to the skin in, 203–207
herpes labialis in, 36, 38
skin bends in, 295–296
Sea anemone stings, 327–328
Seabather's eruption (sea lice), 311–314, 315
Sea creature-related abrasions, 337
Sea creature-related stings, 323–336
Sea lice (seabather's eruption), 311–314, 315
Sea water exposure
  as allergic contact dermatitis cause, 157–158
  as irritant contact dermatitis cause, 168–169
  as *Staphylococcus aureus* infection cause, 4
Seaweed dermatitis, 169–170
Shin and knee guards, as contact dermatitis cause, 137–138
Shingles, 39
Shoes, athletic. *See* Footwear
Shotguns, as irritant contact dermatitis cause, 175–176
Shot putters
  acne mechanica in, 282, 283, 284
  anabolic steroid use by, 297
Showers, communal, 52, 58
Shrimp picker's disease (erysipeloid), 21–22
Skate bite, 102
Skaters
  ice. *See* Ice skaters
  in-line. *See* Rollerbladers
Skater's toenail, 278–279
Skiers. *See also* Lugers
  abrasions and chafing in, 203–207
  black palm in, 247, 248
  exercise-induced angioedema/anaphylaxis in, 195–198
  friction injuries to the skin in, 203–207
  lacerations in, 204
  Mogul, black palm in, 247–249
  skier's toenail in, 275–277
  sunscreen use by, 107, 108, 121
Skier's cold purpura, 306–307
Skier's toenail, 275–277
Ski jumpers. *See also* Lugers
  abrasions and chafing in, 203–207
  friction injuries to the skin in, 203–207
Skin bends, 295–296
Skin cancer, 106
  basal cell carcinoma, 106, 115–118
  heat exposure-related, 300
  melanoma, 106, 111–115, 245, 246, 274
  squamous cell carcinoma, 82, 106, 118–122, 300

Smallpox, 35
Snorkelers. *See also* Boaters
   allergic contact dermatitis in, 131, 132–133
      swim fin-related dermatitis, 131–132
      underwater mask-related dermatitis, 132–133
      wet suit dermatitis, 130
   coral-related abrasions in, 337
   impetigo in, 4
Snowboarders. *See also* Lugers
   sunscreen use by, 107, 108, 121
Snowmobilers. *See also* Lugers
   hot-tub folliculitis in, 24, 25
Soccer players. *See also* Outdoor sports athletes
   abrasions and chafing in, 203–207
   allergic contact dermatitis in
      photolichenoid, 156–157
      shin and knee guard-related, 137–138
   black heel in, 245–246
   cement burns, 165–167
   friction injuries to the skin in, 203–207
   gram-positive infections in, 4
   herpes simplex virus infections in, 38
   impetigo in, 4
   irritant contact dermatitis in, 165–167
   lacerations in, 204
   nodules in, 95, 103, 104
   pads in, 95, 103, 104
   soccer toenail in, 277–278
   sunscreen use by, 110, 117, 121
   tinea pedis in, 57, 59
Soccer toenail, 277–278
Softball players. *See* Baseball players
"Spaghetti and meatballs," 70
Splints, elbow, as contact dermatitis cause, 153
Sponge dermatitis, 170–171, 337
Sponge-diver's disease, 327
Sports equipment
   as acne mechanica cause, 282–283, 284, 285
   as allergic contact dermatitis cause, 127–147
   as molluscum contagiosum cause, 50
Squamous cell carcinoma, 82, 106, 118–122, 300
   verrucous, as swimming pool granuloma mimic, 82
Squash players
   allergic contact dermatitis in, 144
      ball-related, 144–145
      racquet-related, 141–143
   callosities (calluses) in, 218
   racquet sport patches in, 258–260
   stringer's fingers in, 235–236
Staphylococcus aureus infections
   folliculitis, 8–11
   furunculosis, 4, 11–16
   impetigo, 4, 6, 7
   jazz ballet bottom, 224
   methicillin-resistant, 6, 7, 9, 10, 11–16
   otitis externa (swimmer's ear), 29
Starfish, 333
Steroids, anabolic, 297–299
Stingrays, 336
Stings
   insect-related, 321–322
   sea creature-related, 323–336
Strawberry (abrasion), 205
Streptococcus infections, 4
Striae distensae, 298
Stria migrans, 259–260
Stringer's fingers, 235–236
Sunburn, 106–111, 114, 121
   prevention of, 114, 117
Sun exposure. *See* Ultraviolet radiation (UV) exposure
Sunscreen, 38, 106, 107, 109, 110, 114, 117, 190
   as sunburn risk factor, 117
   water-resistant, 314
Surfers. *See also* Boaters
   coral-related abrasions in, 337
   impetigo in, 4
   irritant contact dermatitis in, 170, 174–175
      rafts and boogie boards-related, 174–175
   nodules in, 95, 98–100
   wet suit-related dermatitis in, 130
Surfer's knots. *See* Surfer's nodules
Surfer's nodules, 98–100
Surfer's ulcers. *See* Surfer's nodules
Sweating, as sunburn risk factor, 108, 117, 121
Sweaty sock syndrome, 18
Swim fins, as contact dermatitis cause, 131–132
Swim goggles
   as contact dermatitis cause, 127–130
   as purpura cause, 257–258
Swimmers. *See also* Outdoor sports athletes
   allergic contact dermatitis in
      nose clips and earplugs-related, 134–135
      seaweed-related, 157–159

Index 349

swim fins-related, 131–132
swim goggles-related, 127–130
swimming cap-related, 133–134
underwater masks-related, 132–133
wet suit-related, 130–131
aquagenic urticaria in, 190–191
atypical mycobacterial skin infections in, 81–83
bleached swimmer syndrome, 158–159
bikini bottom in, 20–21
cold urticaria in, 184–186
contact urticaria in, 191–192
coral-related abrasions in, 337
cutaneous myiasis in, 85–86
erysipeloid in, 21
furunculosis in, 11–16
gram-positive infections in, 4
green hair in, 293–294
hot-foot syndrome in, 27–28
impetigo in, 4
irritant contact dermatitis in
   pool water dermatitis, 167–168
   red tide dermatitis, 168–169
   seaweed dermatitis, 169–170
   swimmer's shoulder, 178–179
molluscum contagiosum in, 36, 47, 49
onychomycosis (tinea unguium) in, 65
otitis externa (swimmer's ear) in, 28–30
pool palms in, 229–230
pool water dermatitis in, 158–160
pruritus in, 180–181, 180–182
purpura gogglorum in, 257–258
seabather's eruption (sea lice) in, 311–314
sea creature-related abrasions in, 337
sea creature-related stings in, 323–336
sea water dermatitis in, 157–158
seaweed dermatitis in, 169–170
sponge dermatitis, 170–171
Staphylococcus aureus infections in, 4
swimmer's itch in, 314–316
swimmer's shoulder, 165, 178–179
swimming pool granuloma in, 81–83
tinea corporis in, 76
tinea pedis in, 57, 59, 60, 62
tinea unguium (onychomycosis) in, 65–68
verrucae in, 36
Vibrio infections in, 30–31
warts (verrucae) in, 51, 52
Swimmer's ear (otitis externa), 28–30
Swimmer's itch, 24, 26, 314–316
Swimmer's shoulder, 165, 178–179
Swimming caps, as contact dermatitis cause, 133–134

Swimming equipment, as contact dermatitis cause, 127–134
Swimming pool granuloma, 81–83
Swimming pools
   contact dermatitis in, 158–159, 167–168
   copper deposits in, 293–294
   hot-tub folliculitis transmission in, 25
Swimming pool water dermatitis, 158–159, 167–168
Sycosis barbae, 77
Synchronized swimmers. *See also* Outdoor sports athletes
   aquagenic urticaria in, 190–191
   allergic contact dermatitis, 127–163
      nose clips and earplugs-related, 134–135
      swim goggles-related, 127–130
      swimming cap-related, 133–134
   atypical mycobacterial infections in, 81–83
   bikini bottom in, 20–21
   blonded or dried hair in, 294–295
   cold urticaria in, 184–186
   contact urticaria in, 191–192
   green hair in, 293–294
   hot foot syndrome in, 27–28
   molluscum contagiosum in, 8, 47–51
   onychomycosis (tinea unguium) in, 65
   otitis externa (swimmer's ear) in, 28–30
   pool water dermatitis in, 158–160, 167–168
   pruritus in, 180–182
   purpura googlorum in, 257–258
   swimming pool granuloma in, 81–83
   tinea pedis in, 3, 57, 58–65
   warts (verruca) in, 51, 52

T

Table tennis players, ping-pong patches in, 252–253
"Talon noire," 245, 247. *See also* Black heel
Tape, athletic, as contact dermatitis cause, 147–148
Tennis players. *See also* Outdoor sports athletes; Table tennis players
   abrasions and chafing in, 203–207
   acne mechanica in, 282–283, 284
   allergic contact dermatitis in, 141–142
   athletic shoes-related, 135–137
   tennis racquet-related, 141–143
   black heel in, 245–247
   black palm in, 247–248
   bullae (blisters) in, 209
   callosities (calluses) in, 216–219

Tennis players (*cont.*)
exercise-induced angioedema/anaphylaxis in, 195–198
friction injuries to the skin in, 203–207
lacerations in, 204
onychocryptosis (ingrown toenail) in, 266–268
pitted keratolysis in, 18
stringer's fingers in, 235–236
tennis thighs in, 236
tennis toe in, 262–264
Tennis racquets, as contact dermatitis cause, 141–142
Tennis thighs, 236
Tennis toe, 262–264
Testosterone, synthetic derivatives of. *See* Anabolic steroids
Tetanus immunization, 207
Thermal reactions/injuries, 300–310
bicyclist's nipples, 208
Tinea corporis, 76–77
Tinea corporis gladiatorum, 3, 6, 73–76, 285
differential diagnosis of, 43
Tinea cruris, 3, 17, 71–73
Tinea gladiatorum. *See* Tinea corporis gladiatorum
Tinea pedis, 3, 57, 58–65
Tinea unguium (onychomycosis), 64, 65–68
confused with center's callosities, football toenail, jogger's toe, skater's toenail, skier's toenail, soccer toenail, tennis toe, windsurfer's nail, 265–266
Tinea versicolor, 69–71
Tobogganers. *See* Lugers
"Toe jam," 280–281
Toes, traumatic injuries to, 262–268
Tongue depressors, color plate III
Topical anesthetics, as contact dermatitis cause, 150–151
Topical anti-inflammatory agents, as contact dermatitis cause, 149–150
Track and field athletes. *See also* Runners
acne mechanica in, 282–285
allergic contact dermatitis in, 147
athletic tape-related, 148
anabolic steroid use in, 297–299
callosities (calluses) in, 216–219, 218
friction injuries to the skin in, 203–207
lacerations in, 204
Track bites, 237
Trapshooters, irritant contact dermatitis in, 175–176
Trapshooter's stigma, 175–176

Trauma-related skin conditions
combined factors-related, 282–292
friction injuries, 203–244
in the nails and toes, 262–289
pounding-related, 203
pressure-related, 203, 245–261
Treadmill tracks, 237–238
Triathlon athletes. *See also* Cyclists; Outdoor sports athletes; Runners; Swimmers
Trichophyton equinum, 73
Trichophyton mentagrophytes, 59, 65, 71
Trichophyton rubrum, 60, 65, 71, 73, 77–78
Trichophyton tonsurans, 73, 75–76
Trichophyton verrucosum, 73
Trichophytosis gladiatorum. *See* Tinea corporis gladiatorum
Tropical ulcers, 31–32

U
Ulcers
surfer's (surfer's nodules), 98–99, 100
tropical, 31–32
Ultraviolet radiation (UV) exposure, 300
as herpes labialis cause, 35–36, 37, 38
herpes simplex virus infection-reactivating effects of, 35–36
as photolichenoid dermatitis cause, 155–157
prevention of, 38, 109–111, 114–115
with photoprotective clothing, 108, 109, 111, 114–115, 117–118, 121–122
with sunscreens, 38, 106, 107, 109, 110, 114, 117, 190, 314
as skin cancer cause, 106, 111–122
basal cell carcinoma, 115–118
melanoma, 106, 111–115, 245, 246, 274
squamous cell carcinoma, 82, 106, 118–122, 300
as solar urticaria cause, 181, 187–190
Underwater masks, as allergic contact dermatitis cause, 132–133
Urticaria, 127, 180
aquagenic, 181, 190–191
cholinergic, 181, 182–184
differentiated from exercise-induced angiodema/anaphylaxis (EIA), 196–197
cold, 181, 184–186
contact, 191–192
dermatographism, 186–187
exercise-induced angioedema/anaphylaxis (EIA)-related, 196
solar, 181, 187–190
traumatic plantar, 192–194

V

Vastus medialis muscles, hypertrophic, 236
Verrucae (warts), 36, 50, 51–54
  differentiated from callosities (calluses), 53, 217
  return-to-play guidelines for, 50
Vibratory angioedema, 197
Vibrio infections, 22, 30–31
Viral skin infections, 35–56. *See also names of specific viruses*
  herpes labialis, 35–38
  herpes simplex, 36, 38–47
  molluscum contagiosum, 36, 47–51
  warts (verrucae), 36, 51–54
Volleyball players. *See also* Outdoor sports athletes
  bikini bottom in, 20
  cutaneous larva migrans in, 84
  molluscum contagiosum in, 47, 50

W

Warts. *See* Verrucae (warts)
Water polo players. *See* Synchronized swimmers
Water-skiers. *See also* Boaters
  waterskiing welts in, 238–239
  wet suit dermatitis in, 130
Water-skiing welts, 238–239
Waterslide/waterpark users. *See also* Synchronized swimmers
  aquaslide alopecia in, 241–243
  hot-tub folliculitis in, 24, 25
Water sports participation. *See also specific water sports*
  as basal cell carcinoma risk factor, 115
  as melanoma risk factor, 111–112, 112
  as squamous cell carcinoma risk factor, 118
Water tubers. *See also* Boaters
  abrasions and chafing in, 203–207
  contact dermatitis in, 170
  friction injuries to the skin in, 203–207
Weightlifters
  abrasions and chafing in, 230–231
  acne mechanica in, 282, 283, 284
  allergic contact dermatitis in, 145
    chalk-related, 145–146
    metal weights-related, 145–146
  anabolic steroid use in, 297
  black heel in, 245–246
  black palm in, 247–248
  callosities (calluses) in, 216–219
  furunculosis in, 11
  irritant contact dermatitis in, 171
  powerlifter's patches in, 230–231
  powerlifter's purpura in, 255–256
  stria migrans in, 260
  warts (verrucae) in, 51
  weightlifter's nail in, 271–272
Weightlifter's nail, 271–272
Weights, metal, as allergic contact dermatitis cause, 145
Wet suit dermatitis, 130
Wet suits, as allergic contact dermatitis cause, 130–131
Whirlpools
  Pseudomonas folliculitis transmission in, 25, 27
  sanitation equipment for, 7
  Staphylococcus infection transmission in, 9
Wind sailors, sunburn in, 106
Wind surfers. *See also* Boaters
  allergic contact dermatitis in, 140–141
    wet suit-related, 130
    wishbone-related, 140–141
  lacerations in, 228
  wind surfer's nail in, 280–281
Wind surfer's nail, 280–281
Winter sports athletes. *See* Lugers
Wishbone, as contact dermatitis cause, 140–141
Women athletes
  anabolic steroid use by, 297
  bikini bottom in, 20
  jogger's nipples in, 225, 226
  molluscum contagiosum in, 47
  pulling boat hands in, 286
  solar urticaria in, 187
Wrestlers
  abrasions and chafing in, 203–207
  acne mechanica in, 282, 283, 284
  folliculitis treatment in, 10–11
  friction injuries to the skin in, 203–207
  folliculitis in, 13
  furunculosis in, 8, 13
  gram-positive infections in, 4
  herpes gladiatorum in, 39, 40, 41
  herpes simplex virus infections in, 36, 38, 39, 41, 43, 44, 45, 46
  impetigo in, 4, 5, 7
  incorrect skin disease diagnoses in, 45
  molluscum contagiosum in, 47, 50
  pediculosis in, 86–88
  scabies in, 88–92
  tinea corporis gladiatorum in, 73–76
  warts (verrucae) in, 51, 54

X

Xerosis (dry skin), 180–182, 217